Introduction

Dear readers.

This book is aimed to be easily understandable book for ordinary people, and also for medical doctors, nurses, students, researchers and sportsmen.

The population of the World is increasing at a very high rate, and especially the population in cities is increasing tremendously. This means, that the food intake and physical activity has also changed a lot, especially during the last 40 years. In older times people made a lot of hard physical work, they had a lot of sports activity and the food was simple and very low caloric but healthy. Obesity was very rare among people. But nowadays obesity is increasing at an alarming rate all over the World. There are over 1000 million overweight persons and over 300 million obese persons in the World at the moment.

At the same time several obesity related diseases have increased tremendously, especially hypertension, high cholesterol levels, type 2 diabetes, metabolic syndrome, cardiovascular diseases and asthma. The amounts of daily calories, refined foods, fat, high glycemic index carbohydrates, alcohol and salt have increased strongly in the diet, in many parts of the World. For example the amount of average daily calories in a typical US diet has increased by several hundreds of kilocalories, during the last 40 years. At the same time, the amount of hard physical work and exercise has reduced very strongly.

Obesity is a miss balance between daily caloric intake and daily energy expenditure. In simple terms: people become obese, because they eat too much
energy dense food, and at the same time they lack physical work, physical exercise and other energy consuming daily physical activities.
There are some other, minor reasons for obesity also, such as genetic, hormonal, aging, medical reasons, psychiatric reasons etc., but overeating and lack of exercise and daily physical activity are the 2 main reasons of obesity.

The World famous German physicist, Albert Einstein, made the discovery of the very famous mathematical equation

$$E = mc^2$$

where:
E = Energy
m = Mass
c = constant, the velocity of light.

From this equation we can get a simple idea about the reason for obesity:
if the system (human) energy content E is increased, then the system (human) mass (or body weight) m is also increased. And if energy E is decreased, then the mass m must also decrease.

So: The excessive intake of food and at the same time the lack of hard work, exercise and daily energy consuming activities are the 2 main reasons of obesity. All excess daily food and thus excess energy, be it from fat, carbohydrates, proteins or alcohol, is stored in the body as fat. But if the energy expenditure is increased over the daily energy intake with the help of exercise, hard work, or other physical daily activities, then the stored excess fat is used as a fuel for these physical activities, and the person will lose both weight and body fat mass.

As a rule of thumb, you must reduce your energy intake by 7700 kcal, to reduce your body weight by 1 kg. So if you are really an obese person, you will really need a strict low caloric diet and a strongly increased daily energy expenditure from different physical activities, to lose as much weight in as short time period as possible.

Losing weight is not necessary the biggest problem. Keeping the achieved body weight is very often very hard. This means, you have to permanently change your lifestyle, if you are going to stay at your lower body weight. ALL improvements in your body composition depend on your own brains only!

Besides diet and exercise, there exists a large number of edible plants, spices, medicinal plants, nutrients and pure chemical compounds extracted from these plants, which a helpful in increasing fat burning, decreasing fat storage, or decreasing fat and carbohydrate absorption. For example there are tens of known plants, which decrease the activity of Lipase enzyme, and thus decrease the absorption of fat. Also there are many plants, which decrease the activity of alfa-Amylase enzyme, and thus decrease the absorption of carbohydrates. And there are tens of plants, which decrease of activity of enzymes, such as FAS (=Fatty Acid Synthase), which are responsible for fat storage. And there are tens of plants and chemical compounds, which stimulate the activities of enzymes responsible for fat oxidation. Altogether this book shows over 380 diets, physical methods, edible plants, spices, medicinal plants, nutrients and natural chemical compounds, which by research have been shown to have body fat and body weight decreasing properties.

This book is based strictly on modern scientific research about obesity, and each research reference can be looked at the reference list, at the end of this book. Totally there are over 3000 research references in this book.

Stig Froberg   02/2013, Naantali, Finland.

About the author

Stig Froberg was born 1955 in city Turku, Finland. He graduated as a physicist in Turku University 1983. The last 24 years he has been working with Neste Oil, the Naantali facility unit laboratory. His specialties are laboratory analysis methods and physical properties of liquids and gases.

He has researched over 35 years of nutrition, sports nutrition, sports medicine and herbal medicines. He has knowledge of over 2000 medicinal plants. His hobby is cultivation of food and medicinal plants.

He has 20 years of experience as a competition sportsman, and he is a former Finnish champion in 50 kilometers race walking.

He is the author of the book "Decrease hypertension and cholesterol naturally" available from Amazon.co.uk.

Index

General

Common abbreviations.

p-value: This figure exists again and again in the text, when there is a comparison between the test group and the control or placebo group, using statistical mathematical methods. The difference in measured value is statistically significant between the test group and placebo group, if $p < 0.05$, or if p-value is less than 0.05.

The difference in measured value is more significant, the less the p-value is, between the groups. For example, if $p < 0.001$, the difference in the measured value between test group and placebo group is much more, than if $p < 0.05$. For example, if $p < 0.01$, there is only 1% probability, that the difference in the measured value between groups did happen by accident. If $p < 0.05$, there is only 5% probability, that the difference in the measured value between the groups did happen by accident.

TC = Total Cholesterol
TG = Triglycerides
LDL-cholesterol = "Bad" low density cholesterol
HDL-cholesterol = "Good" high density cholesterol
VLDL-cholesterol = "Very bad" very low density cholesterol
SBP = Systolic blood pressure
DBP = Diastolic blood pressure

Energy
Humans oxidise (or metabolise) carbohydrates, proteins, fats and alcohol to produce energy, needed for all living cells. In this book we use the old unit for energy, kilocalories (kcal). The new unit for energy is kilojoules (kJ). Kilocalories can be converted to kilojoules by the formula 1 kcal = 4.184 kilojoule.

Leptin
Leptin is a peptide hormone, secreted by fat tissue. Leptin was discovered just 1994. The name Leptin comes from Greece language word Leptos (=thin). Leptin gives information to brains about the status of body fat reserves. Obese persons have much more Leptin in blood than non-obese persons. Leptin increases insulin resistance and blood pressure, so it is a harmful hormone. Females have higher Leptin concentrations in serum than males. Alcohol, cortisol and insulin increase Leptin. Body weight reduction and exercise decrease Leptin.

Adiponectin
Adiponectin is a peptide hormone, secreted by fat tissue. It was discovered just 1995-1996 by several research groups. Obese persons have less Adiponectin in serum, than non-obese persons. Females have more Adiponectin than males. Adiponectin increase the basal metabolic rate, so it is a useful hormone, by increasing fat oxidation, without increasing hunger feeling. Body weight reduction increases serum Adiponectin levels. Also fish oil and dietary fiber increases Adiponectin levels.

Inflammatory cytokines
Fat cells are living cells, and not just passive fat storage cells. These cells secrete a number of hormones (Leptin, Adiponectin etc.), and also many inflammatory markers, such as cytokines TNF-alfa, IL-6 etc. So obesity is in reality an inflammatory disease.

Body fat or Adipose tissue
Adipose tissue or body fat is composed of cells, adipocytes. The main function of adipose tissue is to store energy in the form of lipids. It also produces several hormones, such as Leptin and Adiponectin, and also many inflammatory cytokines, such as TNF-alfa and IL-6. In humans, adipose tissue is located beneath the skin (subcutaneous fat), around internal organs (abdominal fat) and in breast tissue. The total fat measured in units of kg is the body fat mass.

Body fat percentage
The body fat percentage is the total weight of fat divided by total body weight, and multiplied by 100%. For example: A person weights 100 kg, and his total body fat mass is 30 kg. Then his body fat percentage is 30 kg/100 kg*100%=30%.

Body mass index BMI
Body mass index BMI is body mass in units of kg divided by the square of height, where height is given in units of meters. For example: A person weights 100 kg, and his height is 180 cm. Then his BMI = $100 \text{ kg}/(1.80 \text{ m})^2 = 30.8 \text{ kg/m}^2$.

Metabolic syndrome
Metabolic syndrome is a clustering of several cardiovascular and metabolic risk factors, including dyslipidemia, hyperglycemia, insulin resistance, hypertension and obesity. There are several slightly different definitions of metabolic syndrome by WHO and other organizations, so we give here an "average" definition of metabolic syndrome. An individual is said to have metabolic syndrome, if he or she has at least 3 of the following symptoms:
  – Insulin resistance
  – triglycerides over 1.7 mmol/L and HDL-cholesterol under 1.0 mmol/L
  – blood pressure: SBP over 140 mmHg and DBP over 90 mmHg
  – plasma glucose over 5.6 mmol/L
  – obesity: BMI>30.0 or waist circumference >102 cm (males) and >88 cm (females).

BW = Body Weight

Extract
Normally when testing different plants for anti-obesity properties, the plant is dried, made into flour, and the effective compounds are extracted with a suitable solvent, many often with water or ethanol or methanol. Then these extracts are given to animals in standardized doses, such as 10 mg/kg BW, which means, that the extract is given to test animal at a dose of 10 milligrams to each kg of body weight.

RQ = Respiratory Quotient.
RQ is the amount of CO2 removed from the body divided by the amount of O2 inhaled during respiration. It gives a figure, how much fat is burned. For carbohydrates RQ=1, for proteins RQ is between 0.8-0.9 and for fat RQ=0.7.

Lipolysis
Lipolysis is the breakdown of lipids. Triglycerides are hydrolyzed to free fatty acids, which are degraded into acyl groups by beta oxidation.

Lipolysis inducing hormones
Lipolysis inducing hormones induce lipolysis. These are: Norepinephrine, ghrelin, growth hormone and testosterone.

Obesity and overweight

Obesity is a medical condition in which excess body fat has accumulated into body and which can be seen often clearly visually. Obesity has adverse effects leading to increased health problems and reduced life expectancy by up to 4-10 years.

Obesity is not a new phenomenon, it has always existed. A good example is the very famous statue Venus of Willendorf, which shows an obese female. The statue is made 24 000 -26 000 years ago.

But now obesity and overweight have increased dramatically all around the World, also in underdeveloped countries. According to the World Health Organization WHO estimates, over 1000 million adults are overweight and of these over 300 million are obese. In many countries obesity has increased three fold since 1980. Childhood obesity is already epidemic in some areas, and according to WHO there are over 18 million obese children, under age of 5 years.

According to WHO, the most important reasons for obesity are increased use of fat, especially saturated fat, sugar and other carbohydrates and energy dense foods, and too little physically demanding work and exercise, together with too little eating of vegetables, fruits, nuts, fish, dietary fiber and whole grains.

Obesity is a strong risk factor in more than 50 different diseases and symptoms, such as: Type 2 diabetes, high cholesterol levels, high triglyceride levels, hypertension, asthma, stroke, myocardial infarction, infertility, impotency, liver diseases, sleep apnea, snoring, depression, osteoarthritis, low back pain, cellulitis, different forms of cancer, hypogonadism and small penis size, low testosterone and growth hormone levels, chronic renal failure, menstrual disorders, low physical endurance and working capability, metabolic syndrome, COPD , skin problems etc.

According to WHO, obesity is defined by using Body Mass Index BMI. When a person´s body weight is expressed in units of kilograms (kg) and height is expressed in units of meters (m), the BMI can be calculated from the formula

$$BMI = body\ weight(kg)/height(m)^2$$

In other words: Body weight in units of kilograms is divided by the square of height, where the unit of height is expressed in meters.

Example: a person´s weight is 80 kg and his height is 175 cm or 1.75 meters.
Then the calculated BMI $= 80\ kg/(1.75m)^2 = 26.12\ kg/m^2$.
Normally the units are dropped off and we say, that the person´s BMI is 26.12.

For adults WHO defines underweight, normal weight, overweight and obesity according to the following table.

BMI	Classification
< 18.5	underweight
18.5 - 24.9	normal weight
25.0 - 29.9	overweight
> 30.0	obese

Adult mean BMI in Africa and Asia is between 22-23 kg/m^2 and in North-America, Europe, Latin America and Pacific island countries it is between 25-27 kg/m^2. This means, the Africans and Asians are generally leaner and less obese.

The most obese countries at the moment are USA, Samoa, Mexico, New Zealand, Chile, Australia, Canada, United Kingdom, Ireland, Luxembourg and Finland.

Obesity is very rare in the following countries: India, Indonesia, China, Korea, Japan and some African countries.

Country	Obesity in units of percentage of total population
USA	35.7%
Mexicoko	30.0%
New Zealand	26.5%
Chile	25.1%
Australia	24.6%
Canada	24.2%
United Kingdom	23.0%
Ireland	23.0%
Luxembourg	22.1%
Finland	20.2%
Iceland	20.1%
Hungary	19.5%
Greece	18.1%
Estonia	18.0%
Russia	16.2%
Sweden	11.2%
Italy	10.3%
Norway	10.0%
Switzerland	8.1%
Japan	3.9%
Korea	3.8%
China	2.9%
Indonesia	2.4%
India	2.1%

(Source: OECD Obesity update 2012).
In some urban areas of Samoa the obesity rate can be up to 75%
(Source: WHO Obesity and overweight)

In USA 68.8% of adults are either overweight or obese. In USA 31.8% of children are either overweight or obese. Of these children 16.9% are obese
(Source: FRAC: Food Research and Action Center)

Total daily energy expenditure TDEE

The 24 hour total daily energy expenditure TDEE is composed of 3 separate parts:

1) Resting energy expenditure, REE.

    This makes typically 60 – 70% of the total daily energy expenditure.
    It is also called resting metabolic rate, RMR.

2) Thermic effect of food, TEF.

    When eating a lot of protein, part of the protein energy content is lost in the body due to digestion etc. The thermic effect of protein may be between 25 – 35% of the protein total energy content. The thermic effect of carbohydrates is between 5 – 15% and the thermic effect of fat is between 0 – 5%. TEF makes typically 10 – 15% of total daily energy expenditure.

3) Physical activity energy expenditure, PAEE.

    PAEE is made of all other energy expenditures, but not sleeping. It is composed of work, exercise, cleaning, speaking etc. PAEE makes the rest of daily energy expenditure, typically 15 – 30%.

Total daily energy expenditure TDEE = REE + TEF + PAEE.

The REE value will decrease, due to aging. This means, the daily energy need is reduced during aging. REE value can be measured by calorimetry. But it can also be calculated, if either weight, height and age or fat free mass FFM are known.

Normally the Harris-Benedict equation from year 1919 is used, but the recent Mifflin (Mifflin et.al. 1990) equations are more accurate.

For men the REE value is calculated from the equation
REE = 10 x weight(kg) + 6.25 x height(cm) – 5 x age(years) + 5

For females the REE values is calculated from the equation
REE = 10 x weight(kg) + 6.25 x height(cm) – 5 x age(years) – 161

Example: Person is female, weight 65 kg, height 170 cm and age 50 years.

Then we can calculate her REE value from
REE = 10 x 65 + 6.25 x 170 – 5 x 50 – 161 = 1301.5 kcal/24 hours.

This is the energy she will need daily, even if she would not do anything else than sleep.

The REE value can be calculated also, when only the person's weight and body fat-% BF% are known, from the equation
REE = 19.7 x FFM + 413

Where: FFM = weight(kg) – BF% / 100% x weight

Example: Body weight is 100 kg and BF% = 30%.

Then the FFM value is: FFM = 100 kg – 30% / 100% x 100 kg = 70 kg
and the REE value can be calculated as
REE = 19.7 x 70 + 413 = 1792 kcal/24 hours.

Energy expenditure in different physical activities

The energy expenditure in different sports activities depends on the sport, the person´s body weight and the average speed of the activity. The higher is the person´s body weight, and the higher is the average speed in that specific activity, the higher is the energy expenditure in 1 hour.

The energy expenditure in different physical activities can be easily calculated with the aid of the known MET values. MET comes from the words Metabolic Equivalent Task. It is a multiple of basal metabolic rate. One MET corresponds to the energy used, when a person is sitting still. MET= 1 kcal/kg*h. If a person weights 70 kg, and he is sitting still 1 hour, he will use 70 kcal of energy.

The MET value of sleeping is 0.9. The MET value is normally within the range between 0.9 (sleeping)-23.0 (fast running).

Generally the energy expenditure in a specific physical activity can be calculated from the formula

E = M*T*MET,

Where:
E = used energy in units of kcal
M = body weight, in units of kg
T = time used in activity, in units of hour
MET = the MET value of the specific activity, at the specified speed. These values are tabulated.

Example:
A person weights 70 kg, and he is running for 1 hour, at a speed of 12 km/hour.
Then the MET value is 11.7 and the total energy expenditure can be calculated as E= 70*1.0*11.7 kcal= 819 kcal.

If the time used is 45 minutes, then T=0.75. If the time used is 30 minutes, then T=0.5 and if the time used is 15 minutes, then T=0.25.

In the following we give the average MET values as a function of speed for the most common physical sports activities. You can easily calculate your energy expenditure with these MET values and the above formula.

Activity	MET-value
Running	
6.0 km/hour	5.3
8.0 km/hour	8.2
10.0 km/hour	10.0
12.0 km/hour	11.7
14.0 km/hour	12.4
15.0 km/hour	13.3
16.0 km/hour	14.4
18.0 km/hour	16.6
20.0 km/hour	19.3
22.0 km/hour	21.9
Walking	
4.0 km/hour	3.1
5.0 km/hour	4.0
6.0 km/hour	5.0
7.0 km/hour	5.9
8.0 km/hour	7.6
9.0 km/hour	9.2
10.0 km/hour	10.9
11.0 km/hour	12.6
12.0 km/hour	14.2
Bicycling	
10.0 km/hour	3.9
15.0 km/hour	5.7
20.0 km/hour	7.0
25.0 km/hour	9.6
30.0 km/hour	11.8
35.0 km/hour	15.8
Bicycling, stationary	
power 50 w	3.0
power 100 w	5.5
power 150 w	7.0
power 200 w	10.5
power 250 w	12.5
Swimming	
20 meters/minute	4.1
30 meters/minute	5.6
40 meters/minute	7.1

50 meters/minute	10.1
60 meters/minute	13.2

Skiing cross country
5 km/hour	7.3
7 km/hour	7.8
10 km/hour	8.4
12 km/hour	8.9
15 km/hour	9.6

Top athletes may use very large amounts of energy during competition. If a Marathon runner weights 60 kg, and he runs Marathon in a time of 2 hours and 6 minutes, he will use 2432 kcal energy during competition!

Practical advice to decrease obesity and overweight

Before we show the excess body weight and body fat decreasing properties of over 380 foodstuffs, diets, medicinal plants, nutrients and physical methods, we give some practical advice to decrease overweight. With this knowledge, each person can easily make a suitable personal diet and exercise program to decrease his or her obesity.

Here is one detailed list of different possibilities.

Exercise
- make at least 3-5 times weekly, 45 minutes -1.5 hours of aerobic exercise, such as walking, Nordic walking, running, swimming, bicycling, ice skating, squash, tennis, ice hockey, football, basketball, volley ball, roller skating, cross country skiing, water polo, ping-pong, badminton, orienteering, hiking, hard physical work, paddling, rowing etc.
- or make at least 3-4 times weekly supervised resistance training in gym, 45-60 minutes each time.
- best method is the combination of aerobic exercises and resistance exercises, at least 4-5 times weekly.
- high intensity interval (HIT) training is also very good. It can even be made at home, with stationary bicycling etc.

Eating frequency
Eat many times daily small size meals, so you do not feel hunger at all.

Meal energy density
Use a lot of vegetables, root vegetables, mushrooms, fruits, berries, whole grains, sprouts, beans, peas, hot and thermogenic spices, low fat meat, lean fish, chicken breast, turkey breast, soaps, cottage cheese, fat free milk products, fiber etc., which have low energy density and low glycemic index GI.

Water
- drink several liters of water daily, especially cold water.
- drink 2-4 dl water before each meal.

Butter, cream and other saturated animal fats
- replace butter and cream by margarine or preferably TOTALLY by vegetable oils (Extra virgin olive oil, Sesame oil, Flaxseed oil, Safflower oil, Amaranth oil, Rice bran oil, Ground nut oil, Pumpkin seed oil).

Sugar
- replace sugar by Honey, preferably by dark honey.

Alcohol
- reduce alcohol consumption to max. 30 grams daily, or stop using it totally.
- replace alcohol and beer with red wine, 2-3 dl daily.

Meat
- use only fat free meat, chicken breast and turkey breast.

Shellfish and mussels
- these have lots of protein, and their energy content is low.

Fish
- eat a lot of different fish (Salmon, Rainbow Trout, Trout, Atlantic Herring, Cod, Anchovies, Mackerel, Tuna, Bonito, Haddock, European Sprat, Halibut etc.).

Coffee and other refreshing drinks
- drink coffee without sugar and cream
- drink green tea
- drink Oolong tea
- drink Pu-Erh tea
- drink Mate tea
- drink Rooibos tea
- drink Honeybush tea
- drink Cacao (without sugar and cream)
- drink Hibiscus tea
- drink Luobuma tea (Apocynum Venetum)
- drink Du-Zhong tea (Eucommia Ulmoides)
- drink Java tea (Orthosiphon Stamineus)
- drink Kuding tea (Ilex Kudingcha)
- drink Nomame tea (Cassia Mimosoides, syn. Chmaecrista Nomame)
- drink Siberian tea (Bergenia Crassifolia)
- drink Jiaogulan tea (Gynostemma Pentaphyllum).

Food and salad oils
Use the following vegetable oils:
- Extra virgin olive oil
- Sesame oil
- Flaxseed oil
- Safflower oil
- Rice bran oil
- Amaranth oil

–   Pumpkin oil.

Nuts

You can use daily the following nuts:
–   Almonds
–   Groundnuts (non-salted)
–   Pistachio nut
–   Cashew nuts.

Milk products

Use daily a lot of fermented, fat free, sugar free milk products with different lactic acid bacteria such as Lactobacillus Casei, Lactobacillus Bulgaricus, Lactobacillus Acidophilus etc.
–   Yoghurt
–   sour milk
–   fat free milk.

Soymilk
–   you can use soymilk instead of milk
–   soymilk can be drank as such or put instead of milk to different foods.

Berries

Eat a lot of the following berries:
–   Black chokeberries
–   Blueberries
–   Red grapes
–   Black raisins, Corinthian raisins
–   Goji berries (Lycium Barbarum)
–   Amla, Indian Gooseberries (Emblica Officinalis)
–   Raspberries (Red Raspberry, Blackberry)
–   Mulberries
–   Schisandra berries (SchisandraChinensis)
–   Seabuckthorn berries
–   Rose hips (also dried flour)
–   Barberries
–   Hawthorn (Crataegus Oxyacantha, C. Pinnatifida).

Fruits

Eat a lot of the following fruits:
–   Water melon (Seeds also)
–   Apple (skin also)
–   Tart cherry (Prunus Cerasus)
–   Bergamot
–   Kumquat (Fortunella Japonica, whole fruit)
–   Clementine
–   Mandarin
–   Red grapefruit
–   Orange
–   Lemon

- Pomelo
- Lime fruit (Citrus Aurantifolia)
- Sudachi, fruit and peel (Citrus Sudachi)
- Guava
- Papaya
- Mango
- Mangostan (Garcinia Mangostana)
- Marolo (Annona Crassiflora, fruit pulp and seeds also)
- Passion fruit (use skin also, grind into flour or put to different foods)
- Persimmon
- Kiwi
- Pepino (Solanum Muricatum)
- Tamarind
- Pitahaya fruit
- Pomegranate (seeds also)
- Prunes and black plums
- Atemoya fruit, Annoona (Annona Atemoya)
- Cantaloupe melon (Cucumis Melo)
- Buddha fruit, Luo Han Guo (Siraitia Grosvenori)
- Dates
- Figs
- Pineapple
- Prickly pear, fruit and seeds (Opuntia Ficus Indica)
- Cornelian cherry (Cornus Mas)
- Japanese Cornelian cherry (Cornus Officinalis).

Root vegetables
Eat a lot of the following vegetable roots:
- dark or red potatoes (Kongo, Inca Red, Shetland Black etc.).
- sweet potatoes (Ipomoea Batatas)
- carrots
- purple carrots
- Jerusalem artichoke
- celery (roots, leaves, stalks, seeds)
- Chinese Bellflower (Platygodon Grandiflorum)
- Jicama (Pachyrhizus Erosus)
- Yacon (Smallanthus Sonchifolius)
- Giant potato (Ipomoea Digitata)
- Lotus, root (Nelumbo Nucifera)
- Turnips (Brassica Rapa)
- Kudzu root (Pueraria Lobata)
- Tiger nut (Cyperus Esculentus)
- Greater burdock, edible burdock (Arctium Lappa).

Vegetables
Eat daily a lot of the following vegetables:
- Tomato

12

- Red cabbage
- Green cabbage
- Broccoli
- Broccolini, Petit Vert (B.Oleracea var. Italica x B. Oleracea var. Alboglabra)
- Kale
- Kimchi (Fermented Chinese cabbage, Brassica Rapa var. Pekinensis)
- Cauliflower
- Purslane
- Peppermint
- Garlic
- Red onions
- Chives (Allium Schoenoprasum)
- Shallot (Allium Ascalonicum)
- Chinese Chives (Allium Tuberosum)
- Welsh onion (Allium Fistulosum)
- Alpine leek (Allium Victorialis)
- Ramsons (Allium Ursinum)
- Society garlic (Tulbaghia Violacea)
- Eggplant
- Gilo (Solanum Gilo)
- Bottle Gourd (Lagenaria Siceraria)
- Wax Gourd (Benincasa Hispida)
- Pointed Gourd (Trichosanthes Dioica)
- Ivy Gourd, fruit (Coccinia Indica)
- Asparagus (Asparagus Officinalis, A. Racemosus, A.Cochinchinensis)
- Bitter melon (Momordica Charantia)
- Egyptian Luffa
- Parsley
- Dill
- Olives (black and green)
- fresh Ginger
- fresh Galangal root (Alpinia Galangal)
- Ashitaba (Angelica Keiskei)
- Rucola (Eruca Sativa)
- Chicory, leaves
- vegetable Sesame, Benniseed (Sesamum Radiatum, leaves)
- Capillary Wormwood, YIN CHEN HAO (Artemisia Capillaris)
- Iwayomogi wormwood (Artemisia Iwayomogi)
- Yomogi (Artemisia Princeps)
- Radish, leaves (Raphanus Sativus)
- Red beet, leaves
- Jute Mallow, leaves (Corchorus Olitorius)
- Fennel bulbs, leaves, stalks, seeds (Foeniculum Vulgare).

Mushrooms
Eat a lot of mushrooms from the following list:
- Shiitake (Lentinus Edodes)

- White button mushroom
- Maitake
- Himematsutake
- Oyster mushroom (Pleurotus Ostreatus)
- King oyster mushroom (Pleurotus Eryngii)
- Jew´s ear mushroom (Auricularia Auricula-judae)
- Bunashijemi (Hypsizigus Marmoreus)
- Cordyceps (Cordyceps Chinensis)
- Monkey head mushroom (Hericium Erinaceus).

Sprouts
Eat the following sprouts:
- Broccoli sprouts
- Mung bean sprouts
- Alfalfa sprouts
- Fenugreek sprouts
- Adzuki bean sprouts
- Soybean sprouts
- Black soybean sprouts
- Pinto bean sprouts
- Red kidney bean sprouts
- Quinoa sprouts
- Buckwheat sprouts
- Tartary buckwheat sprouts
- Broad bean sprouts
- Brown rice sprouts
- Black rice sprouts
- Sesame seed sprouts
- Black Sesame seed sprouts
- Rye sprouts
- Wheat sprouts.

Beans and peas
Eat a lot of beans and peas:
- Soybeans
- Black soybeans
- Pinto beans
- Adzuki beans
- Red kidney beans
- Chickpeas
- Broad beans
- Horse gram (Dolichos Biflorus)
- fresh or frozen peas.

Whole grains
Eat a lot of WHOLE grains:
- whole grain barley

- whole grain oat
- whole grain rye
- whole grain wheat
- whole grain Wild rice (Zizania Latifolia, Zizania Sp.)
- Red rice
- Brown rice
- Black rice
- Purple corn
- Black sesame
- Buckwheat
- Tartary buckwheat (Fagopyrum Tataricum)
- Quinoa (Chenopodium Quinoa)
- Canihua (Chenopodium Palllidicaule)
- Proso millet (Panicum Miliaceum)
- Foxtaill millet (Setaria Italica)
- Sorgum or Durra (Sorghum Bicolor)
- Amarath seeds.

Bran and germs
Use daily a lot of bran and germs in yoghurt, bread etc.:
- rice bran
- oat bran
- barley bran
- rye bran
- sugar beet bran (FIBREX, 73% fiber content!!!)
- wheat germ.

Grass flour
Eat the following grass flours:
- wheat grass
- barley grass.

Sweeties
- replace all sweeties by DARK Chocolate.

Algae
Eat the following algae:
- Wakame
- Chlorella
- Spirulina
- Kelp
- ALL other edible seaweeds.

Salt
- reduce strongly the use of salt. Normally and during winter, the daily need of salt is only between 1-2 grams. The Yanomani Indians in Venezuela Amazon region get only 0.2 grams salt per day, and they have the lowest blood pressure values in the whole World.
- replace salt by spices and spice mixtures, which you can easily make yourself.

Polyunsaturated fatty acids and oils.
Use the following oils in capsule or liquid form:
- Fish oil (EPA+DHA)
- GLA, gamma-Linolenic Acid (from Primrose oil, black currant oil etc.)
- CLA, Conjugated Linolenic Acid
- MCT oil (Medium Chain Triglycerides) Fish oil, CLA and MCT oil should be used between 2-6 grams daily.

Spices.
Most of spices have DODY FAT decreasing properties.
Use the following spices, and make also your own body fat decreasing spice mixture:
- Garlic
- Red onion
- Ginger
- Kencur (Kaempferia Galanga)
- Lesser Galangal (Alpinia Officinarum)
- Indian ginger (Alpinia Calcarata)
- Chinese ginger (Boesenbergia Pandurata)
- Mioga, Japanese ginger (Zingiber Mioga)
- Shampoo ginger, Lempoyang (Zingiber Zerumbet)
- Black ginger, Krachai Dam (Kaempferia Parviflora)
- Taiwan Galangal (Alpinia Pricei)
- Chili (Capsicum Annuum)
- Curcuma (Curcuma Longa)
- Rosmarin
- Parsley
- Dill
- Basil
- Curry
- Cinnamon
- Black pepper
- Long pepper (Piper Longum)
- Javanese long pepper, fruits (Piper Retrofractum, syn. Piper Chaba)
- Hops (Humulus Lupulus)
- Capers
- Clove
- Coriander (seeds and leaves)
- Guinean pepper (Xylopia Aethiopica)
- Fennel
- Nutmeg
- Black cumin (Nigella Sativa)
- Saffron
- Lemon grass
- Sage
- Pineapple sage (Salvia Elegans)
- Tsao-ko Cardamon, seeds (Amomum Tsao-ko)
- False Cardamom, seeds (Amomum Villosum)

- Caraway (Carum Carvi)
- Mustard (seeds)
- Ketchup, crushed tomatoes, tomato puree.

Cheese
- use fat free cottage cheese.

Diets
The following diets are excellent for decreasing obesity, overweight, excess body fat, waist circumference, hypertension, cholesterol, triglycerides, insulin resistance, blood sugar, type 2 diabetes and metabolic syndrome:
- Ketogenic diet
- Protein diet, hypocaloric
- Vegetarian diet
- Lactovegetarian diet
- Stoneage diet
- Mediterranian diet
- Okinawa diet
- VLCD or Very Low Caloric Diet (Under 800 kcal daily).

Acupuncture, electroacupuncture, Shiatshu, Moxibustion, Electrical Stimulation.
- with different acupuncture types body weight can be decreased typically between 3-5 kg, using special acupuncture points.
- at the same time you can treat many other chronic diseases, such as asthma, hypertension, high cholesterol etc. with other acupuncture points. Acupuncture is easy, cheap and safe treatment, used over 5000 years in China, and accepted by World Health Organization, WHO.

Minerals
- increase your daily Calcium by 800-1200 mg
- increase your daily Chromium by 200-400 micrograms
- eat algae for more Iodine
- increase your daily Zinc by 15-30 mg
- if you have no kidney disease, increase your Phosphorous intake by 500-1000 mg.

Protein
The following proteins have excellent fat decreasing properties:
- Soy protein
- Soy protein isolate
- Whey protein
- Fish protein

You can add these to drink, food etc.
Use these proteins ESPECIALLY BEFORE and AFTER each training, to burn more fat, to increase anabolic hormones, to increase immunity to infections and to speed recovery from exercise. Add a little honey or glucose to the AFTER exercise protein drink, to increase Insulin response.

Vinegar
Vinegar has body fat decreasing and immunity stimulating properties.

- use a lot of Vinegar in food, either Apple Vinegar or Vinegar from Black Rice, Kurosu.
- drink daily the following: 2 dl water+ 1 teaspoon Vinegar+1 teaspoon dark honey. Mix well and drink, 2-3 times daily.

Seeds

The following seeds can be eaten as such or added to food:

- Flaxseeds
- Sesame seeds
- Black Sesame seeds
- Fenugreek seeds
- Garden Cress seeds
- Pumpkin seeds (Cuciurbita Pepo)
- Water melon seeds (Citrullus Vulgaris, Citrullus Lanatus)
- Radish seeds (Raphanus Sativus)
- Adlay seeds (Coix Lacryma-Jobi)
- Psyllium seeds (Plantago Ovata).

Dietary supplements.

The following NATURAL supplements have been shown by research to have body fat and body mass decreasing properties:

- Caffeine
- Lipoic acid
- Chromium Picolinate
- Ferulic acid
- Chlorogenic acid
- Indole-3-Carbinol
- Capsaicin
- Capsinoids (Capsiate, Dihydrocapsiate, Nordihydrocapsiate)
- Carvacrol
- Inositol
- Choline
- Corosolic acid
- Quercetin
- Kaempferol
- Apigenin
- Luteolin
- Rutin
- Myricetin
- Isorhamnetin
- Nobiletin
- Resveratrol
- Propolis
- Lycopene
- Astaxanthin
- Mangiferin
- Melatonin
- L-Carnitine

- Acetyl-L-Carnitine
- Propionyl-L-Carnitine
- Genistein
- Daidzein
- Puerarin
- Berberine
- Pycnogenol and Flavangenol
- Grape seed extract (GSE)
- Green coffee extract (GCE)
- Green tea extract (GTE)
- vitamin C (at least 3 grams daily)
- vitamin D3
- Ellagic acid
- Diosgenin
- Apocynin
- beta-Glucan
- Fucoxanthin
- beta-Cryptoxanthin
- Cyanidin-3-Glucoside
- DHEA (Dehydroepiandrosterone)
- Ecdysterone, 20-hydroxyecdysterone
- Lactoferrin
- Oleanolic acid
- Ursolic acid
- Pyruvic acid
- Betulinic acid
- HCA, Hydroxy citric acid
- Curcumin
- Osthole
- Phillyrin
- Pectin
- Cirsimarin
- Inulin and fructo-oligosaccharides
- Guar gum (Cluster bean, Cyamopsis Tetragonoloba).

Amino acids
The following amino acids have body fat and body weight decreasing properties:
- GABA
- L-Arginine
- Glutamine
- L-Citrulline
- Taurine
- BCAA amino acids (Leucine, Valine, Isoleucine)
- HMB (beta-Hydroxy-beta-Methylbutyrate)
- 5-Hydroxytryptophan
- L-Tryptophan
- L-Carnosine

- L-Histidine
- NAC (N-Acetyl-L-Cysteine)
- Glycine.

Herbs and medicinal plants
There are very many medicinal plants, which have body fat and body weight decreasing properties. Please, look at the main text.

DO NOT EAT THE FOLLOWING JUNK FOODS, which contain large amounts of salt, sugar, fat, high glycemic index carbohydrates, calories and very large amount of food adddadditives:
- pizza
- Hamburgers
- French fries
- chips
- ALL sausages
- fatty cheese
- fatty milk
- butter
- cream
- mayonnaise
- ALL convenience food
- wheat flour
- white bread, cookies, pastry, meat pies, cakes
- sugar
- potatoes
- white rice
- rice cakes
- fatty meat
- alcohol
- ALL sugar containing drinks
- ALL sweeties
- white chocolate
- egg yolks
- Yoghurt with sugar.

Diet therapy against obesity and overweight

Diet therapy is very effective in reducing obesity and overweight. It is clearly more efficient than exercise alone. However, diet and exercise together is the most efficient method to decrease obesity and overweight. With a strictly controlled diet, the body weight can be decreased by 1.0 – 2.5 kg per week, and 5 – 10 kg per month, without feeling hunger.

The daily energy from food is totally dependent of the relative amounts of fat, carbohydrates, protein, alcohol, dietary fiber and water, and the total amount of food in grams.

Nutrient	Energy content, kcal/1 gram
water	0
dietary fiber	1.5 – 2.5
protein	4
carbohydrates	4
alcohol	7
fat	9

From the above table, it is clear, that the amount of especially saturated fat and alcohol should be minimized, and the amount of food with high water content, high dietary fiber content, high protein content and high low glycemic index GI carbohydrates content should be increased. Also one should drink a lot of water before meals and reduce the total amount of food at meals. Soups are excellent, because their energy density is very low.

The most efficient food groups to reduce obesity and overweigh are:
- water
- fresh fruits
- fresh berries
- vegetables
- root vegetables
- mushrooms
- peas and beans
- whole grains and dietary fiber products
- fat and sugar free milk, yoghurt and sour milk products
- fat free cheese products
- breast meat of chicken and turkey
- fish and crabs, lobster, mussel
- low fat wild animal meat
- honey
- nuts and seeds, especially sunflower seeds, sesame seeds, flaxseeds, almonds, groundnuts
- whey protein
- fat free soy protein and soy protein isolate

If we look at the mean average energy content of separate food groups, then we can calculate the following average energy content values:

- fresh fruits (not olive and avocado)   46 kcal/100g
- fresh berries (not rose hips)   44 kcal/100g
- vegetables (not basil)   20 kcal/100g
- root vegetables (not garlic, potatoes, sweet potatoes)   31 kcal/100g
- potatoes and sweet potatoes   80 kcal/100g
- mushrooms   24 kcal/100g
- fruit juices, 100%   50 kcal/100g
- fat free fish (perch, pike, pike perch, flounder, burbot, whitefish, Baltic herring, sea trout, tuna)   82 kcal/100g
- fish, all   156 kcal/100g
- crab, lobster, mussel, snail   83 kcal/100g
- chicken and turkey, breast meat   113 kcal/100g

− eggs	143 kcal/100g
− wild animal meat (moose, rabbit, reindeer)	123 kcal/100g
− low fat meat (steak, ham)	109 kcal/100g
− meat products, all	147 kcal/100g
− seeds and nuts	603 kcal/100g
− whole grains	324 kcal/100g
− butter	725 kcal/100g
− vegetable oils	884 kcal/100g
− sugar (sucrose, fructose, glucose)	406 kcal/100g
− honey	330 kcal/100g
− cheese	326 kcal/100g
− far free cottage cheese	84 kcal/100g
− fat free milk, sour milk, yoghurt	32 kcal/100g
− beer	44 kcal/100g
− red wine	70 kcal/100g

We can clearly see from the above list the following things:

1. Fresh fruits, fresh berries, vegetables, root vegetables, mushrooms and fat free milk products can be eaten very large amounts daily, and still the energy intake is very low. If man eats for example 500 grams vegetables and 500 grams fruits daily, and drinks 1 liter fat free milk products daily, the total energy intake is still very low, about 650 kcal/day.

2. From 20 grams of butter man gets the same amount of energy as from 700 grams of fruits, 500 grams of root vegetables or 300 grams of fruits.

3. If man drinks 5 large glasses of beer (0.5 liters, 4.5% alcohol content) daily, he gets 1100 kcal extra energy daily.

4. If man drinks 2 glasses (2.5 dl) of red wine daily, he gets 350 kcal extra energy daily.

With strictly controlled, low calorific value diet man can achieve very large weight reductions in just few months.

When 10 obese volunteers were on a controlled 600 – 800 kcal daily diet, for 3-4 months, the average body weight reduction was 23.2% (106.0 kg → 83.0 kg) (Weigle et.al. 1988).

When 7 obese volunteers were on a controlled 830 – 1120 kcal daily diet for 10 – 16 weeks, the average body weight reduction was 13.4% (95.4 kg → 82.8 kg; $p < 0.01$), body fat mass decreased by 9.2 kg ($p < 0.01$) and body fat-% decreased by 5.5% (38.0% → 32.5%; $p < 0.01$) (Ravussin et.al. 1985).

The following facts hold generally, when trying to decrease obesity by diet:

1. The greater the initial body weight, the greater the body weight reduction is in a certain time period.
2. The less calories in daily diet, the greater weight reductions can be achieved.
3. The longer the diet lasts, the greater is the weight reduction.

4. The longer the diet lasts, the less is the weekly weight reduction. This is because of the reduction of the daily basal metabolic rate.
5. If the diet is stopped, and the original diet is restarted, the weight will normally come back to the original level.
6. If the weight reduction is wanted to stay, then man must change his lifestyle: the food composition has to have less calories, the amount of food has to be reduced and more exercise has to be done.

The following small list contains the most common food items in Western daily food, and their energy, fat, carbohydrate, protein and dietary fiber contents.

NUTRIENTS TABLE

This table gives the energy content (kcal), and fat, carbohydrates, protein and dietary fiber contents in units of grams per 100 grams edible portion of the most common food items in typical Western daily diet. OBSERVE: The values are typical, average values.

Food item, 100g	kcal	fat	carbohyd.	protein	fiber
FRESH FRUITS					
Pineapple	53	0.4	11.2	0.5	1.4
Orange	43	0.3	8.9	0.6	2.1
Apricot	47	0.1	10.0	1.1	1.9
Banana	84	0.4	18.3	1.1	1.8
Guava	68	1.0	14.3	2.5	5.4
Grapefruit	32	0.3	6.5	0.6	1.4
Honeydew	32	0.1	7.0	0.6	0.8
Kiwi fruit	42	0.6	7.1	0.0	2.7
Plum	47	0.3	8.4	0.8	1.7
Mandarin	42	0.3	8.3	0.5	1.9
Mango	57	0.4	10.7	1.0	2.1
Olive	110	11.0	1.8	1.4	4.4
Apple	35	0.1	8.2	0.2	1.5
Papaya	39	0.1	9.8	0.6	1.8
Peach	41	0.3	7.8	1.1	2.1
Persimmon	70	0.2	18.6	0.6	3.6
Pear	36	0.1	8.0	0.3	3.9
Lemon	36	1.1	2.2	0.6	2.8
Cantaloupe	20	0.1	4.1	0.6	0.9
Red grapefruit	36	0.1	6.9	0.8	1.6
Watermelon	35	0.1	7.1	0.9	1.1
Fig	74	0.8	19.0	1.0	3.3
FRESH BERRIES					
Cranberry	22	0.7	3.5	0.4	3.3
Gooseberry	29	0.4	5.4	0.9	3.4
Cherries	52	0.1	11.8	0.9	1.5
Strawberry	43	0.2	8.4	0.5	1.9
Blackcurrant	48	0.4	7.8	1.1	5.8

Blueberry	33	0.6	6.4	0.5	3.3
Rowan berry	32	0.0	6.3	0.7	6.0
Redcurrant	47	0.4	7.5	1.4	5.0
Lingonberry	34	0.5	6.8	0.4	2.6
Rose hips	94	0.5	16.0	3.6	6.1
Cloudberry	54	0.5	7.8	1.4	5.8
Buckthorn berry	79	5.0	6.3	0.7	6.0
Raspberry	34	0.8	4.1	1.0	3.7
Grapes	72	0.4	15.5	0.8	1.1

VEGETABLES

Alfalfa sprouts	24	0.7	0.3	4.0	3.0
Bamboo shoots	11	0.2	0.7	1.5	1.4
Pickle	17	0.1	3.3	0.7	1.1
Sauerkraut	24	0.2	3.7	1.1	2.0
Cabbage	24	0.2	3.4	1.2	2.1
Zucchini	17	0.4	2.5	0.6	0.7
Chinese cabbage	18	0.3	2.3	1.6	0.9
Cauliflower	20	0.3	2.2	1.8	2.3
Cucumber	10	0.1	1.4	0.6	0.7
Pumpkin	12	0.1	2.0	0.7	2.0
Kohlrabi	24	0.2	4.2	1.3	1.9
Kale	25	0.6	3.4	3.4	2.0
Lettuce	12	0.2	1.2	1.1	1.0
Celery, leaf	11	0.2	1.1	1.1	1.0
Swiss chard	15	0.3	1.5	1.4	1.4
Eggplant	20	0.2	3.1	1.3	2.5
Mungbean sprouts	30	0.2	5.9	3.0	1.8
Nettle	17	0.7	1.3	5.9	4.1
Bell pepper, yellow	26	0.2	5.1	0.9	2.0
Bell pepper, red	26	0.4	4.6	0.9	2.0
Bell pepper, green	17	0.3	2.5	0.9	1.8
Asparagus	26	0.6	2.0	2.9	3.5
Broccoli	30	0.3	2.0	4.6	2.5
Parsley	12	0.2	1.1	1.4	8.0
Spinach	11	0.3	0.4	1.6	1.3
Red cabbage	22	0.2	3.5	1.6	1.9
Leek	19	0.2	2.4	1.8	2.1
Chives	27	0.6	3.8	1.4	1.1
Fennel, bulb	17	0.2	1.8	0.9	2.4
Dill	26	0.8	1.0	3.7	2.1
Tomato	21	0.3	3.8	0.6	1.4
Garden cress	21	1.4	0.7	1.4	3.3

ROOT VEGETABLES

Sweet potato	81	0.0	16.8	1.6	3.0
Beetroot in vinegar	32	0.1	6.7	1.0	1.8
Ginger	82	0.8	15.8	1.8	2.0
Rutabaga	25	0.3	4.6	1.0	1.8
Jerusalem artichoke	40	0.2	8.2	1.3	4.0

Black salsify	51	0.4	10.5	1.3	7.3
Turnip	24	0.3	4.2	1.0	1.9
Parsnip	35	0.4	6.2	1.3	4.5
Potato, new	75	0.2	16.1	1.7	1.0
Potato, old	83	0.2	17.6	1.8	1.0
Carrot	28	0.2	5.3	0.6	2.5
Beetroot	34	0.1	2.0	1.4	2.5
Radish	15	0.1	2.0	1.4	1.6
Celery	31	0.2	4.8	1.3	1.7
Garlic	104	0.6	16.3	7.9	2.1

MUSHROOMS

Champignon	25	0.3	3.0	2.1	1.5
King bolete	22	0.5	1.0	3.2	6.0
Milk-cap	19	0.5	1.5	2.1	2.0
Chanterelle	24	0.5	3.0	1.8	1.9
False morel	23	0.5	2.7	1.8	1.9
Oyster mushroom	26	0.3	2.6	2.0	2.4
Shiitake	28	0.3	4.5	1.8	3.3

PEAS AND BEANS

Pea	63	0.4	9.4	5.1	3.1
Broad bean	341	1.5	58.3	26.1	25.0
Chickpea	123	2.0	17.6	8.4	5.0
Lentil	293	1.0	45.7	24.4	8.9
Mung bean	347	1.1	62.6	23.8	16.3
Soy bean, boiled	178	8.0	7.1	16.1	7.1
Fresh green beans	32	0.2	4.1	1.9	2.4

FRESH FRUIT JUICE, 100%

Pineapple	59	0.1	13.4	0.5	0.0
Orange	45	0.1	10.0	0.3	0.0
Grapefruit	41	0.2	9.0	0.4	0.0
Apple	45	0.0	10.7	0.2	0.0
Grapes	63	0.0	14.0	1.0	0.0

FISH

Perch	84	1.7	0.0	17.1	0.0
Anchovis	257	11.4	9.6	28.9	0.0
Eel	363	33.0	0.0	17.5	0.0
Pike	84	1.1	0.0	18.3	0.0
Flounder	96	4.0	0.0	15.0	0.0
Rainbow trout	259	23.4	2.7	10.2	0.2
Rainbow trout, fillet	165	11.0	0.0	16.8	0.0
Pike perch	72	0.7	0.0	16.2	0.0
Bream	106	4.0	0.0	17.3	0.0
Salmon, fillet	195	13.5	0.0	18.7	0.0
Burbot	68	0.5	0.0	15.7	0.0
Mackerel, smoked	292	24.3	0.0	18.9	0.0
Vendace	108	3.4	0.0	19.1	0.0

River lamprey	305	26.4	0.0	17.5	0.0
Redperch	114	5.2	0.0	16.8	0.0
Sardine	191	12.2	0.3	20.0	0.0
Whitefish	100	3.4	0.0	17.2	0.0
Pollock, frozen	78	0.7	0.0	17.6	0.0
Baltic herring	129	7.1	0.0	16.2	0.0
Herring, salted	222	19.0	0.0	13.2	0.0
Halibut	190	13.6	0.0	17.3	0.0
Sea trout	110	3.8	0.0	18.7	0.0
Tuna in water	96	1.5	0.0	22.4	0.0
Tuna in oil	153	9.0	0.0	18.2	0.0
Cod	76	0.7	0.0	17.3	0.0

SHELLFISH AND MUSSELS

Lobster	84	0.9	0.0	18.8	0.0
Shrimp	71	1.1	0.7	14.4	0.0
Cuttlefish	84	1.3	0.0	17.9	0.0
Snail	86	1.3	2.0	16.1	0.0
Mussel, in water	89	2.0	1.9	15.6	0.0

POULTRY AND EGG PRODUCTS

Broiler, leg	294	22.7	0.0	23.0	0.0
Chicken, breast fillet	103	1.5	0.0	23.1	0.0
Turkey	196	7.7	0.0	31.4	0.0
Turkey fillet	146	3.0	0.0	29.4	0.0
Turkey, breast fillet	124	2.2	0.0	25.6	0.0
Chicken	188	12.0	0.0	20.3	0.0
Egg	143	10.3	0.3	12.5	0.0
Egg, yellows	285	25.0	0.2	15.5	0.0
Egg, whites	42	0.1	0.4	9.8	0.0

MEAT

Horse meat	219	13.3	0.0	25.0	0.0
Moose meat	112	3.0	0.0	21.1	0.0
Rabbit	130	5.0	0.0	21.1	0.0
Kebab meat	218	13.2	0.0	24.9	0.0
Ham, boiled	107	4.5	0.0	16.4	0.0
Tongue, cow	202	15.0	0.4	16.7	0.0
Liver, cow	132	3.7	5.8	18.4	0.0
Kidney	126	6.7	0.9	15.6	0.0
Steak, cow	111	2.6	0.0	21.7	0.0
Reindeer	127	4.5	0.0	21.6	0.0
Terderloin, pork	108	2.6	0.0	21.0	0.0
Steak, pork	163	5.5	0.0	28.0	0.0

SEEDS AND NUTS

Sunflower	582	49.5	12.6	23.0	6.0
Cashew nuts	597	46.3	26.0	20.0	3.5
Hazelnut	644	61.0	3.5	14.1	17.5
Groundnuts	535	43.0	12.5	25.6	15.8

Almond	602	54.0	6.6	24.1	7.2
Flaxseed	506	41.9	1.0	19.8	26.4
Walnut	639	64.0	3.3	14.7	15.9
Brazil nut	670	66.4	2.6	14.3	7.5
Pecan nut	710	72.0	4.4	9.2	9.6
Pistachio	581	46.0	16.7	21.4	10.3
Sesame seeds	563	48.2	6.9	26.9	12.3

OIILS AND FATS

Sunflower oil	884	100.0	0.0	0.0	0.0
Margarine, 40% fat	361	40.0	0.3	1.0	0.0
Maize oil	883	99.9	0.0	0.0	0.0
Olive oil	884	100.0	0.0	0.0	0.0
Rape oil	883	100.0	0.0	0.0	0.0
Soy oil	883	100.0	0.0	0.0	0.0
Butter	725	81.3	0.4	1.2	0.0

MILK PRODUCTS

Bulgarian yoghurt	64	3.9	3.4	3.0	0.0
Cheddar cheese	413	34.4	0.1	25.6	0.0
Emmenthal cheese	379	30.0	0.0	27.9	0.0
Feta cheese, cow	227	18.0	1.7	14.0	0.0
Feta cheese, goat	299	25.0	1.2	18.0	0.0
Feta cheese in oil	328	28.8	1.1	17.1	0.0
Gefilus sour milk, 1%	40	1.0	3.7	3.4	0.0
Gouda cheese	375	31.0	0.0	23.5	0.0
Yoghurt, fat free	34	0.1	5.0	3.1	0.0
Mozzarella cheese	261	20.3	0.0	18.6	0.0
Cottage cheese, fat free	84	0.3	2.0	18.0	0.0
Milk, fat free	34	0.1	4.9	3.1	0.0
Milk flour, fat free	356	1.0	52.9	32.4	0.0
Sour milk, fat free	30	0.1	3.6	2.9	0.0
Milk, 1% fat	43	1.0	4.8	3.4	0.0

CEREAL PRODUCTS

Graham flour	328	2.2	60.7	10.6	9.9
Millet	140	1.2	27.5	4.5	1.3
Oat flakes	355	7.3	57.0	14.5	10.0
Oat bran	326	7.7	45.6	18.0	17.5
Fiber, sugar beet	60	0.3	5.5	9.0	73.0
Maize grain	137	2.4	25.6	2.8	3.7
Maize, dried	353	6.7	55.4	12.7	9.2
Barley flakes	313	2.0	64.4	8.3	9.1
French roll	273	1.5	54.9	9.1	3.1
Rye flakes	269	2.5	52.0	8.8	13.9
Rye bread	180	1.2	35.7	5.9	11.0
Rye bran	205	4.3	26.0	15.0	39.0
Crisp bread	298	1.9	57.8	11.4	15.6
Buckwheat flakes	312	2.0	60.5	11.9	5.8
Macaroni, dark	310	3.0	59.4	10.4	5.9

Brown rice	341	2.3	72.0	7.0	4.0
Wheat flakes	301	2.2	58.7	10.6	12.9
Wheat bran	156	4.5	15.4	13.3	37.5
Wheat germ	334	10.0	31.0	29.4	14.0
Wheat roll	284	6.2	49.0	7.3	2.5

SUGARS

Fructose	405	0.0	99.8	0.0	0.0
Honey	330	0.0	80.8	0.5	0.0
Glucose	406	0.0	100.0	0.0	0.0
Sugar	406	0.0	99.9	0.0	0.0

ALCOHOLIC DRINKS

Beer, 5.5%	47	0.0	3.4	0.5	0.0
Beer, 4.5%	42	0.0	4.1	0.4	0.0
Red wine	70	0.0	0.0	0.3	0.0
Vodka, 33%	220	0.0	0.0	0.0	0.0

CONVENIENCE FOOD AND JUNK FOODS

Balkan sausage	266	23.0	2.2	13.1	3.0
Doughnut	423	22.5	48.5	6.0	1.3
Grilled sausage	260	23.0	3.0	10.9	0.3
Hamburger, cow meat	162	4.7	19.2	10.5	1.3
Hamburger, chicken meat	291	19.0	20.7	9.4	1.2
Ice cream	192	12.0	17.3	3.9	0.0
Bologna sausage	211	16.0	8.0	9.3	0.2
Liver casserole	141	4.5	18.7	6.0	0.6
Liver sausage	223	19.0	2.2	11.3	0.0
Chips	520	33.0	50.6	5.3	4.7
French fries	346	19.3	38.6	4.0	0.9

Exercise training against obesity and overweight

Question: What is the "Medicine", which
- decreases body weight and makes the body slim
- decreases body fat mass
- decreases body fat-%
- increases fat free muscle mass
- decreases blood pressure
- increases good HDL-cholesterol
- decreases total cholesterol
- decreases bad LDL-cholesterol
- decreases triglycerides
- improves insulin resistance
- improves metabolic syndrome

- decreases heart rate
- increases heart stroke volume
- slows down aging
- increases lifetime
- keeps the body youthfull
- decreases stress
- increases testosterone, growth hormone GH and beta-endorphin levels
- decreases Leptin and increases Adiponectin levels
- increases aerobic endurance
- increases muscle strength
- increases max. VO2
- it does not have any side effects, when taken regularly several times weekly, all around the year
- it does not cost anything

Answer: Aerobic and resistance training, made at least 3-5 times weekly, at least 45-60 minutes/exercise, all around the year.

The positive effects of aerobic exercise and resistance training on the above mentioned variables has been studied for several tens of years in thousands of scientific research papers, all around the World.

The positive effects of both aerobic exercise and resistance training to the before mentioned variables has been 100%:tly verified in these numerous scientific research papers, most of which are double blind experiments. The amount of physical work as a physical exercise has been reduced to minimum level, especially in industrialized countries. This is the reason, that only exercise and physical training are the only possibilities to keep up a good body composition, endurance and strength. Without regular training, the muscle strength and endurance, the heart pumping capacity, body composition and the overall body physical condition will go down very rapidly, especially during aging, when also the levels of the anabolic hormones testosterone, growth hormone GH, DHEA etc. go rapidly down.

The positive effects of aerobic exercise and resistance training on excess body weight, body fat mass, body fat-% and fat free muscle mass has been researched in so extremely many research papers, that in this book only a very few example research results are given.

Besides the classical low intensity aerobic exercise and resistance training, nowadays also the high intensity aerobic interval training (HIT= High Intensity Training) has become under intensive research, because it has many positive effects on body composition, hormones and exercise performance. With this exercise method you do not need to spend a lot of time doing exercise, because the total exercise time spent is normally from few minutes up to 40 minutes totally. However, you must train at high aerobic level, typically over 70% of your VO2max. High intensity interval training has large positive effects on maximal oxygen uptake VO2max., body anabolic and lipolytic hormones such as testosterone, growth hormone GH, noradrenaline, adrenaline, beta-endorphin, Leptin and Adiponectin and both body fat and fat free muscle mass.

It is well known, that aerobic exercise with low intensity level (typically 40-60% of VO2max.) for a longer time at each exercise period significantly improves the muscles capacity to use fat as energy source, instead of carbohydrates. When comparing non-trained and endurance trained volunteers on bicycle tests, it has been verified, that depending on the power level, endurance trained volunteers burn up to 80-200% more fat, compared to non-trained volunteers (Stisen et.al. 2006).

Due to this fat oxidation enhancing effect of low intensity aerobic exercise, endurance trained athletes have extremely low body weight, body fat mass and fat-%. Or has anybody seen a top level Marathon runner, who has a body weight of 100 kg and has over 20% body fat? Hardly. The average body weight of Marathon runners is, depending of height and gender, between 45 -65 kg.

These same facts hold also for ordinary, overweight persons. When they start regular, typically 3-5 times per week, aerobic exercise, both body weight, body fat mass and body fat-% decrease steadily during each training week. The more time is spent weekly on aerobic exercise, the more is the net energy expenditure and the more fat will be burnt during exercise.

When 25 obese (BMI=32.18) females trained 5 times aerobically per week, at intensity level of 50% of their VO2max., for 12 weeks, body weight decreased by 5.9% or 5.2 kg (88.5 kg->83.3 kg; $p<0.01$) and body fat mass decreased by 6.4% ($p<0.01$). Waist circumference decreased by 3.6 cm (92.9 cm->89.3 cm; $p<0.01$), hip circumference decreased by 3.5 cm (114.5 cm->111.0 cm; $p<0.01$) and plasma Leptin decreased by 25.5% ($p<0.001$) (Polak et.al. 2006).

When 22 obese boys (body fat-%>30%) trained aerobically 3 times per week, 50 minutes during each exercise, for 12 weeks, body fat-% decreased by 4.6% and body fat mass decreased by 5.4%, compared to 10 person control group (Song et.al. 2012).

When comparing the effects of different exercises on reduction of body weight and body fat mass in obese volunteers, then aerobic exercise is the most effective in reducing both body weight and body fat mass, but the combination of both aerobic exercise and resistance exercise decrease also body weight and fat mass, but it is more effective in reducing waist circumference, blood pressure, and triglycerides, and more effective in increasing fat free muscle mass, VO2max., growth hormone GH and testosterone (Ho et.al. 2012; Willis et.al. 2012; Seo et.al. 2010; Ha et.al. 2012).

When 10 obese (fat-% 36.5%, BMI=26.3, age 40 years) female volunteers made combination training for 1 hour, 3 times weekly, for 12 weeks, body weight decreased by 2.7 kg (64.9 kg-> 62.2 kg; $p<0.001$), fat-% decreased by 3.1% (36.5%->33.4%; $p<0.001$), diastolic blood pressure decreased by 3.4 mmHg (78.6 mmHg->75.2 mmHg; $p=0.041$), triglycerides decreased by 12.2% ($p=0.02$) and blood sugar decreased by 6.5% ($p=0.001$), but HDL-cholesterol increased by 13.9% ($p=0.028$) in test group. There were no changes in the 10 person control group. The combination training was as follows: First 30 minutes running at intensity of 60-70% of VO2max., and after this resistance training with 5 different muscle groups (bench press, lat-pull down, shoulder press, leg press, sit ups), involving 3 sets of 10 repetition maximum (10RM) for each of the exercises (Seo et.al. 2011).

Fat free muscle mass is very important, if the weight reduction period is very long, because the higher is the fat free muscle mass, the higher is the resting energy expenditure REE. Normally during strict diet the REE will decrease also, and the weight reduction becomes less effective. The REE will increase about 21 kcal/1 kg muscle mass.

Resistance training is very often made in gyms, because they have many different exercise machines to train different muscle groups. Normally 8-10 different exercises are done, with 3 sets in each, and 8-12 repetitions in each set. Normally more than 1 set per muscle group is done, because it is known, that 3 sets is superior to only 1 set, when trying to develop strength and other muscle properties. The energy expenditure in resistance training varies typically between 6-11 kcal/min (Meirelles et.al. 2004). To this we have to add the very long lasting increased resting energy expenditure REE due to the resistance training. This effect may last between 15-24 hours.

Resistance training decreases significantly body fat mass, but it also increases significantly fat free muscle mass, resting energy expenditure REE after exercise and the levels of fat burning hormones (growth hormone GH, testosterone, noradrenaline, adrenaline) and VO2max. (Pratley et.al. 1994; Schjerve et.al. 2008; Strasser et.al. 2011; Kirk et.al. 2009).

When female volunteers (BMI=28.0) made resistance training 3 times weekly, for 3 years, the resting energy expenditure REE increased by 110 kcal/day or 9%, and fat free muscle mass increased by 10%. There were no changes in control group (Trevisan et.al. 2010).

Walking, Nordic walking and race walking are very popular and very effective aerobic training methods to increase energy expenditure and to decrease body weight, body fat mass and body fat-%. For example the energy expenditure of race walking is higher than in running, when the speed increases over 10 km/hour (Hagberg et.al. 1984).

When using walking, Nordic walking or race walking as an exercise for body weight and body fat mass reduction, it is wise to use interval training method. The following research is a very good example. When type 2 diabetes volunteers made aerobic walking for 60 minutes, 5 times weekly, for 4 months, either by steady speed walking, or by interval walking, 3 minutes fast, 3 minutes slow etc., the following changes were noticed in the interval group, compared to the steady walking speed group: body weight decreased by 3.5 kg ($p<0.001$), fat mass decreased by 3.0 kg ($p<0.001$), VO2max. increased by 10.9% ($p<0.01$), relative oxygen uptake (=VO2max divided by body mass) increased by 16.2% ($p<0.001$), triglycerides decreased by 16.6%, LDL-cholesterol decreased by 12.5% ($p<0.001$), Insulin decreased by 19.5% ($p<0.01$) and blood sugar decreased by 8.5% ($p<0.05$) (Karstoft et.al. 2012).

Now we have shown the positive effects of aerobic exercise, resistance exercise and aerobic plus resistance combination exercise on excess body weight, body fat mass, body fat-%, waist circumference, hormones, blood pressure, blood sugar and blood lipid values. Lastly we look at the positive effects of the HIT method (HIT= High Intensity Training), which is aerobic interval training with high intensity.

This exercise method is very good for lazy people, who do not want to spend long times in gyms or doing long lasting aerobic exercises. This method is a combination of high intensity and reasonable long total exercise time, in minimum total time spent on one exercise. This exercise can be easily done at home using stationary bicycle, treadmill, own dumbbells or own weightlifting barbell.

In interval training, normally several exercise repeats between 10 seconds – 4 minutes duration are done, with equal or longer rest periods between each exercise repeat. The total effect of this exercise is aerobic, and can be made for a long time, but because of the high intensity, over 80% of VO2max., there are also anaerobic elements involved in this exercise. Interval training increases significantly Adiponectin, growth hormone GH and testosterone (Moghadasi et.al. 2012; Shing et.al. 2012; Irving et.al. 2009; Meckel et.al. 2011; Wahl et.al. 2010; Rahimi et.al. 2010).

Aerobic high intensity interval training increases significantly fat oxidation during exercise. This effect was unknown earlier, before the latest research studies.

When 8 female volunteers (age 22 years, weight 65.0 kg) made 7 aerobic interval training sessions (10x4 minutes, 90% of VO2max, rest 2 minutes), during 2 weeks, fat oxidation during exercise increased by 36% (p<0.05), compared to values before training. Also VO2max. increased by 13% (p<0.05) (Talanian et.al. 2007).

Typically in different research studies with high intensity aerobic interval training the following changes has been achieved, with exercise durations between 2-24 weeks (Boutcher 2011):
–   body fat mass decreased by 3 kg or more
–   body weight decreased by 1.5-3.0 kg
–   waist circumference decreased by 2-7 cm
–   VO2max. increased by 6%-41%
–   insulin sensitivity increased by 10%-58%
–   growth hormone GH increased after exercise over 1000% or more, compared to baseline before exercise
–   noradrenaline increased after exercise by at least 1400%, compared to baseline before exercise
–   adrenaline increased after exercise by at least 600%, compared to baseline before exercise

In many research experiments it has been verified, that the resting energy expenditure REE after exercise will increase by 5%-20%, when using high intensity interval training with intensity levels of 70% or more of VO2max. This high REE level after exercise will last between 24-48 hours (Hunter et.al. 1998). This means a 100-200 kcal/day higher energy expenditure each day at rest!

Interval training increase significantly the fat oxidation stimulating hormone noradrenaline levels in plasma, and this high level will last up to 24 hours after exercise (Hunter et.al. 1998).

Interval training increases significantly fat oxidation during exercise (Hunter et.al. 1998; Talanianet.al. 2007).

Because high intensity interval training increases very efficiently the VO2max. level, this gives an extra method to increase fat oxidation during exercise and to reduce excess body weight. When a person with 4.0 liters/minute VO2max. is exercising at a 50% VO2max. level, he spends energy at a rate of 10.0 kcal/minute. However a person with 3.0 liters/minute VO2max. level uses only 7.5 kcal/minute energy, when exercising at 50% of VO2max. level. In both cases the persons do exercise at the optimal 50% of VO2max. level, but the person with higher VO2max. level will burn 33% more energy, and mostly as fat, during each minute of the exercise (Hunter et.al. 1998).

High intensity interval training improves all the following parameters (Heydari et.al. 2012; Cho et.al. 2011; Tjonna et.al. 2008; Hottenrott et.al. 2012; Paoli et.al. 2010; Whyte et.al. 2010; Trilk et.al. 2011; Quinn et.al. 2006; Nybo et.al. 2010; Lee et.al. 2012; Irving et.al. 2008; Little et.al. 2010; Yoahioka et.al. 2001; Wisloff et.al. 2007; Ernest et.al. 2008):
–   body weight decreases
–   body fat mass decreases
–   body fat-% decreases
–   waist circumference decreases

- fat free muscle mass increases
- VO2max. increases
- working power in Watts increases
- RQ-value (Respiratory Quotient) decreases (This means a higher fat oxidation capacity)
- resting energy expenditure REE increases
- fat oxidation increases
- carbohydrate oxidation decreases
- heart rate decreases
- heart stroke volume increases
- blood pressure decreases
- triglycerides decrease
- Insulin decreases
- Insulin resistance decreases
- Aerobic endurance capacity increases
- Adiponectin level increases
- growth hormone GH, testosterone, noradrenaline, adrenaline and IGF-1 levels increase in plasma
- HDL-cholesterol increases

Lastly we can make the following notes, regarding different exercise methods:
Aerobic exercise, resistance exercise, combined aerobic and resistance exercise and high intensity interval training are excellent methods to reduce obesity, high body fat mass, high body fat-% and high waist circumference, and to increase fat free muscle mass.

These exercise methods are excellent also against type 2 diabetes, metabolic syndrome, hypertension and high cholesterol levels, together with proper nutrition with large amounts of fruits, vegetables, nuts, whole grains and protein, but low amounts of saturated fats and high glycemic index GI carbohydrates.

Exercise and Diet Therapy Together Against Obesity and Overweight

Exercise training is a very efficient method to increse daily energy expenditure and thus decrease overweight. Strictly controlled diet is however much more efficient. But the most efficient way to decrease overweight and reduce obesity is to combine both regular exercise training and controlled diet.

This is understandable, because increasing the weekly energy expenditure and decreasing the weekly energy intake will decrease body fat and thus obesity much more efficiently, than both methods done singly.

In a large meta-analysis, which consisted of 493 separate research done on human volunteers during 25 years, it was studied the effects of either exercise, diet or exercise and diet combined on body weight reduction. The average weight of the volunteers was 92.7 kg, BMI was 33.2, fat-% was 33.4% and age was 40 years. The average reduction in body weight was 2.9 kg, in body fat mass 3.3 kg and in body fat-% 3.5% in the exercise only group. In the diet only group body weight decreased by 10.7 kg, body fat mass decreased by 7.8 kg and body fat-% decreased by 6.0%. But in the combined exercise and diet group body weight decreased by 11.0 kg, body fat mass decreased by 9.0 kg and body fat-% decreased by 7.3%. And 1 year after the experiments, body weight in the combined exercise and diet group was significantly lower, compared to either exercise or diet group only (Miller et.al. 1997).

The same kind of results has been achieved also in recent experiments with human volunteers (Foster-Schubert et.al. 2012; Snel et.al. 2012; Volpe et.al. 2008).

As Petrofsky (Petrofsky et.al. 2004; Petrofsky et.al. 2006) has shown, during a very short 7 days experiment with 1200 kcal controlled diet and 6 days per week exercise program, very large decreases in body weight and body fat-% can be achieved. In these experiments the volunteers lost 2.4 kg of body weight, 1.2% in body fat-%, 3.5 cm in waist circumference and also heart rate decreased 4 – 6 beats/minute, systolic blood pressure decreased by 6 – 8 mmHg and diastolic blood pressure decreased by 5 – 6 mmHg. And all these changes just in 7 days.

Acupuncture, electroacupuncture and laser acupuncture

Acupuncture is thousands of years old medical treatment method, which is both cheap and safe. Acupuncture is an official medical treatment method by World Health Organization WHO. In China it has been used over 5000 years, together with medicinal herbs. There are 14 so called Main Meridians, which contain 361 official acupuncture points. Together with EXTRA acupuncture points, the total number of known acupuncute points is over 2000. There are hundreds of books about acupuncture, and just in MEDLINE data files there are over 18500 Scientific research articles about acupuncture.

Acupuncture, electroacupuncture and laser acupuncture have body weight and body fat mass decreasing properties.

When 22 obese (BMI = 39.8) volunteers were given daily 30 minutes electroacupuncture, for 20 days, body weight decreased in test group by 4.2 kg (4.80%: 87.5 kg → 83.3 kg; p = 0.0001), but it did not change in the 12 person (BMI = 32.2) placebo group. Also total cholesterol decreased by 17.5% (222.5 mg/dl → 183.5 mg/dl; p = 0.004), LDL-cholesterol decreased by 19.1% (153,3 mg/dl → 124.0 mg/dl; p = 0.021) and triglycerides decreased by 29.9% (160.5 mg/dl → 112.5 mg/dl; p = 0.038) in test group, but these values did not change in the placebo group. The used acupuncture points were: LI4 (Hegu), LI11 (Quchi), St25 (Tianshu), St36 (Zusanli), St44 (Neiting), Liv3 (Taichong) and Auricular ear points Hungry and Stomach (Cabioglu et.al. 2005).

In a meta-analysis of 44 different research with placebo group, with duration between 2 – 16 weeks, acupuncture decreased body weight in test groups by an average of 2.76 kg, compared to placebo groups (Sui et.al. 2012).

In another meta-analysis with 31 different research with placebo group and 3013 participants, acupuncture decreased body weight in test groups by an average of 1.76 kg, compared to placebo groups (Cho et.al. 2009).

The body weight, body fat mass and Leptin decreasing properties of acupuncture has been verified in very large number of research with human volunteers (Tang et.al. 2009; He et.al. 2008; Jiao et.al. 2008; Wu et.al. 2009; Zhu et.al. 2010; Hu et.al. 2010; Yang et.al. 2010; Zhang et.al. 2011; Chen et.al. 2011; Tong et.al. 2011; Huang et.al. 2011; Rerksuppaphol et.al. 2010; Chien et.al. 2011; Liu et.al. 2012; Qunli et.al. 2005; Kang et.al. 2005; Gao et.al. 2007; Richards et.al. 1998).

The most often used acupuncture points are: LI4 (Hegu), LI11 (Quchi), St25 (Tianshu), St36 (Zusanli), St44 (Neiting), Liv3 (Taichong), Sp6 (Sanyinjiao), Sp9 (Yinlingquan), St40 (Fenlong), Ren6 (Qihai), Ren12 (Zhongwan), Ren4 (Guanyan), St28 (Shuidao), St37 (Shangjuxu) and Auricular ear acupuncture points Hunger, Stomach, Endocrine, Spleen, Lung, Shenmen and Mouth.

Adlay, seeds

(Coix Lachryma-Jobi)

Adlay is also known as Coix or Job`s tears. Adlay is a very important plant in China, Korea, Japan and Taiwan, cultivated for its edible, large seeds. It has also many medicinal properties. It is known to decrease high cholesterol and triglyceride levels. In Asia it is regarded as a functional health food. It is annual, and its cultivation is very easy.

Adlay seeds have body weight and body fat mass decreasing properties.

When obese rats were given high fat diet and Adlay water extract 50 mg/kg BW daily, for 4 weeks, body weight was 24.9% ($p < 0.05$), body fat mass was 22.1% ($p < 0.05$) and total cholesterol was 15.0% ($p < 0.05$) lower in test group, compared to control group (Kim et.al. 2007).

The Adlay seeds body weight, body fat mass, Leptin, total cholesterol, LDL-cholesterol and triglycerides decreasing properties has been verified in great many experiments with rats and hamsters (Yu et.al. 2005; Kim et.al. 2000; Wang et.al. 2012; Huang et.al. 2005; Park et.al. 1988).

In fat cell experiments, Adlay extract inhibits the differentiation of 3T3-L1 fat cells (Ha et.al. 2010) and decreases lipid accumulation into 3T3-L1 fat cells (Kim et.al. 2007).

In the ancient Indian Ayurvedic classical medical textbook Charak Samhita, Adlay is said to have body weight decreasing properties.

When 30 obese (BMI = 29.68) volunteers were given Adlay water mixture (1 part Adlay, 6 parts water) 80 ml daily, for 12 weeks, body weight was 1.25 kg ($p < 0.05$), waist circumference was 1.5 cm ($p < 0.05$) and hip circumference was 0.78 cm ($p < 0.05$) lower in test group, compared to 30 person (BMI = 28.15) control group (Patil et.al. 2012).

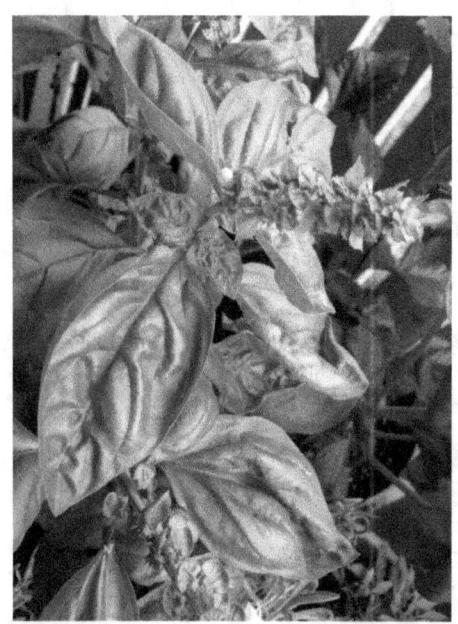

African Basil

(Ocinum Canum)

African Basil is used in Africa as a spice and medicine. It is especially used in diabetes, because it decreases blood sugar.

African Basil has body weight decreasing properties.

When normal and diabetic mice were given daily African Basil water extract, for 13 weeks, body weight was 12% ($p < 0.05$) lower in normal mice group, and 8.3% ($p < 0.05$) lower in diabetic mice group, compared to the control groups (Nyarko et.al. 2002).

When normal and diabetic mice were given daily African Basil water extract for 13 weeks, body weight gain in both groups was significantly ($p < 0.05$) lower, compared to the control groups. Also LDL-cholesterol and total cholesterol in both groups were significantly ($p < 0.05$) lower, but HDL-cholesterol significantly ($p < 0.05$) higher, than in the control groups (Nyarko et.al. 2003).

African Mango

(Irvinga Gabonensis)

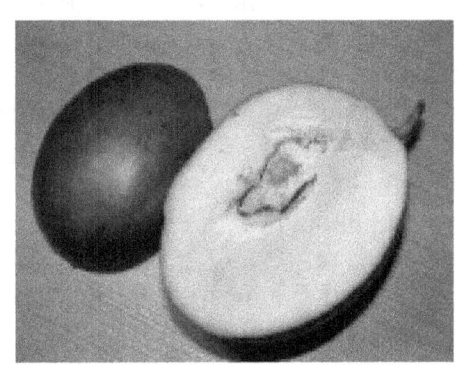

African Mango originates from Central Africa. Its fruit and large seed are edible, and they are an important food item in local cultures. The seeds are very rich in protein.

African mango seeds have body weight decreasing properties.

When 28 volunteers were given 3.15 grams of African Mango seeds daily, for 4 weeks, body weight decreased by 5.6% ($p < 0.0001$) compared to the placebo group (Ngondi et.al. 2005). This was a double blind experiment.

When 61 volunteers were given African Mango seed extract 300 mg daily, for 10 weeks, body weight decreased by 12.8% (97.9 kg → 85.1 kg; $p < 0.01$) and fat-% decreased by 6.3% ($p < 0.05$), compared to the placebo group (Ngondi et.al. 2009). This was a double blind experiment.

When 24 volunteers were given African Mango seed extract 500 mg and Cissus Quadrangularis extract 300 mg daily, for 10 weeks, body weight decreased by 3.0% ($p < 0.05$), compared with the group, which were given only Cissus Quadrangularis extract 300 mg daily (Oben et.al. 2008). This was a double blind experiment. Totally the body weight decreased by 11.86% (99.8 kg → 88.0 kg; $p < 0.001$), compared to the control group, which did get neither extract.

ALCAR

(Alcetyl-L-Carnitine)

and PCAR

(Propionyl-L-Carnitine)

ALCAR or Acetyl-L-Carnitine is the acetylated form of L-Carnitine, which exist in all living animal- and plant cells. PCAR or Propionyl-L-Carnitine is a complex of L-Carnitine and the natural short chain lenght fatty acid, Propionic acid. Both ALCAR and PCAR can be bought as supplements.These are very popular among sportsmen. Both ALCAR and PCAR have many positive health effects.

ALCAR and PCAR have body weight and body fat mass decreasing properties.

When old, 22 month, rats were given 100 mg/kg BW ALCAR daily, for 3 months, body weight was 6.75% (p < 0.01), triglycerides were 25.5% (p < 0.01) and total cholesterol was 20.8% (p < 0.01) lower in test group, compared to control group (Tanaka et.al. 2004).

When human volunteers were given 2 grams ALCAR daily, for 8 months, intramyocellular triglycerides decreased significantly (p = 0.03), serum free fatty acids (FFA) decreased by 19% (p < 0.05) and Respiratory Quotient RQ decreased significantly (p < 0.03) from 0.83 to 0.72. This means that fat oxidation is increased significantly (Benedini et.al. 2009).

When obese mice were given high fat diet and PCAR 200 mg/kg BW daily, for 4 weeks, body weight gain in test group was 81% (p < 0.01) lower, compared to control group. Body fat mass in test group was 28.6% (p < 0.001) lower, compared to control group. Also total cholesterol, blood glucose and Insulin were all significantly (p < 0.05) lower in test group, compared to control group (Mingorance et.al. 2012).

The body weight and body fat mass decreasing properties of PCAR has been verified also in another experiment with rats (Mingorance et.al. 2009).

Alcohol

The use of alcohol has increased all over the World. The energy content of alcohol is 7 kcal/gram, which is the second highest after fat, which has a 9 kcal/gram energy content, compared to the 4 kcal/gram energy content of carbohydrates and protein. The consumption of the recommended 30 grams alcohol per day contributes to approximately 10% of daily energy intake. The addition of this amount of alcohol to daily diet would produce theoretically a 12 kg body weight increase per year. However, this is not so simple matter. It seems to be, that men using moderate amounts of daily alcohol, body weight and body fat mass may increase, but females and alcoholics have a tendency to decrease body fat and body weight, when using alcohol on daily bases. Also with alcohol use, hunger feeling is often increased.

Alcohol increases body weight and body fat mass in men.

Alcohol is known to decrease the contents of the anabolic hormones testosterone, growth hormone GH and melatonin in serum. Alcohol also increases the inflammatory markers igE, IL-1, IL-6 and TNF-alfa in serum, and increases blood pressure.

Alcohol is thermogenic, and increases the 24 hours energy expenditure by 4 – 5%, depending on dose (Suter et.al. 1994; Buemann et.al. 2001).

On the other hand, alcohol significantly decreases fatty acid oxidation (Suter et.al. 1992).

When studying the relations between body weight, alcohol use and diet of 89 538 females and 48 493 males, it was noticed that the total energy intake increased in males drinking more than 50 grams alcohol per day, by 29.6%, compared to abstainers (Colditz et.al. 1991).

The body weight and body fat mass increasing effect of alcohol in males has been verified in many experiments (Wannamethee et.al. 2003; Brandhagen et.al. 2012; Lourenco et.al. 2012).

Aloe

(Aloe Vera, Aloe Ferox)

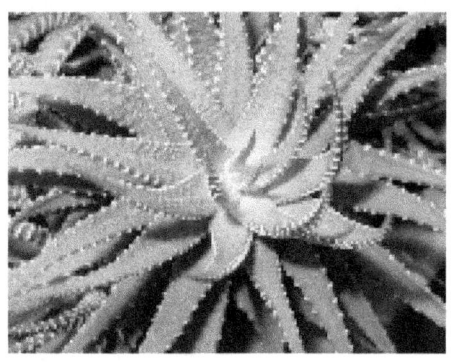

Aloe is a famous medicinal plant. Aloe gel is used in tens of different medicinal ailments and conditions. Aloe is known to decrease blood pressure, blood sugar, triglycerides and cholesterol. Aloe has large number of different Polyphenols, such as Lophenol, Cycloartenol, Aloin, Aloe-Emodin etc.

Aloe has body weight and body fat mass decreasing properties.

When mice were given 350 mg/kg BW daily Aloe Polyphenol extract, for 4 weeks, both body weight (p = 0.008) and blood glucose (p < 0.005) decreased significantly, compared to the control group (Perez et.al. 2007).

When obese mice on high fat diet were given Aloe gel either 50 mg/kg BW or 100 mg/kg BW daily, for 8 weeks, body fat mass decreased by 2.8% and 30%, compared to the control group. Triglycerides decreased by 23.8% (p < 0.05) and 30% (p < 0.01), compared to the control group (Kim et.al. 2009).

The Aloe body weight, body fat mass and triglycerides decreasing properties has been verified in many experiments with rats and mice (Sibuyi et.al. 2007; Misawa et.al. 2012; Misawa et.al. 2008; Nomaguchi et.al. 2011).

Alpha-Linolenic acid and Flaxseed oil

(Linum Usitatissimum)

Flaxseed oil contains large amounts, up to 50 – 60% alpha-Linolenic acid, which is an essential W-3 polyunsaturated fatty acid. From alpha-Linolenic acid the body cells make the famous "fish oil"; EPA (Eicosapentaenoic acid), which is known to decrease body weight and triglycerides. Also Perilla oil and Camelina oil contain large amounts of alpha-Linolenic acid.

Alpha-Linolenic acid and Flaxseed oil have body weight and body fat mass decreasing properties.

When rats were given high fat diet and 1 gram/kg BW Flaxseed oil daily, for 2 months, body weight gain was 32.0% (p < 0.05) lower in test group, compared to control group. Also triglycerides were 67.8% (p < 0.05) and total cholesterol was 70.9% (p < 0.05) lower in test group, compared to control group (Vijaimohan et.al. 2006).

The body weight and body fat mass decreasing properties of alpha-Linolenic acid and Flaxseed oil has been verified in great many animal experiments (Javadi et.al. 2004; Crespo et.al. 2002; Mortise et.al. 2005; Baranowski et.al. 2012).

In animal experiments alpha-Linolenic acid stimulates significantly the activity of fatty acid oxidation enzymes, but inhibits significantly the activity of fatty acid synthesis stimulating enzymes (Ide et.al. 1996; Javadi et.al. 2007; Kabir et.al. 1996; Ide et.al. 2000; Ide et.al. 2000).

When 81 volunteers were given low calorific diet together with either Olive oil or oil mixture with 3.5 grams/day alpha-Linolenic acid, for 6 months, body weight decreased by 7.8 kg in alpha-Linolenic group, which was significantly ($p < 0.05$) more, than the 6.0 kg body weight decrease in the Olive oil group. Also triglycerides ($p < 0.05$) and diastolic blood pressure ($p < 0.05$) decreased significantly more in alpha-Linolenic group, compared to Olive oil group (Baxheinrich et.al. 2012).

The body weight decreasing properties of Flaxseed oil has been verified also in another experiment with human volunteers (Taylor et.al. 2010).

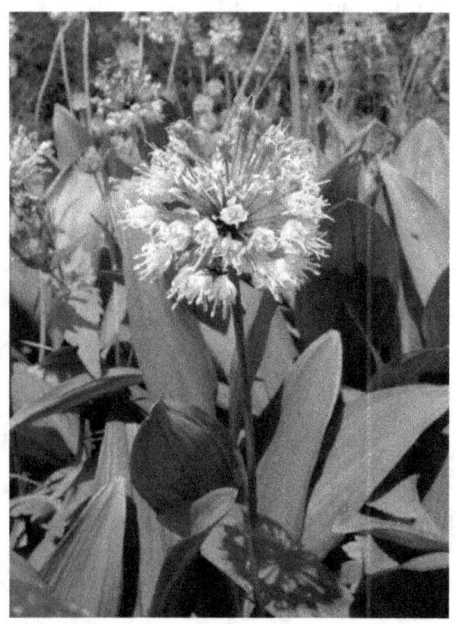

Alpine leek

(Allium Victorialis)

Alpine leek is a very popular edible onion species used as food in Siberia, Korea, Japan and China. Its cultivation is very easy, and it withstands harsh winters.

Alpine leek leaves has body weight, body fat mass, triglycerides, LDL-cholesterol and total cholesterol decreasing properties.

The body weight and body fat mass decreasing property of Alpine leek has been verified in 2 separate experiments with rats and mice (Choi et.al. 2005; Ku et.al. 2011).

Alpine leek decreases triglycerides, LDL-cholesterol and total cholesterol in rabbits, rats and mice (Choi et.al. 2005; Kim et.al. 2000).

American Ginseng, root and leaves

(Panax Quinquefolius)

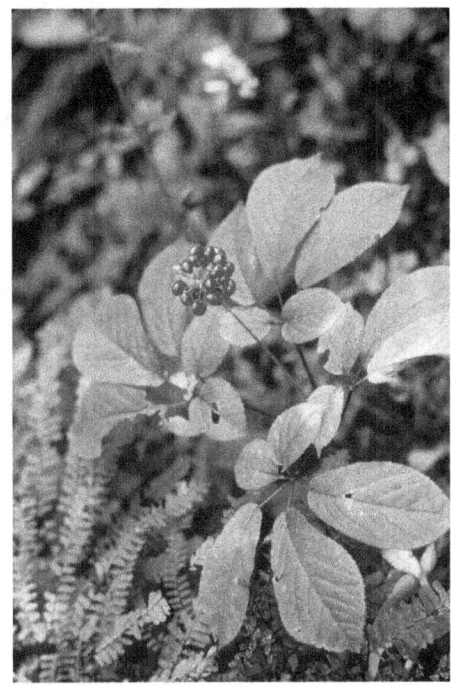

There are many different Ginseng species in the World. In Nort-America there grows the American Ginseng, which has been used as a medicine by native Indians for hundreds of years. All parts of American Ginseng are edible.

American Ginseng roots and leaves have body weight decreasing properties.

When obese mice were given American Ginseng root water extract 300 mg/kg BW daily, for 12 days, body weight in test group was 6.8% (p < 0.01) lower, compared to control group (Xie et.al. 2009).

The body weight decreasing properties of American ginseng leaves has been verified also in another experiment with mice (Liu et.al. 2010).

Amino acids and glucose before and after exercise

Exercise is, together with nutrition, the best possible method to increase daily energy expenditure, and thus decrease body fat mass and body weight. But both pre-exercise and post-exercise amino acids, protein and glucose increase significantly fatty acid oxidation, physical strength, aerobic endurance and speed of recovery from exercise. Normally amino acids and protein is taken 10 – 30 minutes before exercise, and also 5 – 10 minutes after exercise amino acids, protein and glucose is taken, together with water. Instead of amino acids, whey protein, fat free soy isolate or fat free milk can be used.

Pre-exercise and post-exercise amino acids, protein and glucose also significantly increase the concentration of anabolic hormones testosterone, growth hormone GH and IGF-1 in serum, but decrease the catabolic hormone cortisol concentration in serum. The supplements also increase specific resistance against viral diseases during hard training.

Pre-exercise and post-exercise amino acids, protein, creatine, caffeine and glucose have body weight and body fat mass decreasing properties.

When volunteers were given 20 minutes before exercise either 18 grams whey protein or 19 grams carbohydrates, both 24 hours and 48 hours resting energy expenditure REE was significantly (p < 0.05) higher in protein group, compared to carbohydrate group. Both groups had significantly higher REE value, compared to baseline before exercise. Also respiratory exchange ratio RER was after 24 hours significantly (p < 0.05) lower in both group, compared to baseline before exercise. The smaller the RER value, the more body uses fat as fuel (Hackney et.al. 2010).

When volunteers, who trained daily, were given 1.52 grams amino acid mixture 30 minutes before and also immediately after daily exercise, for 12 weeks, body weight was 1.1 kg, fat-% was 1.2% ($p < 0.05$), waist circumference was 1.4 cm, and hip circumference was 1.7 cm ($p < 0.05$) lower in test group, compared to control group. The amino acid mixture consisted of arginine, lysine, proline and alanine. This was a double blind experiment (Michishita et.al. 2010).

The body fat mass and cortisol decreasing, but physical strength, aerobic endurance, testosterone, GH and IGH-1 increasing properties of pre-exercise and post-exercise amino acids, protein, creatine, caffeine and glucose has been verified in great many experiments with human volunteers (Hoffman et.al. 2008; Stark et.al. 2012; Foster et.al. 2012; Byars et.al. 2010; Cribb et.al. 2006; Spillane et.al. 2011; Smith et.al. 2010; Spradley et.al. 2012; Rankin et.al. 2004; Ratamess et.al. 2007; Hoffman et.al. 2010; Bird et.al. 2006).

Angelica, root

(Angelica Gigas, A. Sinensis, A. Acutiloba, A. Dahurica)

In China, Korea and Japan there exists many different Angelica species, which have been used as medicine and food for thousands of years. These are especially: Chinese Angelica, Angelica Sinensis, Japanese Angelica, Angelica Acutiloba, Giant Angelica, Angelica Gigantis and Dahurian Angelica, Angelica Dahurica. The common Angelica, Angelica Archangelis, has been used as food and medicine in Europe for hundreds of years.

Giant Angelica, Chinese Angelica, Japanese Angelica and Dahurian Angelica roots have body weight and body fat mass decreasing properties.

Giant Angelica root and its active compound, Decursin, strongly inhibit the differentiation of 3T3-L1 fat cells, and also strongly inhibit the activation of FAS enzyme. Decursin, when applied to mice on high fat diet at a dose of 200 mg/kg BW daily, for 7 weeks, decrease strongly body weight, body fat mass, triglycerides and total cholesterol (Hwang et.al. 2012).

Also in other experiments with fat cells and rats, Giant Angelica root decreases body weight, body fat mass, Leptin, triglycerides, total cholesterol and inhibits the lipogenesis in 3T3-L1 fat cells (Cha et.al. 2011; Cho et.al. 2005).

Lipolysis is strongly stimulated by 5 Coumarins in the roots of Dahurian Angelica. Also 3 Coumarins strongly inhibit lipogenesis (Kimura et.al. 1982).

Japanese Angelica root extract at a dose of 300 mg/kg BW daily, for 8 weeks, strongly decreases body weight, body fat mass, total cholesterol and triglycerides of rats on high fat diet (Liu et.al. 2012).

In experiments with fat cells, Chinese Angelica root extract inhibits the Triglycerides accumulation into 3T3-L1 fat cells (Guo et.al. 2009).

Apamarga

(Achyranthes Aspera)

The English name of Apamarga plant is Prickly Chaff Flower. Apamarga is an ancient medicinal plant in India, which has been used against obesity. It is known to decrease triglycerides and cholesterol.

Apamarga plant and its seeds have body weight and body fat mass decreasing properties.

When rats were given high fat diet and 120 mg/kg BW of Saponin fraction made from the 70% ethanol extract of Apamarga plant daily, for 8 weeks, body weight in test group was 24.3% ($p < 0.05$) lower, compared to control group. Also fat mass was significantly ($p < 0.05$) lower in test group. Also total cholesterol, triglycerides, LDL-cholesterol and VLDL-cholesterol were significantly ($p < 0.05$ in all parameters) lower, but HDL-cholesterol was significantly ($p < 0.05$) higher in test group, compared to control group (Latha et.al. 2011).

The body weight, body fat mass, triglycerides and total cholesterol decreasing properties of Apamarga has been verified in many other experiments with mice and rats (Rani et.al. 2012; Malarvili et.al. 2011; Latha et.al. 2011; Venkatalakshmi et.al. 2012).

Apocynin

Apocynin is a flavonoid and strong antioxidant, which exists in many famous medicinal plants, such as Apocynum Venetum, Apocynum Cannabium and Picrorrhiza Kurroa, which have been used in cardiovascular diseases for long time in China, USA and India. Apocynin is a specific NADPH Oxidase inhibitor. NADPH Oxidase in an enzyme in cells, which converts oxygen O2, to the Superoxide radical O2-.

Apocynin has body weight decreasing properties.

When mice were given high fat diet and Apocynin 2.4 grams/Liter in their daily drinking water, for 5 weeks, body weight in test group was 9.9% ($p < 0.05$) lower, compared to control group, which got only water (Meng et.al. 2010).

When mice were given high fat diet and Apocynin (5 mM) in their daily drinking water, for 15 weeks, body weight was 14.9% ($p < 0.05$) and systolic blood pressure was 18.2 mmHg (136.6 mmHg $\rightarrow$ 118.4 mmHg; $p < 0.05$) lower in test group, compared to control group (Du et.al. 2010).

Apple

(Malus Domestica)

Apple is a delicious fruit, which contains large amounts of the healthy Quercetin, Pectin and polyphenols. Especially the Apple peel contains large amount of these compounds.

Apple has body weight and fat mass decreasing properties.

When rats were given high fat diet with 5% Apple peels daily, for 3 months, body weight decreased by 24.5% (p < 0.001) in test group, compared to the control group (Tourkostani et.al. 2009).

The body weight and fat mass decreasing properties of Apple and its polyphenols has been verified in many experiments with mice and rats (Li et.al. 2008; Nakazato et.al. 2006; Ohta et.al. 2006).

When human volunteers were given 7.5 dl cloudy Apple juice daily, for 4 weeks, body fat% decreased by 1.0%, and was significantly (p < 0.05) higher, than the 0.2% decrease in control group. There were 68 participants in this experiment (Barth et.al. 2011).

When volunteers were given Apple polyphenols 600 mg daily, for 4 weeks, body weight decreased by 0.9% (p < 0.01) and waist circumference decreased by 2.2 cm (p < 0.05) in test group, compared to the control group. There were 124 volunteers in this experiment (Akamoze et.al. 2010). This was a double blind experiment.

The body weight and fat mass decreasing properties of Apple and its polyphenols has been verified in other experiments too (de Oliveira et.al. 2003; Nagasako-Akazome et.al. 2007).

Arjuna

(Terminalia Arjuna)

Arjuna is a famous medicinal tree. In India Arjuna bark has been used hundreds of years in heart – and cardiovascular diseases and also against obesity. Arjuna decreases high cholesterol and high blood pressure.

Arjuna bark has body weight decreasing properties.

When obese rats were given high fat diet and 50% ethanol extract of Arjuna at a dose of 40 mg/kg BW daily, for 6 weeks, body weight in test group was 20.5% (p < 0.05) lower, compared to control group. Also triglycerides, LDL-cholesterol, VLDL-cholesterol and total cholesterol were significantly lower in test group, compared to control group (Patil et.al. 2011).

Ashitaba

(Angelica Keiskei)

Ashitaba is a famous functional vegetable, which is widely grown in Japan as a health food. It is close relative to the Angelica Archangelica, which is also used as a vegetable plant.

Ashitaba has body weight and body fat mass decreasing properties.

When 9 obese volunteers were given 12.4 grams dried Ashitaba daily, for 8 weeks, body weight decreased by 1.4 kg (87.3 kg → 85.9 kg; $p < 0.05$) and body fat-% decreased by 2.1% (35.3% → 33.4%; $p < 0.01$) (Ohnogi et.al. 2012)

Asparagus, spears and roots

(Asparagus Officinalis, A. Racemosus, A. Cochinchinensis)

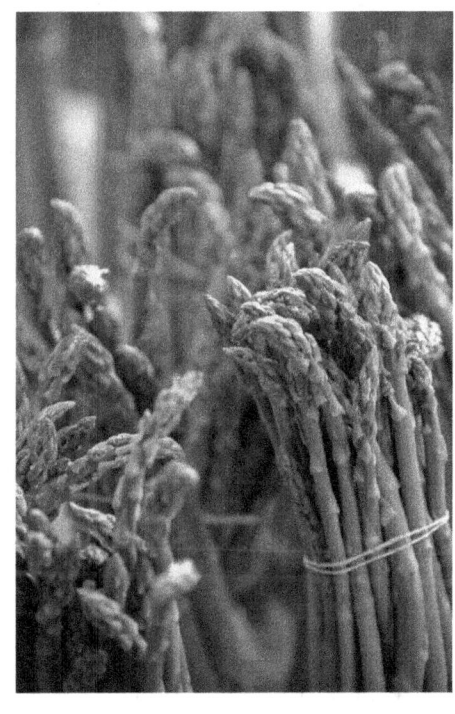

Asparagus, Asparagus Officinalis, is a common delicous spring vegetable. Normally only the spears are used, but the roots are also edible. Also the Chinese Asparagus, Asparagus Cochinchinensis, and Indian Asparagus or Shatavari, Asparagus Racemosus, have edible spears and roots. These Asparagus species roots have been used thousands of years as a medicine.

Asparagus spears and roots have body weight decreasing properties.

Chinese Asparagus, Asparagus Cochinchinensis, root inhibits the 3T3-L1 fat cell differentiation (Choi et.al. 2010).

When obese rats were given high fat diet and 200 mg/kg BW Indian Asparagus, Asparagus Racemosus, root ethanol extract daily, for 15 days, body weight in test group was 29.2% ($p < 0.05$) lower, compared to control group. Also triglycerides, total cholesterol and LDL-cholesterol decreased significantly ($p < 0.05$), but HDL-cholesterol increased significantly ($p < 0.05$) in test group, compared to control group (Komal et.al. 2012).

Also in another experiment with mice, Indian Asparagus root water extract at a dose of 150 mg/kg BW daily, for 45 days, decreased body weight in test group by 7.6%, compared to control group (Sharma et.al. 2012).

When rats were given high amount of cholesterol and 500 mg/kg BW dried Asparagus, Asparagus Officinalis, spears daily, for 5 weeks, body weight in test group was 7% lower, compared to control group. Also total cholesterol, LDL-cholesterol and triglycerides were significantly lower, but HDL-cholesterol was significantly higher in test group, compared to control group (Garcia et.al. 2012).

The Asparagus Officinalis spears body weight decreasing properties has been verified also in experiments with mice (Zhu et.al. 2010; Zhu et.al. 2011) and human volunteers (Chrubasik et.al. 2008).

Assam apple

(Docynia Indica, syn. Pyrus Indica)

Assam apple is a 2 – 3 meters high fruit tree, which originates from Nepal, Sikkim, Bhutan, India and China, in the Himalaya region. The fruits are edible, yellow, 2 – 3 centimeters in diameter and have acidic tase.

Assam apple has body weight decreasing properties.

When obese mice were given 650 mg/kg BW Assam apple ethyl acetate extract daily, for 14 days, body weight was 9.5% (p < 0.05) lower in test group, compared to control group, Total cholesterol was 10.3%, LDL-cholesterol was 28.6%, triglycerides were 31.6% and blood sugar was 14.3% lower in test group, compared to control group (Loan et.al. 2011).

Astaxanthin

Astaxanthin is a red carotenoid, which exists in seaweeds, Chlorella, Spirulina and Wheatgrass. It is sold also as a pure product in markets.

Astaxanthin has body weight and fat mass decreasing properties.

When obese mice were given high fat diet together with 6 mg/kg Bw Astaxanthin daily, for 60 days, body weight decreased in the test group by 11% (p < 0.05), compared to the control group (Bhuvaneswari et.al. 2010).

When obese mice were given high fat diet together with either 6 mg/kg BW or 30 mg/kg BW Astaxanthin daily, for 60 days, body weight decreased in both test groups by 14% (p < 0.05), compared to the control group. Also fat mass decreased in test groups significantly (p < 0.05), compared to the control group. Also triglycerides and total cholesterol decreased significantly in test groups, compared to the control group (Ikeuchi et.al. 2007).

The body weight and fat mass decreasing but fat oxidation stimulating effect of Astaxanthin has been verified in many other experiments too (Hussein et.al. 2007; Ikeuchi et.al. 2006; Aoi et.al. 2008).

Atemoya

(Annona Atemoya)

Annona fruits originate from South-America. Atemoya is a hybrid of 2 different Annona species, Annona Squamosa and Annona Cherimoya. Atemoya is a very delicious fruit, and very popular in Japan, Okinawa and Taiwan.

Atemoya has body weight and body fat mass decreasing properties.

When obese mice were given high fat diet and 500 mg/kg BW Atemoya ethanol extract daily, for 4 weeks, body weight was significantly ($p < 0.05$) lower in test group, compared to control group. Body fat mass was 20% ($p < 0.01$) lower in test group, compared to control group. Also triglycerides were 63% ($p < 0.01$) lower in test group, compared to control group (Beppu et.al. 2009).

Also in experiments with fat cells, Atemoya significantly decreases fat accumulation (Niwano et.al. 2009).

Atractylodes, root

(Atractylodes Lancea, A. Japonica, A. Macrocephala)

Atractylodes have been used in China, Korea and Japan for thousands of years as medicine against obesity, liver diseases etc. Especially CANG ZHU (Atractylodes Lancea) and BAI ZHU (Atractylodes Macrocephala) are very popular in East-Asia. The root is edible.

Atractylodes has body weight decreasing properties.

When diabetic rats were given 10% Atractylodes Lancea root in their daily food, for 4 weeks, body weight in test group decreased by 14.8% ($p < 0.05$), compared to control group. Also total cholesterol ($p < 0.05$), triglycerides ($p < 0.05$) and free fatty acids FFA ($p < 0.05$) decreased significantly in test group, compared to control group (Han et.al. 2009).

The body weight decreasing properties of Atractylodes has been verified in many other experiments (Kim et.al. 2011; Cho et.al. 2004; Han et.al. 2012).

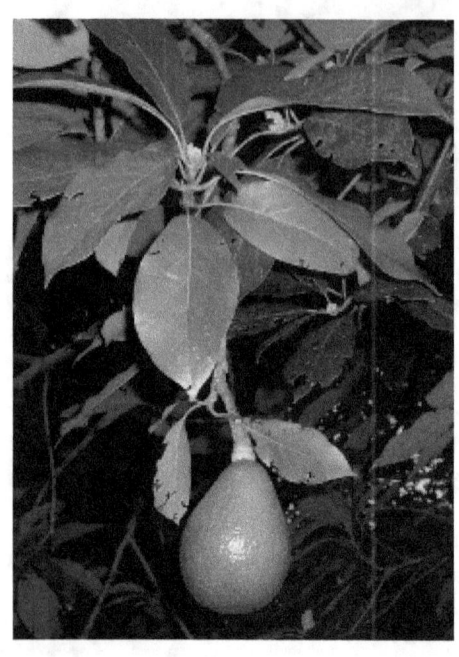

Avocado, leaves and seed

(Persea Americana)

Avocado is a delicious tropical fruit, which is available all year around. Normally only the fruit pulp is used, but especially in Africa the leaves and seeds of Avocado are widely used to decrease high blood pressure and high cholesterol levels.

Avocado leaves and seeds have body weight decreasing properties.

When rats were given high fat and high cholesterol diet and 40 mg/kg BW Avocado leaves methanol extract daily, for 8 weeks, body weight in test group was 12.3% ($p < 0.05$) lower, compared to control group. Also triglycerides were 69.2% ($p < 0.05$), total cholesterol was 60.4% ($p < 0.05$) and LDL-cholesterol was 87.5% ($p < 0.05$) lower, but HDL-cholesterol was 80.0% ($p < 0.05$) higher in test group, compared to control group (Kolawole et.al. 2012).

The body weight decreasing property of Avocado leaves and seeds have been verified also in other experiments with rats (Brai et.al. 2007; Imafidon et.al. 2010).

The blood pressure, cholesterol and triglycerides decreasing properties of Avocado leaves and seeds has been verified in great many animal experiments (Pahua-Ramos et.al. 2012; Imafidon et.al. 2009; Anakaet et.al. 2009; Nwaoguikpe et.al. 2011; Ojewole et.al. 2007).

AyurSlim

AyurSlim is developed in India as a 5 edible herb anti-obesity mixture.
The composition of 1 AyurSlim capsule is as follows:

Guggulu	(Balsamodendrom Mukul), gum resin	70 mg
Garcinia	(Garcinia Cambogia), fruit	300 mg
Haritaki	(Terminalia Chebula), fruit rind	10 mg
Gymnema	(Gymnema Sylvestre), leaves	10 mg
Fenugreek	(Trigonella Foenum-Graecum), seeds	10 mg

All these plants are known to have body weight decreasing, and serum total cholesterol and triglycerides decreasing properties. They have all been used in India for thousands of years either as a food or medicine.

AyurSlim has body weight decreasing properties.

When 32 obese volunteers (BMI = 36.0) were given 4 AyurSlim capsules daily, for 6 months, body weight decreased in test group by 10.4 kg (76.6 kg → 67.2 kg; $p = 0.01$), compared to control value. Also total cholesterol decreased by 36.94% (285.31 mg/dl → 179.89 mg/dl; $p = 0.01$), LDL-cholesterol decreased by 38.4% (166.89 mg/dl → 102.74 mg/dl) and triglycerides decreased by 52.1% (232.73 mg/dl → 11.35 mg/dl; $p = 0.01$) in test group, compared to control values (Singh et.al. 2008).

Azuki bean

(Phaseolus Angularis)

Azuki bean is a very healthy bean. It contains large amounts of protein, fiber and polyphenols. It is the second most used bean in Japan, just after soy bean. Azuki bean is known to lower cholesterol and blood pressure.

Azuki bean has body weight and body fat mass decreasing properties.

When rats were given 1% Azuki bean in their daily food, for 18 weeks, body weight was 8.0% ($p < 0.05$) lower in test group, compared to control group. Leptin was 25.7% ($p < 0.05$) lower, but Adiponectin was 13.0% ($p < 0.05$) higher in test group, compared to control group (Mukai et.al. 2012).

The body weight and fat mass decreasig properties of Azuki bean has been verified in other experiments with rats (Kitano-Okada et.al. 2012; Matsumoto et.al. 2002).

In human volunteers Azuki bean decreases triglycerides and Lipase activity significantly (Maruyama et.al. 2008).

Baical Scullcap

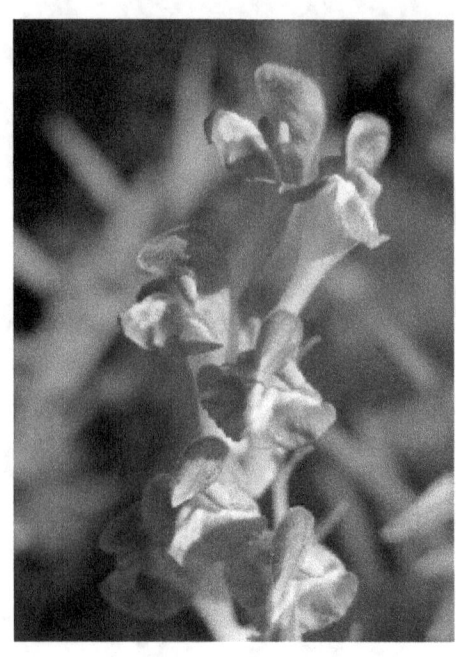

(Scutellaria Baicalensis)

Baical Scullcap is a very famous medicinal plant in China, Korea and Japan. It has been used for thousands of years in different illnesses. It has antiviral, antibacterial and anti-inflammatory properties, and it is also used to decrease high blood pressure and high cholesterol levels. It contains 3 effective flavonoids: Baicalin, Baicalein and Wogonin.

Baical Scullcap, Baicalin and Baicalein have body weight and fat mass decreasing properties.

When obese rats were given high fat diet and 80 mg/kg BW Baicalin daily, for 16 weeks, body weight was 12.17% ($p < 0.05$) lower in test group, compared to control group. Body fat mass was 27% ($p < 0.05$) lower in test group, compared to control group. Also total cholesterol ($p < 0.05$) and LDL-cholesterol were significantly lower, but HDL-cholesterol ($p < 0.05$) was significantly higher in test group, compared to control group (Guo et.al. 2009).

The body weight and body fat mass decreasing properties of Baical Scullcap has been verified in many other experiments with mice (Song et.al. 2012; Pu et.al. 2012; Han et.al. 2011).

Balsam Poplar

(Populus Balsamifera)

Balsam Poplar is a very old medicinal plant, used by Canadian Indian tribest against diabetes. It contains salicylates, populoside etc.

Balsam Poplar has body weight decreasing properties.

When obese mice were given daily 250 mg/kg BW Balsam Poplar 80% ethanol extract, for 8 weeks, body weight in test group was 7.3% ($p < 0.05$) lower, compared to control group (Harbilas et.al. 2012).

Banaba, leaves

(Lagerstroemia Speciosa)

Banaba is a large size tree. The leaves have traditionally been used in East-Asia, especially in Philippines, against diabetes and obesity. The active compound is Corosolic acid.

Banaba leaves have body weight and body fat mass decreasing properties.

When type 2 diabetic mice were given normal diet and 5% Banaba leaves water extract daily, for 12 weeks, body weight was 4.6% (p < 0.01) and body fat mass was 8.5% (p < 0.01) lower in test group, compared to control group (Suzuki et.al. 1999).

Also in other experiments with mice, both Banaba leaves (Tanquilut et.al. 2009) and Corosolic acid from Banaba leaves have been shown to decrease body weight and body fat mass in test groups, compared to control groups.

Barley leaf

(Hordeum Vulgare)

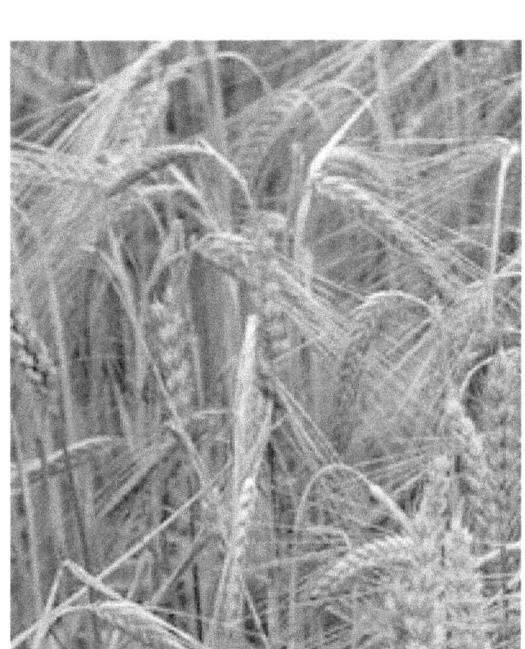

Dried Barley leaf powder is a popular supplement. It contains vitamin E 10.8 mg/100g, vitamin C 100 mg/100g, beta-Carotene 24962 IU/100g and Polyphenols 291.6 mg/100 g (Yu et.al. 2004). Barley leaf powder decreases significantly LDL-cholesterol and total cholesterol, but increases HDL-cholesterol in human volunteers (Yu et.al. 2004).

Barley leaf powder has body weight and body fat mass decreasing properties.

When obese mice were fed high fat diet with 1% Barley leaf powder daily, for 8 weeks, body weight was 10.5% (p < 0.05) lower in test group, compared to the control group. Body fat mass was also significantly (p < 0.05) lower in test group, compared to the control group. Also triglycerides were 28.3% (p < 0.05) and total cholesterol was 25.0% (p < 0.05) lower in test group (Eun-Ju et.al. 2009).

Bauhinia tree, bark

(Bauhinia Purpurea, Bauhinia Variegata)

Bauhinia tree bark has traditionally been used in India and Nepal to decrease high body weight.

Bauhinia tree bark has body weight decreasing properties.

When rats were given high fat diet and either 200 mg/kg BW or 400 mg/kg BW Bauhinia Purpurea tree bark methanol extract daily, for 6 weeks, body weight was 24% (p < 0.05) and 28% (p < 0.05) lower in test groups, compared to control groups. Also triglycerides, LDL-cholesterol and total cholesterol were significantly lower but HDL-cholesterol was significantly (p < 0.05 in all parameters) higher, compared to control group (Ramgopal et.al. 2010).

The body weight decreasing property of Bauhinia Variegata bark extract has also been verified in an experiment with rats (Balamurugan et.al. 2010).

BCAA amino acids

Branched chain amino acids (BCAA) consist of Leucine, Isoleucine and Valine amino acids. These amino acids exist both in human cells and food proteins. BCAA supplements can be purchased from markets.

BCAA amino acids have body weight and fat mass decreasing properties.

When 6 top level sportsmen, who were on hypocaloric (28 kcal/kg BW/day) diet, were given 0.9 grams/kg BW BCAA amino acids, for 19 days, body weight decreased in BCAA group 2.1 kg ($p < 0.05$), compared to the control group. Fat-% decreased in BCAA group 0.5% ($p < 0.05$) more, than in the control group (Mourier et.al. 1997).

When 12 sportsmen were given 14 grams BCAA amino acids daily, for 8 weeks, body fat-% in BCAA group decreased by 2%, which was significantly ($p = 0.039$) higher, than the 1% decrease in control group, which were given 28 grams whey protein daily (Stoppani et.al. 2009). This was a double blind experiment.

When volunteers were given either 0.3 grams/kg BW BCAA amino acids or maltodextrine (placebo) daily, for 3 days, resistance to fatigue was 17.2% better in BCAA group. Also RER value was lower and blood glucose was higher in BCAA group. This means more fat oxidation during exercise (Gualano et.al. 2011). This was a double blind experiment.

Also in another double blind experiment with volunteers, BCAA amino acids decreased RER value and increased workload in ergometer test (Matsumoto et.al. 2009).

In experiments with mice, BCAA amino acids decrease significantly both body weight gain and fat mass (Arakawa et.al. 2011).

Berberine

Berberine is an alkaloid, which exist in many plants, such as Phellodendron Amurense, Coptis Chinensis and Hydrastis Canadensis. Berberine is known to decrease blood pressure and cholesterol.

Berberine has body weight and body fat mass decreasing properties.

When 37 obese volunteers were given 0.9 gram Berberine daily, for 12 weeks, BMI decreased by 13.0% ($31.5 \rightarrow 27.4$; $p < 0.01$), compard to the control group. Waist circumference decreased by 5.2 cm ($p = 0.04$), triglycerides decreased by 38.6% ($p < 0.01$), total cholesterol decreased by 14.2% ($p = 0.03$) and Leptin decreased by 36.0% ($p = 0.04$) in test group, compared to the control group

(Yang et.al. 2012).

When 7 obese volunteers were given 1500 mg Berberine daily, for 12 weeks, body weight decreased by 2.3% and body fat-% decreased by 3.6% in test group, compared to the control group (Hu et.al. 2012).

When 20 obese volunteers were given Phellodendron Amurense extract, standardized to Berberine content, 740 mg daily, for 8 weeks, body weight decreased by 3.0 kg ($p < 0.01$) in test group, compared to the control group. Also triglycerides ($p < 0.01$) and LDL-cholesterol ($p < 0.01$) decreased significantly in test group, compared to the control group (Oben et.al. 200). This was a double blind experiment.

The body weight and body fat mass decreasing properties of Berberine has been verified in many animal experiments (Hu et.al. 2010; Kim et.al. 2009; Xie et.al. 2011; Hu et.al. 2010; Chang et.al. 2012).

Bermuda Grass

(Cynodon Dactylon)

Bermuda Grass is nowadays a cosmopolite plant. It originates from Bermuda islands. It is a very popular medicinal plant, used in diabetes, dysentery, high cholesterol levels etc. Its cultivation is very easy.

When rats, which were given 10% Fructose in the diet, were given Bermuda Grass water extract 2% of their daily diet, for 6 weeks, body weight was 8.4% ($p < 0.05$) lower in test group, compared to control group. Also triglycerides ($p < 0.05$), total cholesterol ($p < 0.05$), blood sugar ($p < 0.05$) and systolic blood pressure ($p < 0.05$) were significantly lower in test group, compared to control group (Bharti et.al. 2012).

beta-Cryptoxanthin

Beta-Cryptoxanthin is a carotenoid, which exists in several food plants. It is known to inhibit cancer and osteoporosis.

Beta-Cryptoxanthin has body weight and body fat mass decreasing properties.

When obese mice were given beta-Cryptoxanthin 0.8 mg/kg BW daily, for 8 weeks, body weight was 13.3% ($p < 0.01$) lower in the test group, compared to the control group. Body fat mass was 19% ($p < 0.01$) lower in the test group, compared to the control group (Takayanagi 2011).

The body weight and body fat mass decreasing properties of beta-Cryptoxanthin has been verified also in other experiments with mice and fat cells (Takayanagi et.al. 2011; Shirakura et.al. 2011).

When human volunteers were given daily juice with 0.25 mg/100 ml beta-Cryptoxanthin, for 12 weeks, body fat was significantly ($p < 0.01$) lower in the test group, compared to the control group (Tsuchida et.al. 2005). This was a double blind experiment.

The following food items contain large amounts of beta-Cryptoxanthin (Source: USDA (US Department of Agriculture) National Nutrient Database Release 22 (SR22)):

Spices, Paprika	7.923 mg/100g
Chili powder	3.490 mg/100g
Winter Squash, raw	3.471 mg/100g
Pumpkin, raw	2.145 mg/100g
Persimmon, raw	1.447 mg/100g
Papayas, raw	0.761 mg/100g
Mandarin oranges, raw	0.407 mg/100g
Mandarin juice	0.214 mg/100g
Kumquat	0.193 mg/100g
Orange juice	0.116 mg/100g
Corn	0.115 mg/100g
Apricots, raw	0.104 mg/100g
Nectarines, raw	0.098 mg/100g
Watermelon, raw	0.078 mg/100g

The largest amounts of beta-Cryptoxanthin are found Chlorella, Spirulina and Kelp (Sullivan et.al. 2011):

Chlorella	49.60 mg/100g
Spirulina	11.20 mg/100g
Kelp	5.00 mg/100g

beta-Glucan

Beta-Glucans are soluble fiber, polysaccharides of Glucose. Beta-Glucans exist in many plants, but barley, oat and mushrooms are the best sources of dietary beta-Glucans. Barley is the best source, it can contain up to 7.5% beta-Glucan. Beta-Glucans have many positive health effects: they decrease high cholesterol and triglycerides, stimulate immunity etc. Germinated barley is included in Chinese pharmacopeia.

Beta-Glucans have body weight and body fat mass decreasing properties.

When 19 volunteers were given 7 grams beta-Glucans daily, for 12 weeks, body mass index BMI decreased by 0.3 kg/m2 (26.2 → 25.9; $p = 0.015$), Waist circumference decreased by 1.2 cm ($p = 0.011$), total cholesterol decreased by 4.6% ($p = 0.037$) and triglycerides decreased by 3.7% ($p = 0.041$) in test group, but there were no changes in the 20 person control group. This was a double blind experiment (Shimizy et.al. 2008).

The body weight, total cholesterol and LDL-cholesterol decreasing, but HDL-cholesterol increasing properties of beta-Glucans have been verified in many human experiments (Pins et.al. 2000; Reyna-

Villasmil et.al. 2007; Reyna et.al. 2003).

In experiments with obese volunteers, beta-Glucans decrease both systolic and diastolic blood pressure (Maki et.al. 2007).

When mice were given high fat diet and 10% beta-Glucans in their daily diet, for 8 weeks, body weight decreased by 37% ($p < 0.01$) and body fat mass decreased by 30% ($p < 0.001$) in test group, compared to control group (Arora et.al. 2012).

The body weight and body fat mass decreasing properties of beta-Glucans have been verified in many experiments with rats and mice (Kang et.al. 2002; Huang et.al. 2011; Choi et.al. 2010).

Betulin, Betulinic acid and Birch, bark

(Betula Sp.)

Birch bark has a long time been used in traditional medicine against different illnesses, such as skin diseases and psoriasis. All different Birch species barks contain pentacyclic triterpenoids, Betulin and Betulinic acid. These can be extracted by alcohol from the bark. Normally the content of Betulin is much higher, but it can easily be oxidized to Betulinic acid. Betulinic acid exists also in many other plants, such as cabbage (Brassica Sp.), mushrooms (Inonotus Obliquus) etc. Betulinic acid is anti-inflammatory, antiviral and anticarcinogenic.

Betulin, Betulinic acid and Birch bark have body weight and body fat mass decreasing properties.

When mice were given high fat diet and 50 mg/liter Betulinic acid in drinking water daily, for 15 weeks, body weight was 13.2% ($p < 0.05$) and body fat mass was 52% ($p < 0.05$) lower in test group, compared to control group. Also triglycerides ($p < 0.05$) and total cholesterol ($p < 0.05$) were significantly lower in test group (de Melo et.al. 2009).

The body weight and body fat mass decreasing properties of Betulin and Betulinic acid has been verified in many other experiments (Tang et.al. 2011; Kim et.al. 2012; Chung et.al. 2006; Choi et.al. 2012).

Big blue lily turf, root

(Liriope Platyphylla)

Big blue lily turf is an ancient medicinal- and edible plant, which is used in China, Korea and Japan against asthma, diabetes and obesity. All parts are edible.

Big blue lily turf root has body weight and fat mass decreasing properties.

When obese rats were given normal diet and 121.7 mg/kg BW Big blue lily turf root water extract daily, for 8 weeks, body weight was 29.9% (p < 0.05), and body fat mass was 42.8% (p < 0.05) lower in test group, compared to control group. Also triglycerides (p < 0.05) and Leptin (p < 0.05) were significantly lower in test group, compared to control group. This was a 4 herb mixture, where most part, 42.86%, was Big blue lily turf root, and the rest were: Platygodon Grandiflorum 28.57%, Schisandra Chinensis 14.29% and Ephedra Sinica 14.28% (Jeong et.al. 2008).

The body weight and fat mass decreasing properties of Big blue lily turf has been verified in many experiments with rats and mice (Kim et.al. 2012; Kim et.al. 2011; Kim et.al. 2012).

Bitter Melon

(Momordica Charantia)

Bitter Melon is an edible vegetable, which has also many medicinal properties. Its cultivation is very easy.

Bitter Melon has body weight and fat mass decreasing properties.

When rats were given Bitter Melon water extract 2 ml daily, for 5 weeks, the following properties decreased significantly (p < 0.05) in the test group, compared to the control group: Body weight by 16.2%, total cholesterol by 20.8%, LDL-cholesterol by 53.2% and triglycerides by 19.0%, but HDL-cholesterol increased by 18.1% (Bano et.al. 2011).

The body weight and fat mass decreasing properties of Bitter Melon has been verified in a large number of experiments with rats and mice (Wang et.al. 2011; Chao et.al. 2011; Huang et.al. 2008; Shih et.al. 2008; Chen et.al. 2003; Chan et.al. 2005).

Black Ginger

(Kaempferia Parviflora)

Black Ginger grows in Thailand, and its name in Thai language is Krachai Dam. The local Thai people call it Thai Ginseng. Black Ginseng root is used as a sex stimulant, against diabetes and to increase blood circulation. Thai people drink commonly Black Ginger tea as a tonic and sex stimulant.

Black Ginger root has body weight and fat mass decreasing properties.

When obese, type 2 diabetic mice were given in their daily food 3% Black Ginger, for 8 weeks, body weight in test group was 15.0% (p < 0.05) lower, compared to control group. Body fat mass was 25% (p < 0.05) lower in test group, compared to control group (Akase et.al. 2011).

Also in another experiment the body weight and body fat mass decreasing properties of Black Ginger has been verified (Shimada et.al. 2011).

Black pepper

(Piper Nigrum)

Black pepper is a very popular spice all around the World. It has also many medicinal uses, against asthma, bronchitis, arthritis etc. The most important compound in Black pepper is Piperine.

Black pepper has body weight and fat mass decreasing properties.

When mice were given Black pepper 1% of their daily diet, for 3 months, body weight decreased by 7.5% ($p < 0.05$), compared to the control group (Longquan et.al. 2007). This corresponds to about 5 grams Black pepper for human daily use.

When obese rats on high fat diet were given daily 40 mg/kg BW Piperine from Black pepper, for 3 weeks, body weight gain was 30% ($p < 0.05$) lower in test group, compared to the control group. Body fat mass decreased by 50% ($p < 0.05$), and triglycerides, total cholesterol and LDL-cholesterol decreased significantly, but HDL-cholesterol increased significantly, compared to the control group (Shah et.al. 2011).

When mice on high fat diet were given daily either 0.03% Piperine, 0.05% Piperine or 1.0% Black pepper on their diet, for 3 weeks, both body weight ($p < 0.05$) and body fat mass ($p < 0.05$) decreased in all test groups, compared to the control group. Also total cholesterol decreased significantly ($p < 0.05$) in all test groups (Okumura et.al. 2010).

Black seed

(Nigella Sativa)

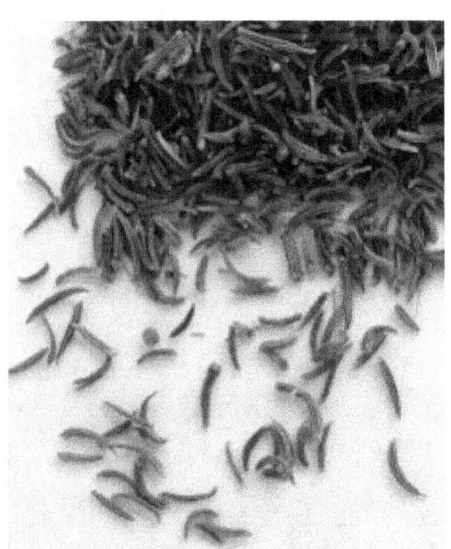

Black seed is an ancient spice and medicinal plant, which has been used in different diseases for hundreds of years. Black seed decreases total cholesterol, triglycerides and blood pressure and it is used also in asthma and diabetes.

Black seed has body weight decreasing properties.

When volunteers were given Black seed oil 2.5 ml daily, for 6 weeks, body weight decreased by 1.2 kg, which was significantly more than the 0.5 kg decrease in the control group (Najmi et.al. 2008). Also blood pressure, total cholesterol and triglycerides decreased significantly ($p < 0.05$), compared to the control group. There were totally 161 volunteers in the experiment.

When 55 female volunteers were given Black seeds 1.6 grams daily, for 12 weeks, body mass index BMI decreased by 0.53 units ($26.31 \rightarrow 25.78$; $p < 0.05$), being significantly more than in the control group (Latiffah et.al. 2012). Also total cholesterol ($p < 0.05$) and blood pressure ($p < 0.05$) decreased significantly, compared to the control group.

When 18 male volunteers were given Black seeds 1.5 grams daily, for 3 months, body weight decreased by 4.5 kg (77.11 kg $\rightarrow$ 72.60 kg; $p < 0.0001$) compared to the control group. In the control group body weight increased by 0.8 kg, from 79.35 kg to 81.14 kg (Datau et.al. 2010). Also systolic blood pressure decreased significantly, compared to the control group.

In many experiments with rats and rabbits, it has been verified, that Black seed decreases body weight, compared to the control groups (Sultan et.al. 2009; Parhizkar et.al. 2011; Buriro et.al. 2011).

Black soy

(Glycine Max var Nigra)

Black soy colour is totally black. The colour pigments of black soy seed coat consist of Cyanidin-3-Glucoside (9.2%), Catechins (6.2%) and Procyanids (39.8%). Black soy is officially a functional food item in China. Cyanidin-3-Glucoside is known to decrease body weight, as do Catechins in green tea. Japanese call black soy "Kokuzui", and it is used in diabetes and as a diuretic.

Black soy has body weight decreasing properties.

When obese mice were given high fat food together with 1% of black soy seed extract in their daily diet, for 14 weeks, body weight was 12.8% ($p < 0.05$) lower in the test group, compared to the control group, which got high fat diet. Also body fat mass was 14.1% ($p < 0.05$) lower in test group, compared to the control group (Kanamotot et.al. 2011).

When obese mice were given high fat food together with either 2%, 5% or 10% of black soy peptide mixture in their daily diet, for 8 weeks, body weight was 5.3% ($p < 0.05$), 12.4% ($p < 0.05$) and 24.3% ($p < 0.05$) lower in the test groups, compared to the control group, which got fat diet (Jang et.al. 2008).

When 35 obese volunteers were given daily black soy peptide mixture, for 12 weeks, body weight ($p < 0.001$), BMI ($p < 0.001$), body fat-% ($p = 0.002$) and body fat mass ($p = 0.001$) were significantly lower in the test group, compared to the 29 volunteer control group. Also Leptin decreased significantly ($p = 0.047$) in the test group (Kwak et.al. 2012). This was a double blind experiment.

Also in other experiments with mice and rats, black soy has significantly decreased body weight ($p < 0.05$), triglycerides ($p < 0.05$), total cholesterol ($p < 0.05$), but increased HDL-cholesterol ($p < 0.05$), compared to control groups (Kwon et.al. 2007; Fukuda et.al. 2011).

Blueberry, berry and leaves

(Vaccinium Myrtillus)

Blueberry is a delicious berry, which grows in Europe, Asia and North America. It can be bought as fresh, dried, in juice form or freezed all around the year. It contains large amounts of healthy Anthocyanides, especially Cyanidin-3-Glucoside up to 100 mg/100g (Jaakola et.al. 2004). Cyanidin-3-Glucoside is known to have weight decreasing properties. But blueberry leaves contain very large amounts of flavonoids, especially Quercetin up to 300 – 1000 mg/100g (Jaakola et.al. 2004). Quercetin is known to have weight decreasing properties. Blueberries have only 33 kcal/100 g energy content. The content of protein is 0.5 kg/100g, fat only 0.6 g/100 g and carbohydrates 6.4g/100g.

Blueberry and blueberry leaves have body weight and fat mass decreasing properties.

Blueberries inhibit Lipase enzyme activity (Slanc et.al. 2009).

Blueberries inhibit adipocyte differentiation (Shiwani et.al. 2012).

Blueberries decrease fat mass, Leptin and total cholesterol in rats and hamsters on high fat diet (Khanal et.al. 2012; Kim et.al. 2010).

When mice were given high fat diet and either water or blueberry juice as a daily drink, for 72 days, body weight was 7.87% and fat-% was 2.6% (32.2% → 29.6%) lower in blueberry juice group, compared to water control group. When mice were given high fat diet and either water or purified blueberry Anthocyanides 0.2 mg/ml as a daily drink, for 72 days, body fat-% was 8.3% (32.2% → 23.9%) lower in test group, compared to water control group (Prior et.al. 2010).

The body weight and body fat mass decreasing properties of blueberries has been verified in many other experiments (Vuong et.al. 2009; Molan et.al. 2008; Seymour et.al. 2011).

Blueberries decreases blood sugar in diabetic mice (Takikawa et.al. 2010).

In experiments with obese volunteers, blueberries decrease both systolic blood pressure by 4.5% ($p < 0.05$) and diastolic blood pressure by 2.8% ($p < 0.05$), compared to control volunteers (Basu et.al. 2010).

In experiments with rats, blueberry leaves decrease triglycerides up to 39% and blood sugar up to 26%, just in 4 days (Cignarella et.al. 1996).

In experiments with diabetic volunteers, blueberry leaves decrease significantly blood sugar (Allen et.al. 1927).

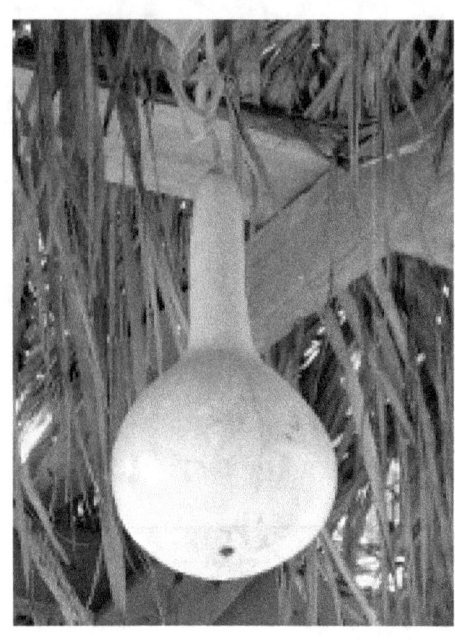

Bottle gourd

(Lagenaria Siceraria)

Bottle gourd is a very popular vegetable in Asia, and its cultivation is very easy. It is known to decrease cholesterol and triglycerides.

When obese rats were given high fat food and Bottle gourd ethanol extract 200 mg/kg BW daily, for 30 days, body weight increased in control group by 3.9% (p < 0.001), but it decreased in Bottle gourd group by 3.74% (p < 0.001). Also total cholesterol (p < 0.001), LDL-cholesterol (p < 0.01) and triglycerides (p < 0.001) decreased in Bottle gourd group significantly, compared to control group (Nadeem et.al. 2012).

The body weight, total cholesterol, LDL-cholesterol and triglycerides decreasing properties of Bottle gourd have been verified also in other experiments with rats (Ghule et.al. 2009; Nainwal et.al. 2011).

Brahmi or Bacopa

(Bacopa Monnieri)

Bacopa is known in Ayurveda as Brahmi. It is a small size, creeping plant, and it is a very famous medicinal plant in India. It can also be eaten as a vegetable. Brahmi increases memory, increases blood flow, decreases blood pressure and it is anti-asthmatic.

Brahmi has body weight decreasing properties.

When rats were given high fat diet and 40 mg/kg BW whole Brahmi plant 90% ethanol extract daily, for 45 days, body weight in test group was 5.1% (p < 0.01) lower, compared to control group (Kamesh et.al. 2012).

Broccoli sprouts

(Brassica Oleracea var. Italica)

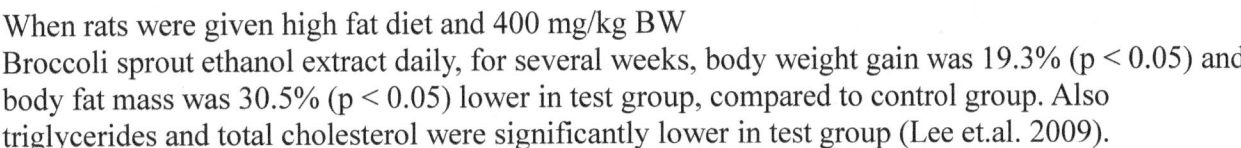

Broccoli sprouts are very popular functional healthy food. They contain large amounts of organic sulfur compounds, which have many positive health effects.

Broccoli sprouts have body weight and fat mass decreasing properties.

When rats were given high fat diet and 400 mg/kg BW Broccoli sprout ethanol extract daily, for several weeks, body weight gain was 19.3% ($p < 0.05$) and body fat mass was 30.5% ($p < 0.05$) lower in test group, compared to control group. Also triglycerides and total cholesterol were significantly lower in test group (Lee et.al. 2009).

In another experiment, where rats were given Broccoli sprout chloroform extract, body weight gain in test group was 53.8% ($p < 0.05$) lower, when compared to green tea control group (Motawee et.al. 2010).

Broccolini

(Brassica Oleracea var. Italica x Brassica Oleracea var. Alboglabra)

Broccolini is a hybrid of the common Broccoli, Brassica Oleracea var. Italica, and Chinese Broccoli or Kailaan, Brassica Oleracea var. Alboglabra. Broccolini is very nutrient rich, and the whole plant is edible. It contains energy only 34 kcal, protein 3 grams, carbohydrates 7 grams and fat 0 grams in 100 grams of edible portion. It has very large amounts of vitamin C, iron, calcium and potassium. Its cultivation is very easy, and cultivation time is 90 days. It is also called Petit Vert, and was developed in 1991 in Japan.

Broccolini has body weight and body fat mass decreasing properties.

When mice were given high fat diet and 5% Broccolini in their daily diet, for 35 days, body weight was 9.1% ($p < 0.05$) and body fat mass was 34.7% ($p < 0.05$) lower in test group, compared to control group. Also FAS enzyme decreased significantly ($p < 0.05$) in test group, compared to control group (Nishida et.al. 2011).

Buckthorn leaves and seeds

(Hippophae Rhamnoides)

Buckthorn berry contains large amounts of functionally healthy compounds. But Buckthorn leaves and seeds contain much larger amounts of flavonoids, tannins and triterpenes, than Buckthorn berry. Tea can be made from Buckthorn leaves.

Buckthorn leaves and seeds have body weight and body fat mass decreasing properties.

When mice were given high fat diet together with either 2% or 5% Buckthorn dried leaves daily, for 6 weeks, body weight in test groups were 6.9% ($p < 0.05$) and 9.9% ($p < 0.05$) lower, than in the control group. Body fat mass was 18.8% ($p < 0.05$) and 24.8% ($p < 0.05$) lower in test group, compared to the control group. Triglycerides were 20.2% ($p < 0.05$) and 25.1% ($p < 0.05$) lower in test groups, and also total cholesterol was 18.5% ($p < 0.05$) and 29.3% ($p < 0.05$) lower in test groups, compared to the control group (Lee et.al. 2011).

The Buckthorn body weight decreasing property has been verified also in another experiment with mice (Nishi et.al. 2007).

Also Buckthorn seeds decrease body weight, body fat mass, triglycerides, LDL-cholesterol and total cholesterol in rats and mice (Yang et.al. 2007; Cao et.al. 2003; Wang et.al. 2011).

Buckwheat

(Fagopyrum Esculentum, Fagopyrum Tataricum)

Buckwheat is a very healthy grain, which contains large amounts of protein and the flavonoid Rutin. Sprouted Buckwheat contains over 10 times more Rutin than the original grain. Buckwheat has cholesterol decreasing properties. Both the ordinary Buckwheat (Fagopyrum Eculentum) and the Tartary Buckwheat (Fagopyrum Tataricum) are easily cultivated. Tartary Buckwheat contains much more Rutin than the ordinary Buckwheat.

Buckwheat has body weight and body fat mass decreasing properties.

When mice were given ethanol extract of sprouted Buckwheat either 100 mg/kg BW or 200 mg/kg BW daily, for 8 weeks, body weight gain was 19.1% ($p < 0.05$) and 60.3% ($p < 0.05$) lower in the test groups, compared to the control group. Also HDL-cholesterol was 66% ($p < 0.05$) higher in the test groups, compared to the control group (Choi et.al. 2007).

When 26 mildly obese (> 10% overweight) and 18 obese (> 20% overweight) volunteers were given Tartary Buckwheat 80 grams daily, for 8 weeks, body weight decreased in the first group by 3.07 kg (76.94 kg → 73.87 kg; $p < 0.01$) and in the other group by 3.50 kg (84.33 kg → 80.83 kg; $p < 0.01$), compared to the control group (Xiping et.al. 1995).

The body fat decreasing properties of Buckwheat flour and protein has been verified in many experiments with rats (Tomotake et.al. 2006; Kayashita et.al. 1995; Kayashita et.al. 1996).

Bunashijemi

(Hypsizigus Marmoreus)

Bunashijemi is a very delicious edible mushroom, which is widely cultivated in Japan and Korea.

Bunashijemi has body weight and body fat mass decreasing properties.

When obese mice were given high fat diet and 5% Bunashijemi in their daily diet, for 8 weeks, body weight was 30.2% (p < 0.05) and body fat mass was 63.5% (p < 0.05) lower in test group, compared to control group. Triglycerides were 75.2% (p < 0.05) and total cholesterol was 58.3% (p < 0.05) lower in test group, compared to control group (Ryu et.al. 2011).

The body weight, body fat mass and total cholesterol decreasing properties of Bunashijemi has been verified also in another experiment with mice (Ohtsuki et.al. 2007).

Burdock

(Arctium Lappa)

Burdock is a popular root vegetable, much cultivated in Asian countries. Its cultivation is very easy.

Burdock root has body weight decreasing properties.

When rats were given 500 mg/kg BW Burdock root daily, for 4 weeks, body weight in test group was 5.9% (p < 0.05) lower, than in the control group (Kuo et.al. 2012).

Burning bush, twigs and bark

(Euonymus Alatus)

Burning bush, or Winged Euonymus, is a very beautiful bush, which young twigs are eaten as vegetable in Korea. The twigs contain very large amounts of polyphenols, up to 235.7 mg/kg (Choi et.al. 2009). The Chinese name is GUI JEON WU and it is used for regulating blood circulation, relieving pain and treating dysmenorrhea.

Burning bush twigs and bark have body weight decreasing properties.

When mice were given high fat diet and 750 mg/kg BW Burning bush bark ethanol extract daily, for 10 weeks, body weight was 12.8% (p < 0.05) lower in test group, compared to control group.

Triglycerides were 12.5% (p < 0.05), total cholesterol was 17.6% (p < 0.05) and LDL-cholesterol was 53.7% (p < 0.05) lower in test group, compared to control group (Park et.al. 2005).

Butter, cream, fatty milk, fatty cheese, saturated fatty acids.

Butter has been used in the World for thousands of years in food and the bread. Butter is composed of saturated fatty acids. It contains large amounts of cholesterol, typically 95 mg/100 g, salt typically 1.5 weight-% and it has very high energy content, 740 kcal/100g. Cream, fatty milk and fatty cheese contain the same type of saturated fatty acids as butter.

Butter, cream, fatty milk, fatty cheese and saturated fatty acids have body weigth and body fat mass increasing properties.

In great many animal experiments it has been verified, that the saturated fatty acids of butter increase body weight and body fat mass most, compared to other fats and oils used normally in cooking (de Wit et.al. 2012; Torres-Rovira et.al. 2012; Hariri et.al. 2010).

In Northern Karelia province, in Finland, there was an exceptionally high mortality from cardiovascular disease in 1970. The most important reason for this was the very large amount of saturated fats, mostly from butter and fatty milk, used by the locals. In 1972 over 90% of population used butter, but nowadays only 5% of population uses butter. This has led to 80% reduction of annual cardiovascular mortality in Northern Karelia province (Puska et.al. 2009).

Whe 19 volunteers were given 40 grams butter daily, for 4 weeks, total cholesterol increased by 8.9% (5.6 mmol/L → 6.1 mmol/L; p < 0.05) and LDL-cholesterol increased by 14.7% (3.4 mmol/L → 3.9 mmol/L; p < 0.05) in test group, compared to control group (Nestel et.al. 2005).

Even very low amounts of butter, 20 – 40 grams daily, increase strongly total cholesterol, LDL-cholesterol, HDL-cholesterol, triglycerides, systolic blood pressure and diastolic blood pressure.

C3G, Cyanidin-3-Glucoside

C3G or Cyanidin-3-O-beta-D-Glucoside is a natural color pigment, which exists especially in dark red and black berries, fruits, grains and legumes. Good C3G sources are: Chokeberry, black currant, blueberry, red grapes, dark plums, purple corn, black corn, cherries, black rice, black rice bran, black soybean, black soybean coat.

C3G has body weight and fat mass decreasing properties.

Black currant contain large amounts of C3G. When rats were given in their daily food either 5% or 10% black currant, for 100 days, body weight decreased by 4% (p < 0.05) and 10% (p < 0.05), compared to the control group, which did not get black currant (Kaume et.al. 2012).

When mice were given in their daily diet 2 grams/1 kg food purple corn extract, for 12 weeks, both body weight ($p < 0.05$) and fat mass ($p < 0.05$) decreased significantly, compared to the control group (Tsuda et.al. 2003). The extract contained 7% C3G.

When pigs were given C3G rich black rice bran, body fat mass decreased significantly, compared to the control group (Kil et.al. 2006).

Also in other experiment C3G decreases significantly both body weight and fat mass (Wei et.al. 2011; Guo et.al. 2011; Guo et.al. 2012).

Caffeine

Caffeine is the well known stimulating component in coffee, tea, Matee and Guarana. Allready from 1915 it has been known, that Caffeine increases the metabolic rate and fatty acid oxidation. There is about 100 – 200 mg of Caffeine in a cop of coffee. Caffeine and Chlorogenic acid are the main lipolytic components in Coffee.

Caffeine has body weight and body fat decreasing properties.

When volunteers were given Caffeine 8 mg/kg body weight, both the metabolic rate and fatty acid oxidation increased significantly, but carbohydrate oxidation decreased significantly, compared to the control group (Acheson et.al. 1980).

When rats were given Caffeine in amounts of 0.025%, 0.050% or 0.100% of daily food, for 21 days, body fat-% decreased according to the following table:

	Body Fat-%
Control	13.4%
0.025% Caffeine	10.6%
0.050% Caffeine	10.3%
0.100% Caffeine	8.9%

(Kobayashi-Hattori et.al. 2005).

The body weight and body fat mass lowering effect of Caffeine has been verified in great many animal experiments (Panchal et.al. 2012; Panchal et.al. 2012; Matsuda et.al. 2011; Lou et.al. 2010).

Calcium

Calcium is an essential macro mineral to humans. It exists especially much in bones. The recommended dietary intake is between 1000 mg – 1500 mg per day for adults. All milk products, including yoghurt, sour milk and cheese, are excellent Calcium sources, as are sesame seeds and sunflower seeds. It has been noticed in many research, that there exist an inverse correlation between dietary Calcium and body weight and Calcium and body fat mass: The more is the dietary Calcium intake, the less is the body weight and body fat mass.

Calcium has body weight and body fat mass decreasing properties.

When mice were given fat rich diet (43% fat) and 1.2 grams/1 kg food Calcium daily, for 60 days, body weight was 14% (p < 0.05) and body fat mass was 53% (p < 0.05) lower in Calcium group, compared to control group without additional daily Calcium. The amount of Calcium was 3.10 mg/1000 kcal in test group and 1.03 mg/1000 kcal in control group (Parra et.al. 2008).

The body weight and body fat mass decreasing properties of dietary Calcium has been verified in many experiments with mice and rats (Marotte et.al. 2012; Sun et.al. 2012; Pilvi et.al. 2007; Sun et.al. 2004; Shi et.al. 2001).

In experiments with 57 volunteers, both body weight (p = 0.03) and body fat mass (p = 0.01) were higher in persons, who had lower daily dietary Calcium intake (Torres et.al. 2011).

When volunteers were given 1500 mg Calcium and 1100 IU D3-vitamin daily, for 3 years, body fat mass increase in test group was 4.0% less (1.4% in test group, 5.4% in control group; p = 0.015), compared to control group. Also fat-% increase in test group was 3.3% less (0.3% in test group, 3.6% in control group; p = 0.01), compared to control group. Body mass index BMI decreased in Calcium group, but increased in control group, the difference being 0.81 kg/m2 units (p = 0.39). This was a double blind experiment with 870 volunteers (Zhou et.al. 2010).

The Calcium body fat mass decreasing and lean body mass increasing properties has been verified also in other double blind experiments with human volunteers (Major et.al. 2009; Rosenblum et.al. 2012; Yin et.al. 2010).

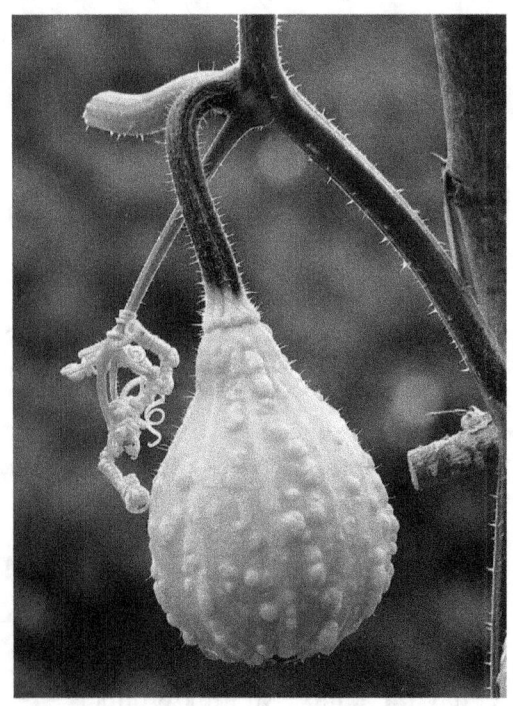

Cantaloupe melon

(Cucumis Melo)

Cantaloupe melon is a delicious melon fruit, which has yellow fruit flesh. Also the peel can be used as food. Peel contains large amount of healthy polyphenols. EXTRAMEL is commercial Cantaloupe melon product made from the fruit flesh extract. It contain large amounts of strong antioxidants, such as SOD (Superoxide dismutase) and Catalase.

Cantaloupe melon fruit and peel have body weight and body fat mass decreasing properties.

When hamsters were given high fat diet and 5.6 mg EXTRAMEL extract daily, for 84 days, body weight decreased by 29% and fat mass decreased by 25% in test group, compared to control group. Also triglycerides decreased by 68%, Leptin decreased by 99%, Insulin decreased by 39%, but Adiponectin increased by 29% in test group, compared to control group (Decorde et.al. 2009).

When rats with high cholesterol levels were given Cantaloupe melon peel methanol extract 500 mg/kg BW daily, for 28 days, body weight, total cholesterol, LDL-cholesterol and triglycerides decreased significantly, but HDL-cholesterol increased significantly in test group, compared to control group (Bidkar et.al. 2012).

Also in other experiments with rats and hamsters Cantaloupe melon peel extract and EXTRAMEL decreased significantly total cholesterol and LDL-cholesterol, but increased significantly HDL-cholesterol and Thyroid hormones in test group, compared to control group (Parmar et.al. 2009; Decorde et.al. 2010).

Capers

(Capparis Spinosa)

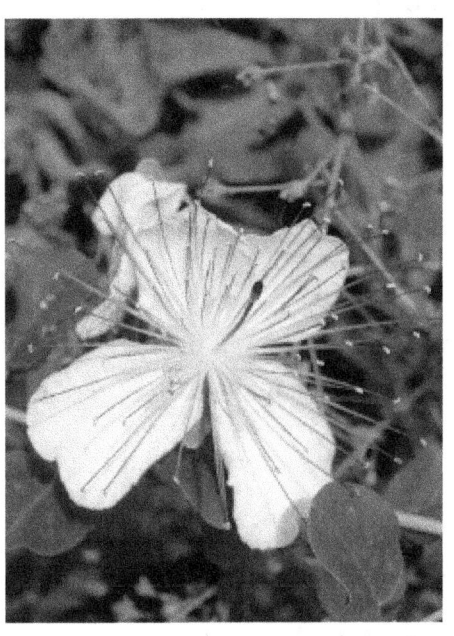

Capers are very popular spice all around the World. Capers contain large amounts of flavonoids, especially Quercetin (180 mg/100g) and Kaempferol (135 mg/100g). These flavonoids have large number of different positive effects on human health.

Capers have body weight decreasing properties.

When obese mice were given high fat diet together with 20 mg/kg BW Capers water extract daily, for 15 days, body weight was 22.2% (p < 0.01) lower in test group, comared to the control group (Lemhadri et.al. 2007).

When diabetic rats were given 20 mg/kg BW Capers water extract daily, for 15 days, body weight was 9.1% (p < 0.05) lower in test group, compared to the control group. Also triglycerides (p < 0.05) and total cholesterol (p < 0.05) were significantly lower in test group, compared to the control group (Eddouks et.al. 2005).

Capsinoids

(Capsiucum Annuum, CH-19 Sweet)

Capsinoids are close relatives of the familiar pungent compound Capsaicin, which exists in Chili peppers. Capsinoids are abundant in the CH-19 Sweet Chili pepper, developed in Japan. But Capsinoids are non-pungent, so they do not give the hot feeling when eaten. The most common Capsinoids are Capsiate, Dihydrocapsiate and Nordihydrocapsiate.

Capsinoids have body weight and fat mass decreasing properties.

When mice were given 10 mg/kg BW Capsinoids daily, for 2 weeks, body weight was 5.5% ($p < 0.05$) and body fat mass was 29.8% ($p < 0.05$) lower in test group, compared to control group (Haramizu et.al. 2011).

When 7 volunteers were given 0.4 grams/kg BW CH-19 Sweet Chili pepper daily, for 2 weeks, body weight decreased in test group by 1.77 kg (69.90 kg → 68.13 kg; $p < 0.05$), when it increased in the 5 person control group by 0.52 kg (68.13 kg → 68.85; $p > 0.5$). Also total fat area decreased in test group by 8.3% (189.0 cm^2 → 173.23 cm^2; $p < 0.05$), but it did not change in the control group (Kawabata et.al. 2006).

The body weight and body fat mass decreasing but energy expenditure, fat oxidation, body temperature and oxygen consumption increasing properties of Capsinoids has been verified in many experiments with human volunteers (Yoneshiro et.al. 2012; Ohnuki et.al. 2001; Inoue et.al. 2007; Snitker et.al. 2009; Reinbach et.al. 2009).

Caralluma

(Caralluma Fimbriata)

Caralluma is an edible cactus, which is used in India besides as a vegetable, to suppress hunger and to increase endurance.

Caralluma has body weight and fat mass decreasing properties.

When rats were given together with high calorific diet Caralluma either 25 mg/kg BW, 50 mg/kg BW or 100 mg/kg BW daily, for 90 days, body weight gain was 29.8% ($p < 0.05$), 35.77% ($p < 0.05$) and 36.30% ($p < 0.05$) lower in test groups, compared to control group. Also triglycerides ($p < 0.0001$), LDL-cholesterol ($p < 0.0001$), total cholesterol ($p < 0.0001$) and Leptin ($p < 0.0001$) were significantly lower but HDL-cholesterol ($p < 0.0001$) was significantly higher in the test groups, compared to the control group (Kamalakkannan et.al. 2010).

When 35 volunteers were given Caralluma water-ethanol extract 1 grams daily, for 60 days, body weight decreased 1.0 kg more in test group, compared to the control group. Waist circumference decreased significantly (96.9 cm → 93.9 cm; $p < 0.0001$) in test group, compared to the control group. Body fat-% decreased by 1.2% ($p = 0.07$) in the test group. Also hunger decreased significantly ($p < 0.001$) compared to the control group (Kuriyah et.al. 2007). This was a double blind experiment. There were 25 volunteers in the control group.

Caraway, seed

(Carum Carvi)

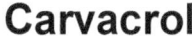

Caraway seed is a very old spice and medicinal plant. It is known to decrease triglycerides and total cholesterol. It is used in diabetes, cardiovascular diseases and hypertension.

Caraway seed has body weight decreasing properties.

When normal rats were given Caraway seed hot water extract 20 mg/kg BW daily, for 15 days, body weight in test group was 8.4% ($p < 0.05$) lower, compared to control group. Also in diabetic rat group, Caraway seed significantly ($p < 0.01$) decreased body weight, compared to control group. Also triglycerides and total cholesterol were significantly lower in both test groups, compared to control group (Lemhadri et.al. 2006).

Also in another experiment with obese rats, Caraway in an herbal mixture decreased significantly the body weight of test group, compared to control group (Gupta et.al. 2012).

Carvacrol

Carvacrol is a natural phenolic compound, found in many aromatic spices, such as Marjoram (Origanum Majorana), Oregano (Origanum Vulgare), Basil (Ocimum Basilicum), Summer Savory (Satureja Hortensis), Winter Savory (Satureja Montana) etc., and especially in oils extracted from these plants. Dried Basil has 111.6 mg/100 g and dried Oregano has 108.3 mg/100 g Carvacrol.

Carvacrol has body weight and fat mass decreasing properties.

When mice were given high fat diet and 0.1% Carvacrol in their daily diet, for 4 weeks, body weight was 24% ($p < 0.05$) and fat mass was 36% ($p < 0.05$) lower in test group, compared to control group (Cho et.al. 2011).

Celery leaves, stalks, seeds

(Apium Graveolens)

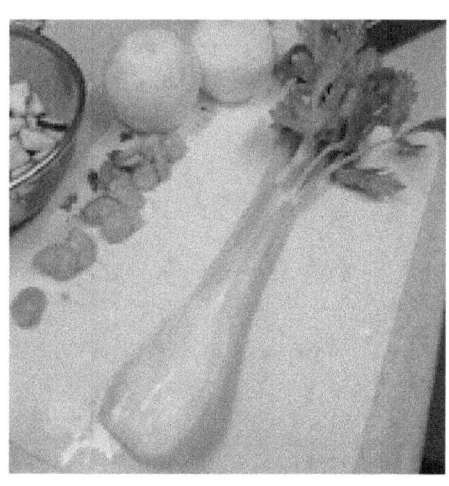

Celery is cultivated as a vegetable all around the World. All parts of Celery can be eaten. Celery is known to decrease blood pressure and cholesterol.

Celery has body weight decreasing properties.

Celery stalks and leaves have only 11 kcal/100 grams energy content, which is one of the least among all vegetables. With such a low energy density, Celery stalks and leaves can be eaten in great amounts, without increasing the daily energy input.

When obese rats were given high fat diet and 5% Celery leaves in daily diet, for 3 months, body weight was 11.9% ($p < 0.05$) lower in test group, compared to the control group (Tourkostani et.al. 2009).

When obese rats were given high fat diet and 10% Celery leaves in daily diet, for 4 weeks, body weight gain in test group was 27.8% ($p < 0.05$) lower, than in the control group. Also LDL-cholesterol, total cholesterol and triglycerides were significantly lower in test group, compared to the control group (Belal 2011).

The body weight decreasing property of Celery stalks and leaves has been verified in other experiments with rats (Nehal et.al. 2011; Tsi et.al. 2000).

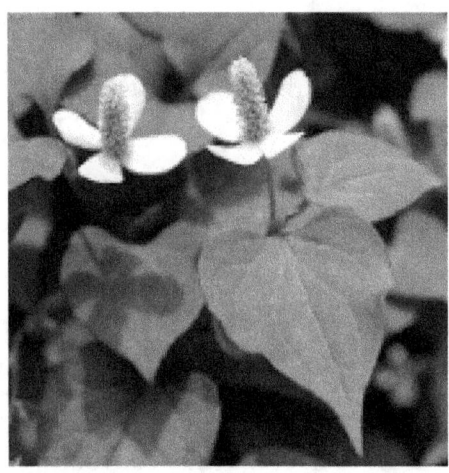

Chamaleon

(Houttuyania Cordata)

Chameleon is a very popular vegetable in East-Asia, especially in Vietnam, China, Japan etc. Its Japanese name is Dokumani. It is antiviral, antibacterial, antihypertensive and anti-inflammatory.

Chamaleon leaves have body weight and body fat mass decreasing properties.

When mice were given high fat diet and 2% on Chamaleon leaves water extract daily, for 11 weeks, body weight was 20.9% ($p < 0.005$) lower in test group, compared to control group. Body fat mass was 49.0% ($p < 0.005$) lower in test group, compared to control group (Miyata et.al. 2010).

The body weight and body fat mass decreasing properties of Chamaleon leaves has been verified also in another experiment with mice (Lin et.al. 2012).

Chickpea

(Cicer Arietinum)

Chickpea is one of the World's most important cultivated legumes. It contains large amounts of protein, carbohydrates and dietary fiber. It has very large amounts of Pangamic acid (Vitamin B15), which decreases strongly high cholesterol and triglyceride levels (Singh et.al. 1893).

Chickpea has body weight and body fat mass decreasing properties.

When rats were given high fat diet and 10% Chickpea daily, for 8 months, body weight decreased by 14% ($p < 0.05$), body fat mass decreased by 28% ($p < 0.05$), Leptin decreased by 17.0% ($p < 0.01$), triglycerides decreased by 44.8% ($p < 0.01$) and LDL-cholesterol decreased by 23.2% ($p < 0.05$) in test group, compared to control group (Yang et.al. 2007).

When chicken were given normal food and 5% Chickpea daily, for 45 days, body weight gain was 15.2% ($p < 0.05$) lower in test group, compared to control group (Algam et.al. 2012).

Chickweed

(Stellaria Media)

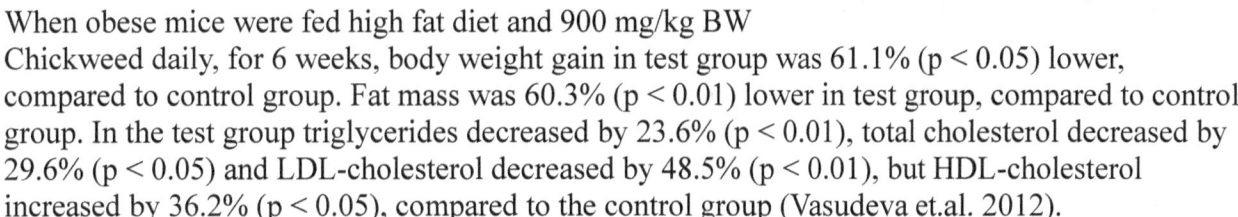

Chickweed is found commonly all around the World, in moist places. It has a very high nutrient content and it is used in India generally as a vegetable. Its cultivation is very easy.

Chickweed has body weight and fat mass decreasing properties.

When obese mice were fed high fat diet and 900 mg/kg BW Chickweed daily, for 6 weeks, body weight gain in test group was 61.1% ($p < 0.05$) lower, compared to control group. Fat mass was 60.3% ($p < 0.01$) lower in test group, compared to control group. In the test group triglycerides decreased by 23.6% ($p < 0.01$), total cholesterol decreased by 29.6% ($p < 0.05$) and LDL-cholesterol decreased by 48.5% ($p < 0.01$), but HDL-cholesterol increased by 36.2% ($p < 0.05$), compared to the control group (Vasudeva et.al. 2012).

In another experiment with mice, Chickweed decreased significantly body weight, fat mass and triglycerides in test group, compared to control group (Chidrawar et.al. 2011).

Chicory

(Cichorium Intybus)

Chicory is a very old vegetable and medicinal plant. Its root has been used instead of coffee, and the leaves are very popular vegetable all over Europe. The root contains 12 – 23% Inulin.

Chicory has body weight decreasing properties.

When obese rats were given high fat diet with 5% Chicory leaves daily, for 4 weeks, body weight gain in test group was 28.8% ($p < 0.05$) lower, compared to control group. Also total cholesterol, LDL-cholesterol, VLDL-cholesterol and triglycerides were significantly lower, but HDL-cholesterol significantly ($p < 0.05$ in all parameters) higher in test group, compared to control group (Ahmed et.al. 2009).

Chili pepper and Capsaicin

(Capsicum Annuum)

Chili pepper is one of the most commonly used spices in the World. The pungent compound in Chili pepper is Capsaicin. Chili is available all around the year as fresh or dried powder, and its cultivation is very easy.

Chili pepper and Capsaicin have body weight and fat mass decreasing properties.

When rats were given normal diet and 3% Chili pepper in their daily food, for 7 weeks, body weight was 15.6% ($p < 0.01$) lower in test group, compared to control group (Akpamu et.al. 2012).

When obese rats were given high fat diet and 0.016% Capsaicin daily, for 8 weeks, body weight was 10.2% ($p < 0.05$), body fat mass was 24.5% ($p < 0.05$), triglycerides were 29.3% ($p < 0.05$) and total cholesterol was 24.7% ($p < 0.05$) lower in test group, compared to control group (Ann et.al. 2011).

The body weight and fat mass decreasing properteis of Chili and Capsaicin has been verified in great many experiments with mice, rats and rabbits (Yo et.al. 2012; Oh et.al. 2003; Yoon et.al. 2005; Sambaiah et.al. 1982; Kang et.al. 2010; Kawada et.al. 1986).

In experiments with human volunteers Chili and Capsaicin increase fat oxidation by up to 38.7% ($p < 0.05$), decrease carbohydrate oxidation by up to 20% ($p < 0.05$) (Yoshioka et.al. 1998; Manuela et.al. 2003) and decrease body fat mass significantly ($p = 0.0373$) compared to control groups (Chang et.al. 2003).

Chili pepper, seed

(Capsicum Annuum)

Except Chili pepper, also the seeds are edible.

Chili pepper seeds have body weight decreasing properties.

When rats were given high fat diet and either 5%, 10% or 15% Red Chili pepper seeds daily, body weight gain in test groups were 5.9% ($p < 0.05$), 7.4% ($p < 0.05$) and 17.2% ($p < 0.05$) lower, compared to control group (Song et.al. 2009).

The body weight, triglycerides, total cholesterol and LDL-cholesterol decreasing but HDL-cholesterol increasing properties of Chili pepper seeds has been verified in many animal experiments (Jeon et.al. 2010; Song et.al. 2010; Song et.al. 2011).

Chinese Bellflower

(Platycodon Grandiflorum)

Chinese Bellflower roots are edible, and they have been used as food and medicine in Asia, especially in China, Korea and Japan, for hundreds of years. As a medicine, it is used in Asthma, Bronchitis, Colds, to loose mucus, against hypertension and high cholesterol levels. Its cultivaton is very easy. Chinese Bellflower contains large amounts of Inulin and Saponins, which are the effective compounds.

Chinese Bellflower roots have body weight decreasing properties.

When slim rats were given Chinese Bellflower root 5% in their daily diet, for 4 weeks, body weight decreased by 10.4% ($p < 0.05$), compared to the control group (Kim et.al. 2000).

When rats were given Chinese Bellflower root 5% in their daily diet, for 8 weeks, body weight decreased by 21.4% ($p < 0.05$), compared to the control group. Triglycerides also decreased ($p < 0.05$) significantly, compared to the control group (Han et.al. 2000).

When hyperlipidemic rats were given Chinese Bellflower root water extract at a dose of 150 mg/kg daily, for 7 weeks, body weight decreased by 33% ($p < 0.05$), compared to the control group (Park et.al. 2007).

When hamsters were given Chinese Bellflower root Saponins either 0.3% or 0.5% of their daily diet, total cholesterol decreased by 13% ($p < 0.05$) and 28% ($p < 0.05$), compared to the control group (Zhao et.al. 2008).

Also in experiments with mice, Chinese Bellflower root Saponins decreased body weight significantly, compared to the control groups (Kim et.al. 2009; Han et.al. 2002). The same has been verified in experiments with rats too (Zhao et.al. 2005; Park et.al. 2005).

Chinese Blackberry

(Rubus Suavissimus)

Chinese Blackberry is also called Sweet tea. It originates from Southern China, an tea made from its leaves is a very popular healthy tea in China and Japan. It is used against obesity, diabetes and asthma. The leaves contain up to 4% a triterpenoid glucoside called Rubusoside, which is over 100 times sweeter than ordinary sugar.

Chinese Blackberry leaves have body weight and fat mass decreasing properties.

When obese rats were given 220 mg/kg BW Chinese Blackberry leaves extract daily, for 9 weeks, body weight gain was 22% ($p < 0.001$) and fat mass was 48% ($p < 0.001$) lower in test group, compared to control group (Koh et.al. 2011).

Chinese Ginger, root

(Boesenbergia Pandurata; Syn. Kaempferia Pandurata)

Chinese Ginger is a popular root vegetable in East-Asia. It is also called Fingerroot, because the roots look like human fingers.

Chinese Ginger root has body weight and body fat mass decreasing properties.

When obese mice were given high fat diet and 200 mg/kg BW Chinese Ginger root ethanol extract daily for 8 weeks, body weight was 14.0% ($p < 0.05$) and body fat mass was 30.5% ($p < 0.05$) lower in test group, compared to control group (Kim et.al. 2012).

Chinese jewel orchid

(Anoectochilus Formosanus)

Chinese jewel orchid is a beautiful orchid, which grows in China and Taiwan. It is a very important medicinal plant in Taiwan and China, and it is used as a functional healthy tea against liver diseases, impotence, hypertension, diabetes, fatigue and cardiovascular diseases.

Chinese jewel orchid has body weight and fat mass decreasing properties.

When mice were given Chinese jewel orchid water extract 1000 mg/kg BW, 5 days per weeks, for 4 weeks, body fat mass was 26% ($p < 0.05$) lower in test group, compared to control group. Swimming endurance increased by 61% ($p < 0.05$) in test group, compared to control group. These changes mean, that Chinese jewel orchid stimulates strongly fat oxidation (Ikeuchi et.al. 2005).

When obese rats were given Chinese jewel orchid water extract 200 mg/kg BW daily, for 12 weeks, body weight gain was 7.96% ($p < 0.05$) lower in test group, compared to control group (Shih et.al. 2001).

The Chinese jewel orchid body weight and fat mass decreasing properties has been verified in many experiments with mice and rats (Du et.al. 2008; Du et.al. 2001; Du et.al. 2003).

When 66 volunteers were given 450 mg Chinese jewel orchid daily, for 6 – 12 months, total cholesterol, LDL-cholesterol and VLDL-cholesterol decreased significantly ($p < 0.05$), compared to baseline values (Du et.al. 2007).

Chinese Lantern Tree, fruit

(Dichrostachys Glomerata)

Chinese Lantern tree grows in Africa, India and Caribbean islands. The fruits and seeds are edible, and the dried fruits are used as spice in Africa.

The Chinese Lantern tree fruits have body weight and body fat mass decreasing properties.

When 23 obese volunteers were given 800 mg Chinese Lantern tree dried fruit Daily, for 8 weeks, body weight decreased in test group by 7.67 kg (98.43 kg → 90.76 kg; $p < 0.05$), when it decreased only by 1.32 kg (102.93 kg → 101.60 kg; $p > 0.05$) in the 23 person control group. Also fat-% decreased by 3.20% (45.64% → 42.44%; $p < 0.05$) in test group, but only by 0.7% ($p > 0.05$) in control group. Waist circumference decreased by 7.2 cm ($p < 0.05$) and hip circumference decreased by 8.9 cm ($p < 0.05$) in test group, but they did not change in control group ($p > 0.05$). Also systolic blood pressure, diastolic blood pressure, triglycerides and total cholesterol decreased significantly ($p < 0.05$), but HDL-cholesterol increased significantly ($p < 0.05$) in test group, compared to control group (Kuate et.al. 2011). This was a double blind experiment.

Chinese plantain, seed

(Plantago Asiatica)

Chinese plantain is a very famous medicinal plant, which has been used in China for thousands of years in different illnesses. The Chinese name of this herbal medicine is CHE QIAN ZI.

Chinese plantain seed has body weight and body fat mass decreasing properties.

When obese rats were given high fat diet and 100 mg/kg BW Chinese plantain seed water extract daily, for 8 weeks, body weight in test group was 14.0% ($p < 0.05$) lower, compared to control group. Total body fat mass was 54.9% ($p < 0.05$) lower in test group, compared to control group. Also triglycerides ($p < 0.05$), total cholesterol ($p < 0.05$) and LDL-cholesterol ($p < 0.05$) were significantly lower in test group, compared to control group (Hwang et.al. 2012).

Also in another experiment with rats Chinese plantain seed decreased body weight ($p < 0.05$), total cholesterol ($p < 0.05$) and LDL-cholesterol ($p < 0.05$) significantly, compared to control group (An et.al. 2003).

Chinese Willow, leaves

(Salix Matsudana)

Chinese Willow originates from China, but it is nowadays cultivated as an ornamental tree in many other northern countries.

Chinese Willow leaves have body weight decreasing properties.

When rats were given high fat diet and 5% polyphenol extract of Chinese Willow leaves daily, for 9 weeks, body weight gain in test group was 20% ($p < 0.05$) lower, compared to control group (Han et.al. 2003).

The active compounds are flavonoids, Apigenin-7-O-Glucoside, Luteoling-7-O-Glucoside etc. (Han et.al. 2003; Zhang et.al. 2000).

Chorella

(Chlorella Vulgaris, Chlorella Sp.)

Chlorella is a very healthy fresh water algae, which contains up to 60% protein, large amounts of w-3 fatty acids and vitamins. It contains also large amounts of the carotenoids Fucoxanthin, Astaxanthin, beta-Cryptoxanthin and Neoxanthin, which stimulate fatty acid beta-oxidation.

Chlorella has fat mass decreasing properties.

When 34 volunteers were given 8 grams Chlorella daily, for 16 weeks, body fat-% decreased by an average of 4% ($p < 0.05$), compared to the control group. Also blood sugar ($p < 0.05$) and total cholesterol ($p < 0.05$) decreased significantly in the Chlorella group, compared to the control group (Mizoguchi et.al. 2008).

The body weight and fat mass decreasing properties of Chlorella has been verified in many experiments with animals and cells (Lee et.al. 2008; Hidaka et.al. 2004; Chon et.al. 2009).

Chlorogenic acid

Chlorogenic acid is a natural polyphenol, which exist especially in green coffee beans. Chlorogenic acid is a strong antioxidant.

Chlorogenic acid has body weight and fat mass decreasing properties.

When 15 volunteers were given along with coffee 1000 mg Chlorogenic acid daily, for 12 weeks, body weight decreased in test group by 5.7 kg (p < 0.05), when it decreased only by 1.7 kg (p < 0.05) in the control group. Also body fat-% decreased significantly by 3.6% (27.2% → 23.6%; p < 0.05) in test group, but only by 0.7% (p > 0.05) in control group (Thom et.al. 2007). This was a double blind experiment.

The same kind of results of seen also in another double blind experiment with human volunteers (Tomonori et.al. 2009).

In volunteers Chlorogenic acid significantly increases fat oxidation (p < 0.05) and oxygen uptake (p < 0.05) (Ota et.al. 2010).

In animal experiments Chlorogenic acid decreases body weight, body fat mass, FAS enzyme, Leptin and Insulin, but increases Adiponectin (Cho et.al. 2010; Murase et.al. 2011; Li et.al. 2009).

Chokeberry

(Aronia Melanocarpa)

Chokeberry is extremely healthy berry. It contains more Anthocyanins than any other berry, and also large amounts of flavonoids and vitamins. It is very cold hardy, that the berries can be eaten also on wintertime. Chokeberry is known to decrease blood pressure and cholesterol.

When rats on a fructose containing diet were given Chokeberry 60% ethanol extract either 100 mg/kg BW or 200 mg/kg BW daily, for 6 weeks, body weight in test groups were 3.36% (p < 0.05) and 4.32% (p < 0.05) and body fat mass were 9.78% (p < 0.05) and 13.04% (p < 0.05) lower, compared to the control group. Also triglycerides, LDL-cholesterol and total cholesterol were significantly lower, but HDL-cholesterol was significantly higher (p < 0.05 in all parameters) in test groups, compared to the control group (Qin et.al. 2012).

Choline

Choline is a vitamin like compound, which exists both in human cells and food. Soya lecithin is a very good Choline source.

Choline has body weight and fat mass decreasing properties.

When rats were given Choline supplement in their daily food, for 24 days, weight gain was 57.6% (p < 0.05) lower in test group, compared to the control group. The liver fat mass was 27.4% (p < 0.05) in Choline group, compared to the control group (Kenney et.al. 1995).

When rats were given in their daily food 0.01% Caffeine, 0.5% Carnitine and 1.15% Choline, for 4 weeks, fat mass decreased by 18.5% (p = 0.0140) and body weight decreased by 3.1% in test group, compared to the control group. Also triglycerides (p = 0.0003) decreased significantly in test group, compared to the control group (Sachan et.al. 2000).

The fat mass and triglycerides decreasing properties of Choline has been verified in other experiments with guinea pigs and rats (Daily et.al. 1998; Hongu et.al. 2000).

Chromium

Chromium is an essential trace mineral for humans. It has a very important role in glucose and lipid metabolism. It is normally used as Chromium Picolinate.

Chromium has body weight reducing properties.

When 62 volunteers were given Chromium Picolinate 400 micrograms daily, for 3 months, body weight decreased by 5.98 kg ($p < 0.001$), fat-% decreased by 5.1% ($p < 0.001$) and total fat mass decreased by 6.18 kg ($p < 0.001$) compared to the control group (Kaats et.al. 1998). This was a double blind experiment.

When 66 volunteers were given Chromium Picolinate 400 micrograms daily, for 72 days, body weight decreased by 1.26 kg ($p < 0.05$), body fat-% decreased by 1.6% ($p < 0.05$) and fat mass decreased by 1.89 kg ($p < 0.05$), compared to the control group (Kaats et.al. 1996). This was a double blind experiment.

The same kind of results have been noticed also in other human experiments (Crawford et.al. 1999; Chen et.al. 2007; Martin et.al. 2006).

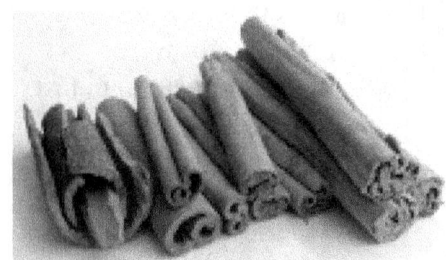

Cinnamon

(Cinnamomum Zeylanicum)

Cinnamon is a very popular spice and medicinal plant all over the World. Cinnamon is known to decrease triglycerides, total cholesterol, blood pressure and blood sugar.

Cinnamon has body weight decreasing properties.

When 15 volunteers were given Cinnamon 2.0 grams daily, for 3 months, body weight decreased by 1.86 kg ($p < 0.01$), compared to the control group. Also triglycerides and total cholesterol decreased significantly (Balasasirekha et.al. 2011).

When 11 volunteers were given Cinnamon extract 500 mg daily, for 12 weeks, the body total fat decreased by 0.7% ($p < 0.02$) and the lean body mass increased by 1.1% ($p < 0.02$), compared to the control group (Ziegenfuss et.al. 2006).

When 19 volunteers were given Cinnamon 3.0 grams daily, for 8 weeks, body weight decreased by 0.9 kg ($p < 0.05$) and body fat content decreased y 0.44% ($p < 0.05$), compared to the control group (Vafa et.al. 2012). This was a double blind experiment.

Also in animal experiments with rats, Cinnamon decreases both body weight and body fat content (Couturier et.al. 2010; El-kewavy et.al. 2011).

Cirsimarin

Cirsimarin is a flavonoid, which exists in many plants, especially in different Thistle (Cirsium Sp.) species. All Thistle species have edible leaves and roots.

Cirsimarin has body weight and fat mass decreasing properties.

When mice were given normal food and Cirsimarin either 25 mg/kg BW or 50 mg/kg BW daily, for 18 days, body fat mass was 45% ($p < 0.05$) and 48% ($p < 0.05$) lower in test group, compared to control group. Body weight decreased by 7.2% and 8.0% in test groups, compared to control group (Zarrouki et.al. 2010).

In another experiment with fat cells, it was verified, that Cirsimarin was 20 times stronger lipolytic agent than the known lipolytic agent Caffeine (Girotti et.al. 2005).

CLA
(Conjugated Linoleic Acid)

Conjugated Linoleic acids are a group of several isomers of the essential fatty acid, Linoleic acid. Conjugated Linoleic acid exist especially in different meat products, but also in different seeds, such as Pomegranate seeds. These Conjugated Linoleic acid isomers are called collectively CLA. They can be bought as dietary supplements in markers. The typical dose is 1-6 grams daily.

CLA has body weight and body fat mass decreasing properties.

When 12 obese volunteers were given 6 grams CLA daily, for 12 weeks, body weight was 3.6 kg ($p < 0.001$) lower in test group, compared to 12 volunteers control group (Test group: 81.1 kg → 78.6 kg; $p < 0.001$; Control group: 76.0 kg → 77.1 kg; $p > 0.05$). Also fat mass decreased in test group by 2.8 kg ($p < 0.001$), compared to control group, and fat-% decreased in test group by 2.3% ($p < 0.001$), when it increased by 0.6% ($p > 0.05$) in control group. This was a double blind experiment (Ha et.al. 2010).

The body weight and body fat mass decreasing properties of CLA has been verified in great many double blind experiments with human volunteers (Chen et.al. 2012; Gaullier et.al. 2007; Thom et.al. 2001; Kamphuis et.al. 2003; Blankson et.al. 2000; Raff et.al. 2009; Riserius et.al. 2001; Racine et.al. 2010; Gaullier et.al. 2004; Gaullier et.al. 2005).

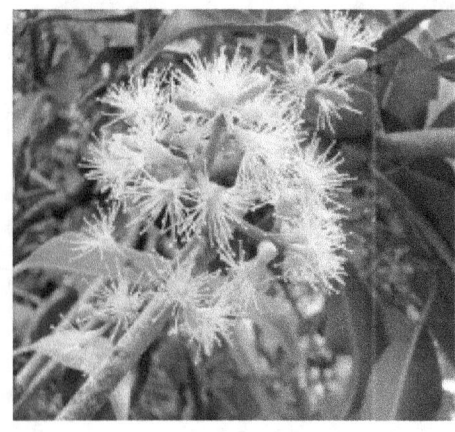

Clove

(Syzygium Aromaticum)

Clove is the very old and common spice from Asia, which is in use all over the World. Besides spice, Clove is also used in Asia in dental pain, headache and respiratory disorders.

Clove has body weight and body fat mass decreasing properties.

When mice on a high fat diet were given Clove ethanol extract 0.5% daily, for 9 weeks, body weight gain was 44.8% ($p < 0.05$) lower in test group, than in the control group. Also body fat mass was 54.0% ($p < 0.05$) lower in the test group, than in the control group. Also serum Glucose, Insulin and Leptin levels were reduced in the test group (Jung et.al. 2012).

Same results were noticed also in another experiment with mice. When mice were given in their daily diet Clove an amount, which would correspond to 5 grams spice in a day for adult human, for 3 months, body weight was 6.7% ($p < 0.05$) in the test group, compared to the control group. Also triglycerides decreased significantly in the test group (Longquan et.al. 2007).

Cocoa

(Theobroma Cacao)

Cocoa is the healthy dark powder of Theobroma Cacao fruit seeds, and the main component in Chocolate. Cocoa contains large amounts of healthy polyphenols. Cocoa is known to decrease high blood pressure and high cholesterol levels.

When rats were given high fat diet together with 12.5% Cocoa powder daily, for 3 weeks, body weight decreased by 8.2% ($p < 0.05$) and relative fat-% by 18.4% ($p < 0.05$) in test group, compared to the control group. Also triglycerides decreased in test group by 23.7%, compared to the control group (Matsui et.al. 2005).

When mice were given in their daily diet either 0.5% or 2.0% of cocoa polyphenols, for 13 weeks, body weight decreased by 13.8% ($p < 0.05$) and 16.4% ($p < 0.05$) and body fat decreased by 34.5% ($p < 0.05$) and 53.7% ($p < 0.05$) in the test group, compared to the control group (Yamashita et.al. 2012).

Cocoa decreased significantly both body weight and body fat mass in obese mice (Sy et.al. 2012).

Coleus, root

(Coleus Forskohlii syn. C. Barbatus)

Coleus is a very old food and medicinal plant, which has been used in India over 3000 years. The root is edible, and it is a source of unique triterpene named Forskolin, which is a specific Adenylate Cyclase activator and increases cAMP levels. Forskolin decreases blood pressure, decreases intraocular pressure in Glaucoma, relaxes smooth muscles in lung pipes and eases asthma symptoms etc. It grows in India, Nepal, Sri Lanka, Egypt, Ethiopia, Brazil and West-Africa.

Coleus and Forskolin have body weight and body fat mass decreasing properties.

When rats were given 5% Coleus extract in their daily food, for 27 days, body weight decreased by 5.3% ($p < 0.05$) and body fat mass decreased by 36.4% ($p < 0.05$) in test group, compared to control group. Also FAS enzyme decreased significantly ($p < 0.05$) in test group (Han et.al. 2005).

Also in other experiments with rats Forskolin decreases body weight (Battochio et.al. 2005).

In experiments with fat cells, Forskolin stimulates significantly lipolysis (Allen et.al. 1986; Okuda et.al. 1992).

When 15 obese men were given 50 mg Forskolin daily, for 12 weeks, body fat mass decreased by 11.23% (4.52 kg; 37.43 kg → 32.91 kg; $p < 0.05$), but it did not change in the 15 person control group. Also testosterone increased in test group significantly ($p < 0.05$) by 16.77%, when it decreased by 1.08% in control group. Systolic blood pressure decreased by 6.27 mmHg (132.743 mmHg → 126.47 mmHg) in test group (Goddard et.al. 2005). This was a double blind experiment.

When 6 obese females were given 50 mg Forskolin daily, for 8 weeks, body weight decreased by 4.16 kg ($p < 0.05$), fat-% decreased by 7.75% (33.63% → 25.8%; $p < 0.05$), diastolic blood pressure decreased by 5.0 mmHg (71.0 mmHg → 66.0 mmHg) and systolic blood pressure decreased by 9.17 mmHg (113.67 mmHg → 104.50 mmHg) (Badmaev et.al. 2002)

Common Ash, seeds

(Fraxinus Excelsior)

Common Ash is a tree, which is familiar to everybody. The seeds are used as a food in Morocco, and they have been earlier also eaten in Europe. The seeds are known to decrease high blood sugar levels.

Common ash seeds have body weight and fat mass decreasing properties.

When mice were given high fat diet and Common Ash seeds hot water extract 0.5% daily, for 16 weeks, body weight was 11.36% ($p < 0.05$) and body fat mass was 17.85% ($p < 0.05$) lower in test group, compared to control group. Also blood sugar was 76.52% ($p < 0.001$) lower in test group, compared to control group (Ibarra et.al. 2011).

Common Reed

(Phragmites Communis)

Common Reed grows all around the World, along seashore. All parts of Common Reed are usable: Roots can be made into edible flour, stems can be used for roofs etc., and young leaves can be eaten like asparagus. Dried young leaves contain up to 19% protein.

Young Common Reed leaves have body weight and body fat decreasing properties.

When rats were given high fat diet and only 1% young Common Reed leaves in their daily diet, for 8 weeks, body weight was 3.4% ($p < 0.05$) lower in test group, compared to control group. Total body fat mass was 11.0% ($p < 0.05$) lower in test group, compared to control group. Also triglycerides were 36.0% ($p < 0.05$) and total cholesterol was 19.6% ($p < 0.05$) lower in test group, compared to control group (Lee et.al. 2010).

Cordyceps

(Cordyceps Chinensis)

Cordyceps is a very famous medicinal mushroom, which has been used thousands of years in China against different illnesses. Cordyceps is aphrodisiac, and it increases testosterone levels. The active compound is Cordycepin (3-Deoxyadenosine). This mushroom is called Dong Chong Xia Cao in Chinese.

Cordyceps has body weight decreasing properties.

When rats were given high fat diet and either 1.5 ml/100 g BW water or 1.5 ml/100 g BW 33% strong Cordyceps in water infusion daily, for 20 weeks, body weight in test group was 15.5% ($p < 0.01$) lower, compared to control group. Also the liver triglycerides ($p < 0.01$) and total cholesterol ($p < 0.01$) were significantly lower in test group, compared to control group (Dai et.al. 2006).

The body weight decreasing properties of Cordyceps has been verified in many animal and fat cell experiments (Guo et.al. 2010; Kan et.al. 2012; Takahashi et.al. 2012; Liu et.al. 2011; Shimada et.al. 2008).

Coriander seeds and leaves

(Coriandrum Sativum)

Coriander is known all over the World as a spice. All parts of Coriander can be used, but normally only the seeds and leaves are used. Coriander seeds are rich source of Flavonoids and Polyphenols, such as Rutin, Quercetin, Isoquercetin, Chlorogenic acid, Ferulic acid etc. Coriander seeds are known to lower triglycerides and cholesterol levels.

Coriander seeds and leaves have body weight decreasing properties.

When mice on a high fat diet were fed daily with either 1% or 3% Coriander seed water extract, for 12 weeks, body weight gain was 28.7% (p < 0.01) and 66.7% (p < 0.001) lower in test groups, than in control group. Also triglycerides and total cholesterol levels were significantly (p < 0.001) lower in test groups, than in control group (Patel et.al. 2011).

When rats with high cholesterol levels were given in their daily food either 10%, 15% or 20% Coriander leaves, for 6 weeks, the body weight in the test group were significantly (p < 0.05) lower, compared to the control group (El-Kherbawy et.al. 2011).

Cornelian cherry, fruit

(Cornus Officinalis, Cornus Mas)

Both Cornelian cherry, Cornus Mas, and Japanese Cornelian cherry, Cornus Officinalis, are delicious fruits. Japanese Cornelian cherry has been used hundreds of years in China, Japan and Korea also as a medicine against diabetes, asthma and impotence. It increases serum testosterone levels in animal experiments.

Cornelian cherry fruit has body weight decreasing properties.

When obese mice were given high fat diet and 0.1% Cornelian cherry anthocyanidin extract daily, for 8 weeks, body weight gain in test group was 24% lower, compared to control group (Jayaprakasam et.al. 2006).

When obese mice were given high fat diet and Japanese cornelian cherry fruit ethanol extract at a dose of 25 mg/liter every second day, for 56 days, body weight in test group was 28.5% (p < 0.05) lower, compared to control group (Hwang et.al. 2011).

Cornelian cherry fruit decreases triglycerides, LDL-cholesterol, and total cholesterol, but increases HDL-cholesterol both in humans (Uasgary et.al. 2012) and in animal experiments (Park et.al. 2009; Gao et.al. 2012; Rafieian-Kopaei et.al. 2011).

Corosolic acid

Corosolic acid is a triterpene, which exists in many plants, such as the leaves of Guava (Psidium Guajava) and Loquat (Eriobotrya Japonica).

Corosolic acid has body weight and body fat mass decreasing properties.

When obese mice were given high fat diet and 0.023% Corosolic acid in their daily food, for 9 weeks, body weight was 10% (p < 0.05), body fat mass was 15% (p < 0.05), triglycerides were 22% (p < 0.05) and serum glucose was 23% (p < 0.05) lower in test group, compared to control group (Yamada et.al. 2010).

In experiments with cells, Corosolic acid inhibits the differentiation of 3T3-L1 fat cells (Zong et.al. 2007).

Costus

(Saussurea Lappa)

Costus is a plant, which belongs to the same genus (Compositae), than the familiar Greater Burdock, Arctium Lappa. Costus grows in Himalaya. The root is used against hypertension, high cholesterol levels and chronic bronchitis in India and China.

Costus has body weight decreasing properties.

When obese rats were given high fat diet and 200 mg/kg BW Costus root ethanol extract daily, for 7 days, body weight in test group was 45.0% (p < 0.01) lower, compared to control group. Also triglycerides, LDL-cholesterol and total cholesterol decreased significantly (p < 0.05), but HDL-cholesterol increased significantly (p < 0.05) in test group, compared to control group (Anbu et.al. 2011).

Also in another experiment with mice, Costus decreased body weight significantly, compared to control group (Yoon et.al. 2011).

Cudrania, leaves

(Cudrania Tricuspidata)

Cudrania is a small size tree, which grows in Korea, China and Japan. It has edible fruits and its leaves and bark has a long time been used against hypertension, inflammation, liver diseases and cancer. Its English name is Chinese Silkworm Thorn.

Cudrania leaves have body weight and body fat mass decreasing properties.

When obese rats were given high fat diet and 10% Cudrania leaves daily, for 5 weeks, body weight gain was 14.0% and body fat mass was 16.8% (p < 0.05) lower in test group, compared to control group (Park et.al. 2012).

The body weight, body fat mass, triglycerides and total cholesterol decreasing properties of Cudrania has been verified also in other experiments with mice (Lee et.al. 2011; Lee et.al. 2012).

Cudrania inhibits very strongly the activity of Lipase enzyme (Kim et.al. 2012).

The blood pressure decreasing property of Cudrania is well documented (Kang et.al. 2002).

Curcuma

(Curcuma Longa)

Curcuma is a very popular spice, used all around the World. It has also many medicinal properties, and it is known to be strongly anti-carsinogenic. The effective compound is Curcumin (Diferuloylmethane)

Curcuma and Curcumin have body weight and body fat mass decreasing properties.

When obese type 2 diabetic rats were given high fat diet and 50 mg/kg BW Curcumin daily, for 8 weeks, body weight in test group was 8.5% ($p < 0.05$) lower, compared to control group. Also triglycerides were 23.4% ($p < 0.05$), total cholesterol was 6.4% ($p < 0.05$), LDL-cholesterol was 9.9% ($p < 0.05$) and VLDL-cholesterol was 12.4% ($p < 0.05$) lower, but HDL-cholesterol was 37.1% ($p < 0.05$) higher in test group, compared to control group (Hussein et.al. 2013).

The body weight and body fat mass decreasing properties of Curcuma and Curcumin has been verified in great many animal experiments (Kim et.al. 2012; Kuo et.al. 2012; Shao et.al. 2012; Srinivasan et.al. 1987; Ho et.al. 2012; Weisberg et.al. 2008; Asai et.al. 2001; Ejaz et.al. 2009).

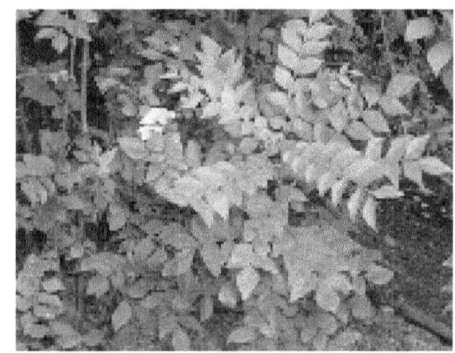

Curry

(Murraya Koenigii)

Curry is a very popular spice all around the World. In Asia it is also used as a medicinal plant.

Curry has body weight decreasing properties.

When obese rats were given Curry ethanol extract 300 mg/kg BW daily, for 2 weeks, body weight gain in test group was 77.2% ($p < 0.05$) lower, than in the control group. Test group rats had an average final weight of 325 grams, and control rats had an average final weight of 387 grams. The initial weight was same. Also triglycerides and total cholesterol decreased significantly ($p < 0.05$) in the test group, compared to the control group (Birari et.al. 2010).

The body weight and triglycerides decreasing and fat oxidation increasing properties of Curry has been verified in many experiments with mice (Xie et.al. 2006; Tembhurn et.al. 2009; Saraf et.al. 2011).

Date

(Phoenix Dactylifera)

Dates are very delicious and nutrient rich fruits.

Dates have body weight decreasing properties.

When obese rats were given high fat diet and Date water extract 100 mg/kg BW daily, for 4 weeks, body weight decreased in test group by 36.8% (p < 0.05), compared to the control group. Also total cholesterol decreased by 46.0% (p < 0.05), triglycerides decreased by 15.2% (p < 0.005), and LDL-cholesterol decreased by 66.6% (p < 0.005), but HDL-cholesterol increased by 42.4% (p < 0.005) in test group, compared to the control group (Vembu et.al. 2012).

In human volunteers, Dates decrease triglycerides by 8-15% (p < 0.05) (Rock et.al. 2009).

DHEA

(Dehydroepiandrosterone)

DHEA is a natural hormone secreted by adrenal cortex. It is a precursorof testosterone. Its concentration in plasma is much higher than any other human hormone. During aging from 25 years to 75 years, DHEA production decreases by 80%. During aging also the other anabolic hormones testosterone, growth hormone GH, IGF-1 and estrogens decrease strongly, but the catabolic hormones cortisol and prolactin increases strongly in plasma. In many countries DHEA is sold as a nutrition supplement. The normally used dose is 25 – 50 mg daily. DHEA has no known negative effects, when used in these dosages daily over 1 year, in double blind experiments. The natural metabolite of DHEA is 3-Acetyl-7-Oxo-DHEA. When given orally to aging volunteers, DHEA increases strongly the concentration of anabolic hormones testosterone, GH, IGF-1, estrogens and DHEA, but decreases strongly the catabolic hormone cortisol. DHEA gives also a strong physical and mental wellbeing feeling because it increases the beta-Endorphin levels.

DHEA has body weight and body fat mass decreasing properties.

When 57 elderly volunteers were given 50 mg DHEA daily, for 12 months, body weight decreased by 1.6 kg (p = 0.008), body fat decreased by 1.6 kg (p = 0.001) and fat-% decreased by 1.3% (p = 0.001) in men in test group, compared to control group. Also the inflammatory cytokines IL-6 (p = 0.02) and TNF-alfa (p < 0.0001) decreased significantly in test group, compared to control group. This was a double blind experiment (Weiss et.al. 2011).

When 13 volunteers were given 3-Acetyl-7-Oxo-DHEA 200 mg daily, for 8 weeks, body weight decreased by 1.91 kg (p = 0.01) and fat-% decreased by 1.23% (p =0.02) in test group, compared to 10 person control group (Kalman et.al. 2000).

The body weight, body fat mass, total cholesterol and LDL-cholesterol decreasing properties of DHEA has been verified in many double blind experiments with human volunteers (Morales et.al.

1998; Gomez-Santos et.al. 2012; Nestler et.al. 1988; Al-Harithy 2003; Villareal et.al. 2000).

The testosterone, estrogens, GH, IGF-1, beta-Endorphin and DHEA increasing but cortisol decreasing properties of DHEA has been verified in many human experiments (Morales et.al. 1998; Genazzani et.al. 2001; Morales et.al. 1994; Kroboth et.al. 2003; Genazzani et.al. 2004; Stomati et.al. 1999; Stomati et.al. 2000; Boxer et.al. 2010; Ostojic et.al. 2010).

In experiments with animals, DHEA strongly decreases body weight, body fat mass and cortisol, but increases testosterone (Sanchez et.al. 2008; Hansen et.al. 1997; MacEwen et.al. 1991; McIntosh et.al. 1999).

Dietary fiber

Dietary fiber is the insoluble complex carbohydrates of plants, such as cellulose, hemicellulose, beta-glucans, lignin, pectin, waxes etc. Dietary fiber increase bulk, soften stool and eases hunger feeling. The recommended daily intake varies typically between 25 – 40 grams. Very good sources of dietary fiber are: Oat bran, rye bran, wheat bran, sugar beet bran, barley bran, rye breads, beans, cocoa flour, fruits, vegetables, nuts and psyllium seeds. Dietary fiber is known to decrease high blood pressure and high cholesterol.

Dietary fiber has body weight and body fat mass decreasing properties.

In cross-sectional studies, dietary fiber in inversely associated with body weight and body fat mass: The less is the daily dietary fiber intake, the more weight and body fat (Slavin et.al. 2005).

When the intake of dietary fiber is increased by 14 grams per day, for 4 months, energy intake decreases by 10% and body weight decrease by an average of 1.9 kg. In obese persons, the weight reduction are even more, up to 2.4 kg (Howarth et.al. 2001).

When 9 obese volunteers were given 14.7 grams extra dietary fiber daily, for 1 – 8 months, body weight decreased by an average of 8.0 kg ($p < 0.01$) and total cholesterol decreased by an average of 46.0% ($p < 0.01$), compared to baseline values (Kaul et.al. 1993).

When obese volunteers were given 4 grams extra dietary fiber daily, for 24 weeks, body weight decreased in test group by 8.0 kg, being significantly ($p < 0.05$) more, than the 5.8 kg weight reduction in control group. This was a double blind experiment with 53 volunteers (Birkevedt et.al. 2000).

The body weight, body fat mass, triglycerides, total cholesterol, LDL-cholesterol and blood pressure decreasing properties of dietary fiber has been verified in many double blind experiments with human volunteers (Ryttig et.al. 1989; Rössner et.al. 1987; Tajik et.al. 2012; Wood et.al. 2007; Pal et.al. 2011; Salas-Salvado et.al. 2008).

Dill and Isoharmnetin

(Anethum Graveolens)

Dill is a very common annual spice and vegetable, cultivated all around the World. It contains very large amount of the flavonoid Isorhamnetin, 43.5 mg/100g fresh weight. Only dried parsley contains more Isorhamnetin, 331 mg/100g dry weight. In Iran Dill is used to lower high cholesterol values.

Dill and Isorhamnetin have body weight decreasing properties.

In experiments with fat cells, Isorhamnetin inhibits 3T3-L1 adipocyte differentiation and fat accumulation into fat cells (Iwashita et.al. 2001; Lee et.al. 2010; Lee et.al. 2009).

When rats with original weight of 220 grams were given high fat diet and 500 mg dried Dill daily, for 30 days, body weight was by average 5% lower in test group, compared to control group. Total cholesterol was 38.7% ($p < 0.05$), LDL-cholesterol was 66.5% ($p < 0.05$) and triglycerides were 33.1% ($p < 0.05$) lower, but HDL-cholesterol was 24.6% ($p < 0.05$) higher in test group, compared to control group (Yazdanparast et.al. 2008).

Dill decreases body weight both in normal and diabetic rats, compared to control groups (Morteza et.al. 2010).

Diosgenin

Diosgenin is a phytoestrogen, which exists in Sweet potato (Dioscorea Batatas) and other yam species, and also in Fenugreek (Trigonella). Diosgenin is known to decrease cholesterol. Also Sweet potato and Fenugreek are known to have body weight decreasing properties.

Diosgenin has body weight decreasing properties.

When diabetic rats were given normal diet and 1% Diosgenin in their daily food, for 3 weeks, body weight in test group was 23.6% ($p < 0.05$) lower, compared to control group (McAnuff et.al. 2005).

When exercising rats were given Diosgenin 15 mg/kg BW daily, for 6 weeks, body weight in test group was 14.2% ($p < 0.05$) lower, compared to exercising group without Diosgenin (Salimeh et.al. 2011).

Dollar Bush

(Zygophyllum Album)

Dollar Bush is a small bush. There are about 50 different Dollar Bush species in the World, mostly in Africa. In Tunisia the local species, Zygophyllum Album is used medicinally against asthma, diabetes and rheumatism.

When rats were given high fat diet and 400 mg/kg BW Dollar Bush (Zygophyllum Album) ethanol extract daily, for 6 weeks, body weight in test group was 12% ($p < 0.05$) lower, compared to control group. Also triglycerides, total cholesterol, LDL-cholesterol and Leptin were significantly ($p < 0.05$) lower, but HDL-cholesterol was significantly ($p < 0.05$) higher in test group, compared to control group (Mnafgui et.al. 2012).

Drumstick tree, fruit

(Moringa Oleifera)

Drumstick tree is extremely important food plant in tropical countries. All parts, leaves, fruits, seeds and flowers, are edible. Leaves contain protein 9.4 g/100g, energy 64 kcal/100g, vitamin C 51.7 mg/100g, iron 4.0 mg/100g, magnesium 147 mg/100g, Calcium 185 mg/100g, potassium 337 mg/100g. Also the leaves have very high levels of flavonoids: Quercetin 89.8 mg/100g and Kaempferol 36.3 mg/100g. India is the biggest producer of Drumstick fruits. Drumstick tree grows very quickly. It can reach 3 meters height in within 10 months.

Drumstick tree fruit has body weight decreasing properties.

When rabbits were given high fat diet together with cholesterol, and 200 mg/kg BW Drumstick fruit dried powder daily, for 4 months, body weight gain in test group was 89.11% ($p < 0.001$) lower, compared to control group. Also triglycerides ($p < 0.01$), total cholesterol ($p < 0.01$), LDL-cholesterol ($p < 0.01$) and VLDL-cholesterol ($p < 0.01$) decreased significantly, but HDL-cholesterol increased ($p < 0.01$) significantly in test group, compared to control group (Mehta et.al. 2003).

Du-Zhong tea

(Eucommia Ulmoides)

Du-Zhong tea is made from the leaves of the Eucommia Ulmoides tree. Du-Zhong tea is extremely popular in China, Japan and Korea, and it has been officially given a functional food status in these countries. Du-Zhong tea is known to decrease blood pressure, triglycerides, total cholesterol and LDL-cholesterol. It contains large amounts of Chlorogenic acid and Asperuloside, which decrease body weight, triglycerides and cholesterol.

Du-Zhong tea has body weight and fat mass decreasing properties.

When obese rats were given high fat diet and 10% dried Du-Zhong leaves in their daily diet, for 4 weeks, body weight was 20% ($p < 0.01$) lower in Du-Zhong tea group, than in the control group, which got high fat diet. Also fat mass was significantly ($p < 0.05$) lower in Du-Zhong group. Triglycerides were also significantly ($p < 0.05$) lower in Du-Zhong tea group (Ando et.al. 2007).

The body weight and fat mass decreasing properties of Du-Zhong tea has been verified in 4 other experiments (Zhang et.al. 2012; Hirata et.al. 2011; Fujikawa et.al. 2010; Lee et.al. 2004).

Du-Zhong tea decreases strongly triglycerides, total cholesterol, LDL-cholesterol, and FAS enzyme activity and stimulates the fatty acid beta-oxidation (Choi et.al. 2008; Park et.al. 2006; Kobayashi et.al. 2012).

East-African olive tree, leaves

(Olea Hochstetteri)

East-African olive tree is a close relative to the familiar European olive tree, Olea Europaea, which has great economic importance. The East-African olive tree is also used medicinally, against diabetes etc.

East-African olive tree leaves have body weight decreasing properties.

When rats were given East-African olive tree leaves water extract either 250 mg/kg BW, 500 mg/kg BW or 1000 mg/kg BW daily, for 3 weeks, body weight in test groups were 36.96% ($p < 0.05$), 43.52% ($p < 0.05$) and 52.21% ($p < 0.05$) lower, compared to control group. Also total cholesterol was significantly ($p < 0.05$) lower in each test group, compared to control group (Aji et.al. 2010).

Ecdysterone or 20-Hydroxyecdysone

Ecdysterone is a natural compound, which exists in insects and many plants. Especially Quinoa (Chenopodium Quinoa) edible seed contains large amounts of Ecdysterone.

Ecdysterone has body weight and body fat mass decreasing properties.

When obese mice were given 10 mg/kg BW Ecdysterone daily, for 13 weeks, body weight was 12.47% ($p < 0.05$) lower in test group, compared to control group. Also Adiponectin was 73.4% ($p < 0.05$) higher in test group, compared to control group (Kizelsztein et.al. 2009).

Also in other experiments with mice Ecdysterone decreases both body weight and body fat mass, compared to control group (Wang et.al. 2011; Foucault et.al. 2012).

When obese volunteers were given 200 mg Ecdysterone daily, for 3 months, body weight decreased by 1.5 kg, fat mass decreased by 5%, waist circumference decreased by 2.5 cm, triglycerides decreased by 42% and LDL-cholesterol decreased by 13%, compared to baseline values (Seidlova-Wuttke et.al. 2012).

Eggplant

(Solanum Melongena)

Eggplant is a common vegetable, which is cultivated all around the World.

Eggplant has body weight decreasing properties.

When obese rats were given high fat diet together with 4% Eggplant in their daily food, for 4 weeks, body weight gain was 42.9% (p < 0.05) lower in test group, compared to the control group. Total cholesterol was 42.9% (p < 0.05), LDL-cholesterol 63.8% (p < 0.05) and triglycerides 42.9% (p < 0.95) lower, but HDL-cholesterol was 17.2% (p < 0.05) higher in test group, compared to the control group (Edijala et.al. 2005).

When obese rabbits were given high fat diet together with 10 ml Eggplant juice daily, for 2 weeks, body weight was 24.7% (2.95 kg → 2.22 kg; p < 0.05) lower in test group, compared to the control group. Also LDL-cholesterol, total cholesterol and triglycerides were significantly (p < 0.05) lower in test group, compared to the control group (Jorge et.al. 1998).

Elephant Creeper

(Argyreia Speciosa, Synonyme Argyreia Nervosa)

Elephant Creeper is a vine like plant, which grows in India, Africa, Hawaii and Caribbean islands. The root is used against obesity, diabetes, rheumatism and cough.

Elephant Creeper root has body weight decreasing properties.

When rats were given high fat diet and 500 mg/kg BW of Elephant Creeper root 70% strong ethanol extract daily, for 6 weeks, body weight was 15.6% (p < 0.01) lower in test group, compared to control group. Leptin was 41.5% (p < 0.01) lower in test group, compared to control group. Also triglycerides, LDL-cholesterol and total cholesterol were significantly (p < 0.01 in all parameters) lower, but HDL-cholesterol was significantly (p < 0.01) higher in test group, compared to control group (Kumar et.al. 2011).

English plantain, leaves

(Plantago Lanceolata)

English plantain is also called Narrow leaf plantain. It is a very old medicinal and culinary plant, which has been used especially against respiratory diseases. The leaves and seeds are edible. Its cultivation is very easy.

When mice were fed high fat diet and 10% dried English plantain leaves in their daily diet, for 4 weeks, body weight was 5.8% ($p < 0.05$) and body fat mass was 55.5% ($p < 0.01$) lower in test group, compared to control group (Yoshida et.al. 2012).

Epimedium, leaves

(Epimedium Sp.)

There are many Epimedium species in the World, most growing in China. Typical species are Epimedium Brevicorum, Epimedium Sagittatum etc. The Chinese name is YING YANG HUO. Epimedium is a very old and famous Chinese medicinal plant. It is especially famous for its aphrodisiac effect, which is caused by the active compound, Icariin. Icariin stimulates testosterone synthesis, and gives a stronger penis erection. For that reason it is also called in English by the name: Horny goat weed. It is widely used against osteoporosis, hypertension, asthma and chronic bronchitis.

Epimedium leaves have body weight decreasing properties.

When mice were given Epimedium leaves water extract at a dose of 40 mg/kg BW daily, for 2 weeks, body weight gain in test group was 26.9% lower, compared to control group (Kim et.al. 2001).

European Fan Palm

(Chamaerops Humilis)

Tea made from the leaves of European Fan Palm has been used traditionally in Morocco against diabetes. The tea is also diuretic and anti-inflammatory.

European Fan Palm leaves have body weight decreasing properties.

When obese rats were given 10 mg/kg BW European Fan Palm leaf water extract, for 30 days, body weight in test group was 28.5% ($p < 0.01$) lower, compared to control group. Plasma glucose was 60% ($p < 0.001$), total cholesterol was 78.5% ($p < 0.001$) and triglycerides were 65.7% ($p < 0.001$) lower in test group, compared to control group (Gaamoussi et.al. 2010).

Evodia, fruit

(Evodia Rutaecarpa)

Evodia fruit is a very old Chinese medicinal plant. The main effective compound is Evodiamine.

Evodia fruit and Evodiamine have body weight and body fat mass decreasing properties.

When mice were given high fat diet and 0.03% Evodiamine in their daily food, for 2 months, body weight gain was 60.0% ($p < 0.01$) and body fat mass was 38.0% ($p < 0.01$) lower in test group, compared to control group (Wang et.al. 2008).

The Evodia fruit and Evodiamine body weight and fat mass decreasing properties has been verified in many experiments with animals and fat cells (Bak et.al. 2010; Kobayashi et.al. 2001; Hu et.al. 2010; Kim et.al. 2009).

When 20 volunteers were given Evodiamine 6.75 mg daily, for 8 weeks, body mass index BMI decreased in test group by 1.1 kg/m2, being significantly ($p = 0.020$) higher, than the 0.6 kg/m2 BMI decrease in the 16 person control group (Kim et.al. 2008). This was a double blind experiment.

Extra Virgin Olive Oil

(Olea Europea)

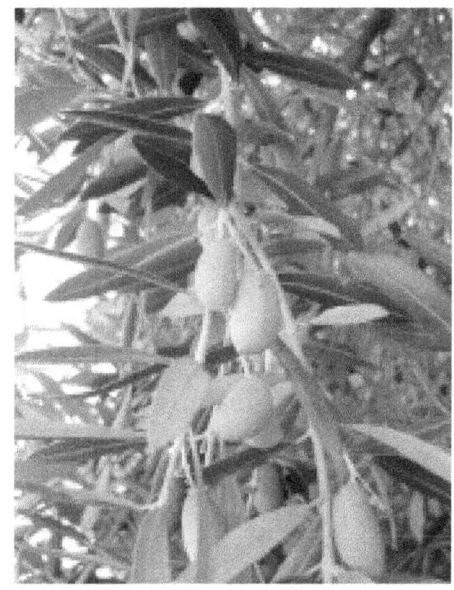

Extra virgin olive oil is cold pressed olive oil, which includes all the healthy polyphenols of olive fruits, especially Oleuropin and Hydroxytyrosol. Olive oil has been used around Mediterranian sea for thousands of years. Olive oil is composed mainly of monounsaturated fatty acids (MUFA), especially Oleic acid.

Extra virgin olive oil has body weight and fat mass decreasing properties.

When 8 obese volunteers were firstly 4 weeks on saturated fat diet (Butter, cream, milk, fat meat: SFA group), and then on monounsaturated olive oil diet (MUFA group) for 4 weeks, body weight decreased by 2.1 kg ($p = 0.0015$) and body fat mass decreased by 2.6 kg ($p = 0.0034$) in the MUFA group, compared to the SFA group (Piers et.al. 2003).

Also in other experiments, with totally 900 persons, it has been noticed, that olive oil decreases body weight (Razquin et.al. 2009; Soriguer et.al. 2009).

When examining fat oxidation difference between olive oil and saturated fat from cream, it has been verified in 2 different experiments, that olive oil significantly increases fat oxidation, compared to saturated fats (Soares et.al. 2004; Piers et.al. 2002).

The most important phenolic compound in extra virgin olive oil, Oleuropin, decreases significantly body weight, body fat mass and stimulates both oxygen consumption and fat oxidation in experiment with rats (Oi-Kano et.al. 2008; Ebaid et.al. 2010).

Also Hydroxytyrosol, which is also an important compound in extra virgin olive oil, increases oxygen consumption and fat oxidation (Hao et.al. 2010).

False Turmeric, root

(Curcuma Comosa)

False Curcuma is a close relative of the common Turmeric, Curcuma Longa. False Curcuma is cultivated especially in Thailand. The root is strongly estrogenic and anti-inflammatory, and it is generally used in different female problems, menopause and vaginal disorders.

False Curcuma root has body weight and body fat mass decreasing properties.

When obese OVX rats were given False Curcuma root hexane extract 250 mg/kg BW, 3 times weekly, for 12 weeks, body weight was 28% ($p < 0.05$) and body fat mass was 27% ($p < 0.05$) lower in test group, compared to control group. Also total cholesterol and LDL-cholesterol were significantly lower in test group (Prasannarong et.al. 2012).

The triglycerides, total cholesterol and LDL-cholesterol decreasing but HDL-cholesterol increasing properties of False Curucma has been verified in many animal experiments (Piyachaturawat et.al. 1997; Piyachaturawat et.al. 1999).

Fennel

(Foeniculum Vulgare)

Fennel is a very common vegetable and spice. All parts of Fennel can be eaten: Bulbs, leaves, stalks, seeds. Fennel is known to decrease blood pressure and cholesterol.

Fennel has body weight and body fat decreasing properties.

When mice were given 1% Fennel in their daily diet, for 90 days, weight gain was 8.4% ($p < 0.05$) lower in test group, compared to the control group (Longquan 2007). This amount corresponds to about 5 grams daily use by humans.

When obese mice were given high fat diet and 300 mg/kg BW Fennel seed methanol extract, for 42 days, body weight was 15.1% ($p < 0.05$) lower in the test group, compared to the control group. Fat mass was 53.7% ($p < 0.05$) lower in test group, compared to the control group (Garg et.al. 2011).

The body weight, triglycerides, LDL-cholesterol and total cholesterol decreasing, but HDL-cholesterol increasing properties of Fennel has been verified in many other experiments with rats and mice (Helal et.al. 2011; Al-Doghachi et.al. 2012; Oulmouden et.al. 2011). In these experiments, Fennel bulb, Fennel herb and Fennel seed oil were used.

Fenugreek

(Trigonella Foenum-Graecum)

Fenugreek seeds and sprouts are used as a food and medicine all around the World. They are known to decrease blood sugar, blood pressure and cholesterol.

Fenugreek has body weight and body fat mass decreasing properties.

When 10 type 2 diabetes patients were given 100 grams of Fenugreek seeds daily, for 2 years, body weight decreased by 2.12 kg in test group, compared to control group. Also triglycerides decreased by 15.1% ($p = 0.025$), total cholesterol decreased by 7.2% ($p = 0.05$) and LDL-cholesterol decreased by 10.6% ($p = 0.05$), but HDL-cholesterol increased by 18.1% ($p = 0.025$), compared to control group (Mitra et.al. 2006).

Fenugreek decreases significantly hunger, fat use and body fat mass in human volunteers (Mathern et.al. 2009; Poole et.al. 2010; Chevassus et.al. 2009).

The Fenugreek body weight and fat mass decreasing property has been verified in great number of experiments with mice and rats (Jette et.al. 2009; Hussein et.al. 2011; Geetha et.al. 2011; Muraki et.al. 2012; Handa et.al. 2005; Parhizkar et.al. 2011; Uemura et.al. 2010; Hamza et.al. 2012; Vijayakumar et.al. 2010; Ramadan et.al. 2011; Muraki et.al. 2011; Ikeuchi et.al. 2006).

Fermented Napa cabbage, Kimchi

(Brassica Rapa var. Pekinensis)

Kimchi is fermented Napa cabbage, and it has been used in Korea as a food for hundreds of years. It is very easy to make Kimchi. The healthy properties of Kimchi have been studied in many scientific articles in Korea.

Kimchi has body weight and fat mass decreasing properties.

When rats were given high fat diet and 10% Kimchi daily, for 8 weeks, body weight decreased by 7.2% ($p < 0.05$) and body fat mass decreased by 21.3% ($p < 0.05$) in test group, compared to control group. Also plasma triglycerides and LDL-cholesterol decreased significantly in test group (Kong et.al. 2007).

The body weight, fat mass, triglycerides and LDL-cholesterol decreasing properties of Kimchi has been verified in many experiments with rats and mice (Kwon et.al. 2004; Park et.al. 2012; Yu et.al. 2005; Sheo et.al. 2004).

When 24 volunteers were given 300 grams Kimchi daily, for 4 weeks, body weight decreased by 1.5 kg (73.0 kg → 71.5 kg; $p < 0.05$) in test group, compared to control group. Also total cholesterol decreased by 5.8% ($p < 0.05$), triglycerides decresed by 39.8% ($p < 0.05$), Leptin decreased by

22.2% (p < 0.05), systolic blood pressure decreased by 4.8 mmHg (126.1 mmHg → 121.3 mmHg; p < 0.05) and diastolic blood pressure decreased by 4.2 mmHg (76.9 mmHg → 72.7 mmHg; p < 0.05) in test group, compared to control group (Kim et.al. 2011).

The total cholesterol, LDL-cholesterol and triglycerides decreasing but HDL-cholesterol increasing properties of Kimchi has been verified in other human experiments too (Kim et.al. 2012; Choi et.al. 2001).

Ferulic acid

Ferulic acid is a natural organic compound, which exists in citrus fruit, banana, bamboo shoots, eggplant, cabbage, broccoli, rice bran, apple seed, oat bran, and barley bran. It is a strong antioxidant and increases swimming endurance in animal experiments.

Ferulic acid has body weight decreasing properties.

When mice were fed high fat diet and 0.5% Ferulic acid in their daily diet, for 7 weeks, body weight in test group was 16.2% (p < 0.05) lower, compared to control group. Triglycerides were 24.3% (p < 0.05), total cholesterol was 20.4% (p < 0.05) and FAS enzyme activity was 24.6% (p < 0.05) lower, but HDL-cholesterol was 20.0% (p < 0.05) higher in test group, compared to control group (Son et.al. 2010).

The body weight decreasing property of Ferulic acid has been verified also in experiments with rats (Srinivasan et.al. 1987).

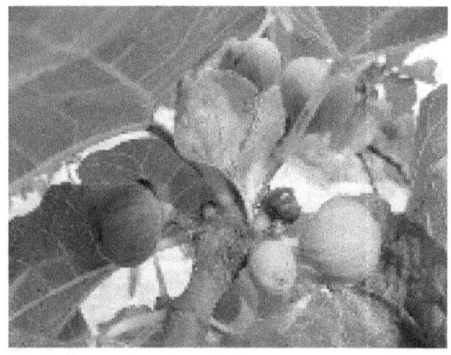

Fig, fruit

(Ficus Carica)

Figs are delicious fruits, which are especially grown around the Mediterranian countries. Figs are very healthy fruits. Dried figs contain up to 12% dietary fiber, and fresh figs have 1100 mg/100g polyphenols, which is much more than in any other fruit, berry or vegetable.

Fig fruit has body weight decreasing properties.

When rats were given normal food and 1% dried fig powder daily, for 4 weeks, body weight in test group was 8% (p < 0.05) lower, compared to control group (Lee et.al. 2012).

In experiments with diabetic rats, figs decrease significantly triglycerides, total cholesterol, LDL-cholesterol and VLDL-cholesterol, but increase significantly HDL-cholesterol in test group, compared to control group (El-Shobaki et.al. 2010).

Fish meat and fish protein

Fish contains large amounts of high quality protein and healthy Omega-3 fatty acids. It is known, that Omega-3 fatty acids increase fat oxidation, decrease body weight, decrease body fat mass and decrease serum triglycerides. But fish protein also lowers body weight and body fat.

Fish meat and fish meat protein has body weight and fat mass decreasing properties.

Low-fat fish like Cod have a very low energy content, approximately 80 kcal/100 grams. This is about 20% lower, than Chicken or Turkey meat or low-fat beef.

When 80 volunteers were given 3 times per week low-fat Cod 150 grams portion, for 4 weeks, body weight decreased about 1 kg more in the Cod group, compared to the 80 person control group, which got equal amount of Sunflower oil (Thorsdottir et.al. 2007).

When 17 obese volunteers were given by average 4.5 grams Cod protein daily, for 8 weeks, body fat-% decreased from 40.5% to 39.4% being significantly ($p < 0.05$) lower, than in the control group, which was given placebo (Vikoren et.al. 2012).

When rats were given either Casein or fish protein from Salmon daily for 28 days, both body weight ($p < 0.01$) and body fat mass ($p < 0.05$) decreased significantly more in the Salmon protein group, compared to the Casein protein group (Pilon et.al. 2011).

Fish oil

Fish contains large amounts of polyunsaturated Omega-3 or W-3 fatty acids, especially EPA (Eicosapentaenoic acid) and DHA (Docosahexaenoic acid). These fatty acids decrease blood pressure and they strongly reduce plasma triglyceride content. Fish oil stimulates the fatty acid beta-oxidation.

Fish oil has body weight and body fat mass decreasing properties.

When 68 young, obese volunteers were given W-3 fish oil 4.1 grams daily, for 4 wees, body weight decreased by 5 kg during this time, being 1 kg more, than in the control group, which did not get the W-3 fish oil (Thorsdottir et.al. 2007). Body fat mass decreased by 0.7 kg more in the experimental group, compared to the control group.

When 6 volunteers were given W-3 fish oil 6 grams daily, for 3 weeks, the body fat mass decreased by 0.54 kg ($p < 0.05$) compared to the control group. The basal fat oxidation increased by 21.8% ($p < 0.05$), compared to the control group. The RER-value decreased from 0.834 to 0.815 ($p < 0.05$), which means a higher fat oxidation in the fish oil group (Couet et.al. 1997).

When 22 volunteers were given 4 grams fish oil daily, for 6 weeks, the body fat mass decreased by 0.7 kg ($p = 0.03$), compared to the control group, which was given 4 grams Safflower oil daily (Noreen et.al. 2011). This was a double blind experiment.

The body fat mass decreasing properties of fish oil has been verified also in other experiments with humans (Hill et.al. 2007; Kabir et.al. 2007).

In experiments with mice and rats, fish oil decreases significantly both body weight and body fat mass (Nakatani et.al. 2003; Hassanali et.al. 2010).

Fish oil should be used 3 – 6 grams daily for effectively to reduce body fat mass.

Flaxseed

(Linum Usitatissimum)

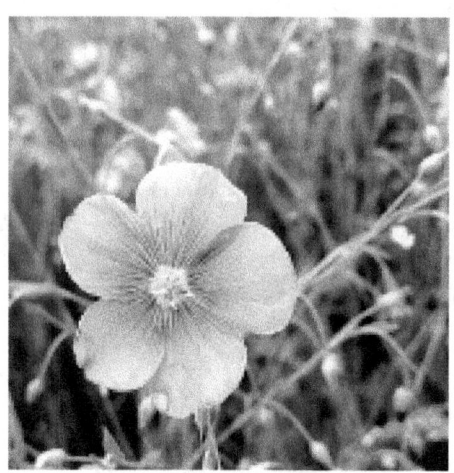

Flaxseed is a very popular, healthy seed. It is known to decrease cholesterol and blood pressure. Flaxseed oil contains up to 60% alpha-Linolenic acid, and Flaxseed has very high content of Lignans, especially SDG.

When 13 type 2 diabetic volunteers were given 32 grams Flaxseed daily, for 12 weeks, body weight in test group was 4% ($p < 0.05$) lower, compared to the control group (Taylor et.al. 2010).

In another, double blind experiment with 179 human volunteers, Flaxseed also decreased body weight significantly ($p = 0.016$), compared to the control group (Dodin et.al. 2008).

In an experiment with 283 human volunteers, Flaxseed also decreased body fat significantly (Wu et.al. 2010).

When rats were given in their diet 25% Flaxseed daily, for 160 days, body weight in test group was 27.0% ($p < 0.05$) lower, compared to the control group. Also LDL-cholesterol decreased by 22%, triglycerides decreased by 23% but HDL-cholesterol increased by 47% in test group, compared to the control group (Daleprane et.al. 2010).

The body weight and body fat mass decreasing properties of Flaxseed has been verified in many experiments with rats and mice (Tominaga et.al. 2012; Fukumitsu et.al. 2008; Park et.al. 2012; Brant et.al. 2012; Cardozo et.al. 2010).

Foetid Cassia, seed

(Cassia Tora)

Foetid Cassia is a small, annual plant. Its leaves are eaten as vegetable in Asia, and its roasted seeds are used for healthy tea, which is used against several diseases. The seed is known to lover cholesterol and blood pressure, and it is diuretic and hepatoprotective. The seed is a very important medicine in Chinese pharmacopeia.

Foetid Cassia seeds have body weight decreasing properties.

When obese rats were given high fat diet and 300 mg/kg BW Foetid Cassia seed ethanol extract daily, for 8 weeks, body weight was 11.3% ($p < 0.05$) lower in test group, compared to control group. Also total cholesterol was 35.9% ($p < 0.01$), LDL-cholesterol was 52.5% ($p < 0.01$) and triglycerides were 30.1% ($p < 0.01$) lower, but HDL-cholesterol was 42.7% ($p < 0.01$) higher in test group, compared to control group (Tzeng et.al. 2013).

The body weight decreasing properties of Foetid Cassia seed has been verified in many other animal experiments (Junbao et.al. 2004; Tzeng et.al. 2013; Nam et.al. 2008).

Food energy density

By definition, food energy density is the calorific content of 100 grams foodstuff. The unit is thus kcal/gram. The energy density of fat is 9 kcal/g, alcohol 7 kcal/g, protein 4 kcal/g, carbohydrates 4 kcal/g, dietary fiber 1.5 – 2.5 kcal/g and water 0 kcal/g. The energy density greatly affects body weight: The less is the energy density, the less is the intake of calories and fat, and the less is the body weight and body fat mass, when the volume of food in meals is kept constant. The simplest way to reduce energy content in meals is to increase the amount of fruits, vegetables, soups, protein, complex carbohydrates, dietary fiber and water intake. The amount of energy in meals can be reduced significantly, without hunger feeling and without reducing the volume of the meal.

When 54 volunteers were given in laboratory conditions, in randomized way, 8 lunch during 2 weeks, of which 4 contained meat, but in 4 the meat was replaced by mushrooms, the energy intake from meat lunch was 730 kcal, but only 310 kcal in mushroom lunch, although satiety, appetite, satiation and palatability were the same. This means, the volunteers got 57.5% ($p < 0.0001$) less energy from mushroom lunch, compared to meat lunch. The average energy intake during 24 hours in mushroom lunch group was 18.5% (1639.5 kcal versus 2013.5 kcal; $p < 0.0001$) lower, compared to meat lunch group. Also the 24 hours fat intake was 28.2 grams or 31.7% ($p < 0.0001$) lower in mushroom group, compared to meat group (Cheskin et.al. 2008).

When 85 volunteers were given normal food and also 127 grams of either water, Grapefruit juice or Grapefruit before breakfast, lunch and dinner, for 12 weeks, body weight decreased by average of 7.1%, BMI decreased by average of 1.86 kg/m2, fat mass decreased by average of 2.7 kg, body fat-% decreased by average of 1.1% and waist circumference decreased by average of 5.0 cm, compared to original values, althought the weight of food in grams did not change, only the energy density decreased by 20 – 29% (Silver et.al. 2011).

The same kind of results has been achieved also in other experiments with human volunteers (Ello-Martin et.al. 2007).

Frequency of eating

Eating frequency affects directly to the feeling of hunger and energy intake, and thus to body weight and body fat mass.

Large eating frequency has body weight and body fat mass decreasing properties.

When obese (BMI = 40.02) volunteers were given 980 kcal breakfast either as a single meal, or divided to 5 smaller meals, given every 1 hour, energy intake at lunch was 27% ($p < 0.05$) smaller in the multiple feeding group, compared to the single meal group. The amount of breakfast was 33% of the daily calorie intake (Speechly et.al. 1999).

Exactly the same kind of results has been achieved in experiments with lean (BMI = 23.11) volunteers (Speechly et.al. 1999).

So when trying to decrease body weight, it is important to divide the daily amount of food to 5 – 6 small portions, and eat them evenly, from morning to evening.

Fucoxanthin

Fucoxanthin is a carotenoid, which exist in all seaweeds, like Wakame (Undaria Pinnatifida), and also in Chlorella, Spirulina and Wheat grass.

Fucoxanthin has body weight and body fat mass decreasing properties.

When 151 volunteer were given 2.4 mg Fucoxanthin daily, for 16 weeks, body weight decreased in test group by an average of 5.2 kg ($p < 0.05$) and body fat mass decreased by an average of 3.55 kg ($p < 0.05$), compared to the control group. Also triglycerids decreased significantly ($p < 0.05$) in the test group (Abidov et.al. 2010). This was a double blind experiment.

The body weight and body fat mass decreasing properites of Fucoxanthin has been verified in a very large number of experiments with rats and mice (Okada et.al. 2011; Kang et.al. 2012; Woo et.al. 2009; Jeon et.al. 2010; Lasi et.al. 2012; Maeda et.al. 2007; Hu et.al. 2012; Maeda et.al. 2007; Maeda et.al. 2009; Woo et.al. 2010; Park et.al. 2011; Maeda et.al. 2005)

GABA

(Gamma-Aminobutyric Acid)

GABA is a very common neurotransmitter. It is made in cells from Glutamate amino acid and B6 vitamin. GABA exists also in food, germinated rice and germinated beans are excellent GABA sources. GABA decreases blood pressure and improves sleep.

GABA has body weight and body fat mass decreasing properties.

When obese mice were given high fat diet and either water or 2 mg/ml GABA daily, for 20 weeks, body weight decreased by 16.6% (p < 0.05) and body fat mass decreased by 20.8% (p < 0.05) in GABA group, compared to the water control group (Tian et.al. 2011).

Also in other experiments with mice GABA decreases body weight, body fat mass, triglycerides and LDL-cholesterol, but increases HDL-cholesterol and Adiponectin (Soh et.al. 2004; Tews et.al. 1981; Ohara et.al. 2011).

When 7 volunteers were given the GABA agonist Baclofen 30 mg daily, for 12 weeks, body weight decreased by 1.6 kg (93.3 kg → 91.7 kg; p < 0.05) and waist circumference decreased by 2.3 cm (107.9 cm → 105.6 cm). Also Leptin decreased by 19.2% (p < 0.05) (Arima et.al. 2010).

Galangal root

(Alpinia Galangal)

Galangal root is very popular food, spice and medicinal plant in Asia. It is known to decrease triglycerides and cholesterol.

Galangal root has body weight and fat mass decreasing properties.

When obese rats were given Galangal root ethanol extract 400 mg/kg BW in their daily diet, for 6 weeks, body weight decreased by 11.58% (p < 0.05) and body fat mass decreased by 41.26% (p < 0.05) in the test group, compared to the control group. Also triglycerides, LDL-cholesterol and total cholesterol decreased significantly (p < 0.01 in all variables) in the test group, but HDL-cholesterol increased significantly (p < 0.01) in the test group, compared to the control group (Kumar et.al. 2010).

Gamma-Linolenic acid, GLA

GLA is an essential polyunsaturated fatty acid in human body. It is made from the Linolenic acid in food. GLA is also abundant in many vegetable oils, such as Evening Primrose seed oil, Black Currant seed oil and Borage, Borago Officinal seed oil. GLA can be purchased from markets in capsule form. GLA has blood pressure and cholesterol decreasing properties.

GLA has body weight and fat mass decreasing properties.

When formerly obese volunteers were given either 890 mg GLA daily (Corresponding 5 grams Borago Officinalis seed oil), or 5 grams Olive oil (Placebo group) daily, for 12 months, body weight increased in GLA group by 2.17 kg, but 8.79 kg in the placebo group. GLA significantly (p < 0.03) decresed the body weight gain compared to the placebo group (Schirmer et.al. 2007). The number of volunteers was 24.

When rats were given in their daily food either 1.5% or 4.0% of GLA rich oil, for 4 weeks, the weight gain in GLA group was significantly by 8.8% ($p < 0.05$) and by 11.2% ($p < 0.05$) lower, compared to the control group, which got Soya oil (Takada et.al. 1994). Also fat mass decreased ($p < 0.05$) significantly, compared to the control group. The GLA content of the used oil was 25.3 grams GLA/100 grams oil. GLA also significantly increased the fatty acid beta-oxidation.

In many experiments with rats, the body weight and fat mass decreasing properties of GLA has been verified (Liu et.al. 2004; Thurmond et.al. 1993; Phinney et.al. 1993; Takahashi et.al. 2000).

Garden cress, seed

(Lepidium Sativum)

Garden cress is a delicious vegetable and salad plant. Also its seeds can be used as spice, and they have many medicinal uses against asthma, hypertension, high cholesterol and water retention.

Garden cress seeds have body weight decreasing properties.

When normal and diabetic rats were given daily 20 mg/kg BW Garden cress seed water extract, for 15 days, body weight in both groups were significantly ($p < 0.05$) lower, compared to control groups. Also blood glucose were significantly ($p < 0.05$) lower in both groups, compared to control groups (Eddouks et.al. 2005).

When hypercholesterolemic rats were on a high fat diet, and were given Garden cress seeds either 5% or 10% of their daily food, for 8 weeks, body weight ($p < 0.05$), total cholesterol ($p < 0.05$), LDL-cholesterol ($p < 0.01$) and triglycerides ($p < 0.05$) were significantly lower, but HDL-cholesterol ($p < 0.05$) was significantly higher in test group, compared to control group (Al Hamedan 2010).

Garden pea

(Pisum Sativum)

Garden pea is a very popular vegetable, which is eaten both raw and cooked. It contains only 63 kcal/100 g energy and 5.1 grams/100 grams protein.

Garden pea has body weight decreasing properties.

Garden pea ihibits Lipase (Slanc et.al. 2009), but stimulates Adinopectin (Okada et.al. 2010).

In experiments with rats, garden pea proteins decrease total cholesterol and triglycerides and inhibits FAS enzyme (Rigamonti et.al. 2010).

Also in experiments with pigs, garden pea decreases both total cholesterol and LDL-cholesterol (Martins et.al. 2004).

In experiments with hamsters, garden pea increases significantly ($p = 0.036$) oxygen consumption

(Marinangeli et.al. 2011).

In experiments with obese volunteers, garden pea decreases Insulin (Marinangeli et.al. 2011), carbohydrate oxidation (Marinangeli et.al. 2011) and food intake (Geraedts et.al. 2011).

When rats were given either 20% garden pea protein or 20% casein in their daily diet, for 16 days, body weight gain was 4.7% ($p < 0.05$) lower in test group, compared to control group (Spielmann et.al. 2008).

The body weight, triglycerides and Insulin decreasing properties of garden pea has been verified also in another experiment with rats (Martinez et.al. 1995).

Garlic

(Allium Sativum)

Garlic is one of the most famous food and medicinal plant in the World. It has been used as a food and medicine for at least over 5000 years. Garlic is known to lower blood pressure, cholesterol and triglycerides. Aged Garlic extract (=AGE) is made easily, by slicing Garlic for several months in concentrated alcohol.

Garlic has body weight and fat mass decreasing properties.

When 8 volunteers were given AGE 80 mg daily, 5 times weekly, for 12 weeks, body weight decreased by 3.0 kg (58.3 kg → 55.3 kg; $p < 0.001$) and fat-% decreased by 1.9% (29.4% → 27.5%; $p < 0.001$), which were significantly more, than the body weight and fat-% decrease in the 6 person control group (1.9 kg; 61.7 kg → 59.7 kg for body weight and 33.9% → 32.4%; $p < 0.05$ for body fat-%). Also in the test group triglycerides decreased by 18.3% and heart rate decreased by 8.3 beats/minute (69.1 beats/minute → 60.8 beats/minute) (Seo et.al. 2012).

In great many experiments with mice, rats, rabbits and Guinea pigs, the body weight and body fat mass decreasing properties of Garlic in test groups, compared to the control groups, has been verified (Cho et.al. 2003; Yoon et.al. 2005; Jung et.al. 2011; Elkayam et.al. 2003; Kang et.al. 2010; Pourkabir et.al. 2010; Iweala et.al. 2005; Kim et.al. 2011; Kim et.al. 2011; Kawada et.al. 1999).

Garlic Vine

(Pachyptera Hymenaea, Synonym: Mansoa Alliaceae)

Garlic Vine originates from South-America. The leaves smell strongly exactly like Garlic. Both leaves and flowers are edible, and they are used as spice, instead of Garlic. Garlic vine is also used medicinally against rheumatism, flu, fever, influenza etc.

Garlic Vine has body weight decreasing properties.

When rats were given high fat diet and 400 mg/kg BW Garlic Vine water extract daily, for 4 weeks, body weight in test group was 18.0% (p < 0.001) lower, compared to control group. Also total cholesterol was 66.1% (p < 0.001). LDL-cholesterol was 60.0% (p < 0.001) and triglycerides were 57.6% (p < 0.001) lower in test group, compared to control group (Verma et.al. 2012).

Genistein and Daidzein

Genistein and Daidzein are isoflavonoids, which exist in many plants, such as red clover and especially in different soy products. Full fat soy flour contains 96 mg/100g, fat free soy flour contains 71 mg/100g, soy beans contain 73 mg/100g and soy protein isolate, extracted with water, contains 55 mg/100g Genistein.

Genistein and Daidzein have body weight and body fat mass decreasing properties.

When rats were given high fat diet and 0.2% (=2000 ppm) Genistein in their daily food, for 12 weeks, body weight was 35.7% (p < 0.05) and body fat mass was 75.0% (p < 0.05) lower in test group, compared to control group. Also triglycerides, total cholesterol and Leptin were significantly lower in test group, compared to control group (Seong et.al. 2007).

The body weight and body fat mass decreasing properties of Genistein has been verified in great many animal experiment (Park et.al. 2006; Yang et.al. 2006; Kim et.al. 2006; Naaz et.al. 2003; Kim et.al. 2006; Kim et.al. 2010).

When 25 volunteers were given 70 mg isoflavonoids daily, for 1 year period, body weight decreased by 3 kg (p = 0.07) and body fat-% decreased by 1.8% (p = 0.053) more in test group, compared to control group (Aubertin-Leheudre et.al. 2007). This was a double blind experiment.

When 30 volunteers were given 40 mg isoflavonoids and 300 mg L-Carnitine daily, for 12 weeks, body weight decreased by 1.2 kg (p < 0.001) and fat-% decreased by 0.9% (p < 0.05) more in test group, compared to 30 person control group (Gwak et.al. 2007).

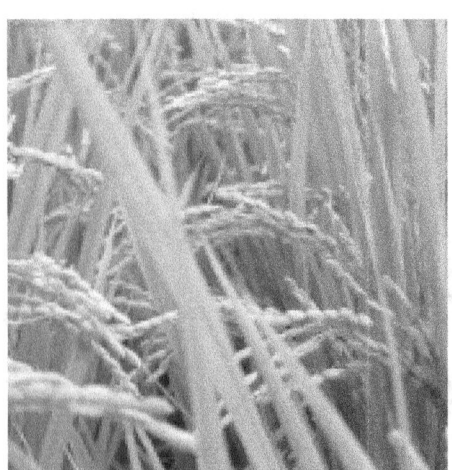

Germinated Brown Rice

(Oryza Sativa)

Rice grain is one of the most often used food item. Germinated brown rice contains large amounts of healthy compounds, such as GABA and gamma-Oryzanol, compared to non-germinated brown rice. GABA decreases blood pressure and gamma-Oryanol decreases cholesterol and triglycerides.

Germinated brown rice has body weight and fat mass decreasing properties.

When mice were given in their daily food 0.15% methanol extract of germinated brown rice, for 7 weeks, body weight was 17.8% (p < 0.05) lower, compared to the control group. Also body fat mass (p < 0.05), total cholesterol (p < 0.05) and triglycerides (p < 0.05) were significantly lower, than in the control group (Ho et.al. 2012).

When rats were given in their daily food either control diet, 50% of brown rice or 50% of germinated brown rice, for 6 weeks, body weight gain was 10.5% (p < 0.05) lower in the germinated rice group, compared to conrtol group or brown rice group. Also systolic blood pressure (p < 0.05) and triglycerides (p < 0.05) were significantly lower in the germinated rice group than in the control group (Choi et.al. 2006).

Also in a third experiment with mice germinated brown rice decreased significantly fat mass (p < 0.05), triglycerides (p < 0.05) and total cholesterol (p < 0.05), compared to the control group (Oh et.al. 2005).

Giant potato

(Ipomoea Digitata)

Giant potato is a close relative to our familiar edible root, Sweet potato, Ipomoea Batatas. Giant potato tubers are edible, and they are used in India to lower high blood pressure.

Giant potato tubers have body weight decreasing properties.

When rats were given high fat diet and methanol extract of Giant potato tubers at a dose of 300 mg/kg BW daily, for 9 weeks, body weight was 22.7% (p < 0.001) lower in test group, compared to control group. Also triglycerides, total cholesterol, LDL-cholesterol and VLDL-cholesterol were significantly (p < 0.05 in all parameters) lower, but HDL-cholesterol was significantly higher in test group, compared to control group (Muthu et.al. 2011).

When 30 hypertensive patients were given dried Giant potato tuber 3 grams daily, for 12 weeks, systolic blood pressure decreased by 38.8 mmHg (157.60 mmHg → 118.8 mmHg; p < 0.001), diastolic blood pressure decreased by 19.2 mmHg (95.2 mmHg → 76.0 mmHg; p < 0.01), total cholesterol decreased by 26.1% (p < 0.05), triglycerides decreased by 16.0% (p < 0.05), LDL-cholesterol decreased by 32.5% (p < 0.05) and VLD-cholesterol decreased by 16.0% (p < 0.05) in test group, but in the 20 person control group there were no significant changes in any parameter (Vartika et.al. 2011).

Gilo

(Solanum Gilo, Synonyme Solanum Aethiopicum)

Gilo is also called Scarlet Eggplant. It is a close relative to the common Aubergine, Solanum Melongena. Gilo is cultivated for its edible green fruits all over the World. It originates from Africa.

Gilo has body weight decreasing properties.

When rabbits were given high fat diet and 10% Gilo fruit in their daily diet, for 6 weeks, nody weight gain in test group was 47.6% (p < 0.05) lower, compared to control group. Also triglycerides, total cholesterol and LDL-cholesterol decreased significantly (p < 0.05 in all parameters) in test group, compared to control group (Odetola et.al. 2004).

Ginger

(Zingiber Officinalis)

Ginger is an ancient food, spice and medicinal plant, which is known all over the World. Ginger lowers cholesterol and triglycerides. It is also used in different inflammatory ailments.

Ginger has body weight and fat mass decreasing properties.

When obese mice were given daily 250 mg/kg either Ginger methanol extract or ethylacetate extract, for 8 weeks, body weight decreased significantly (p < 0.05) compared to the control group. Body weight in control group was 41.6 grams, in methanol extract group 32.5 grams and in ethylacetate extract group 35.8 grams (Goyal et.al. 2006). Methnaol extract group had 21.8% lower body weight than the control group.

When rats, which were fed high fat diet, were given either 250 mg/kg, 500 mg/kg or 1000 mg/kg Ginger daily, for 8 weeks, there was a dose dependent decrease in body weight, compared to the control group. Body weight was 9.3% (p < 0.05) in the 250 mg/kg group, 13.6% (p < 0.05) in the 500 mg/kg group and 15.8% (p < 0.05) in the 1000 mg/kg group lower, than in the control group. Also body fat mass had a dose dependent significant (p < 0.05) decrease, compared to the control group (Malik et.al. 2011).

The body weight and fat mass decreasing properties of Ginger has been verified also in other experiments with mice and rats (Nammi et.al. 2009; Han et.al. 2005; Pulbutr et.al. 2011).

Ginkgo leaf

(Ginkgo Biloba)

Ginkgo is extremely famous medicinal plant, which is widely researched all around the World. It is a strong antioxidant, improves memory, improves blood circulation, inhibits asthma, lowers blood pressure and decreases high cholesterol.

Ginkgo leaf has body weight decreasing properties.

When rats were given cholesterol 500 mg/kg BW daily, and either 10 mg/kg BW, 25 mg/kg BW or 50 mg/kg BW Ginkgo leaf water extract, for 90 days, body weight in test groups were 3.1%, 3.5% and 7.1% lower, compared to control group. Also triglycerides, LDL-cholesterol and total cholesterol were significantly lower in test groups, compared to control group (Gupta et.al. 2006).

The body weight, triglycerides and total cholesterol decreasing properties of Ginkgo has been verified also in experiments with mice (Cong et.al. 2011).

Ginkgo leaf inhibits strongly FAS enzyme (Tian et.al. 2004) and Lipase enzyme (Bustanji et.al. 2011).

Ginseng

(Panax Ginseng; Panax Japonicus; Panax Quinquefolium)

Ginseng is possibly the most researched medicinal and food plant in the whole World. Normally the Ginseng root is used, but also the Ginseng leaves and berries contain the functionally effective Ginsenoids and Saponins. Ginseng increases resistance against stress and bacterial infections. It also increases aerobic endurance by stimulating the fatty acid beta-oxidation.

Ginseng has body weight and body fat mass reducing properties.

There exist large amounts of research papers concerning the antiobesity effect of Ginseng.

When 36 non-insulin dependent NIDDM patients were given Ginseng root 200 mg daily, for 8 weeks, body weight decreased by 1.5 kg ($p < 0.05$), compared to the control group (Sotaniemi et.al. 1995).

When obese volunteers were given Ginseng daily, for 12 weeks, body weight ($p < 0.01$), body fat mass ($p < 0.01$) and fat-% ($p < 0.01$) decreased significantly, compared to the control group (Kim et.al. 2002; Kim et.al. 2002).

The body weight and body fat mass decreasing properties of Ginseng has been verified in a large number of experiments with rats and mice (Lee et.al. 2010; Yun et.al. 2004; Song et.al. 2012; Xiong et.al. 2010; Liu et.al. 2008; Han et.al. 2005; Park et.al. 2011; Yuan et.al. 2010; Kim et.al. 2011).

Glasswort

(Salicornia Herbacea)

There exist many different species of Glasswort in the World. They grow along the seaside. Glassworts are eaten as vegetable in many parts of the World. In Korea the local Glasswort species, Salicornia Herbacea, is regarded as a healthy functional vegetable.

Glasswort has body weigt and fat mass decreasing properties.

When rats were given high fat diet and 5% Glasswort in their daily diet, for 4 weeks, body weight was 9% ($p < 0.05$) and body fat mass was 28% ($p < 0.05$) lower in test group, compared to cotrol group. Triglycerides were 28.2% ($p < 0.05$) and LDL-cholesterol was 41.9% ($p < 0.05$) lower, but HDL-cholesterol was 51.8% ($p < 0.05$) higher in test group, compared to control group (Seo et.a. 2012).

The body weight and cholesterol decreasing properties of Glasswort has been verified also in another experiment with mice (Park et.al. 2006).

Glutamine

Glutamine is a natural amino acid, which exists in ordinary food and muscle cells. Glutamine has an important role as an immunostimulant. Glutamine also increases GH (Growth Hormone) levels in plasma.

Glutamine has body weight decreasing properties.

When 6 obese female (BMI = 32.4) were given Glutamine 0.3 grams/kg bodyweight daily, for 4 weeks, body weight decreased by 2.8 kg or 3.4% (85.0 kg → 82.2 kg; $p < 0.01$), compared to the control group, which got protein. Also waist circumference decreased by 3.8 cm (102.7 cm → 98.9 cm; $p = 0.01$), compared to the control group (Lacaria et.al. 2011).

When mice were given daily dose of Glutamine, which was 2.87% of daily energy consumpton, for 16 weeks, body weight decreased by 28.5% (37.9 kg → 27.4 kg; $p < 0.05$), compared to the control group (Opara et.al. 1996).

In humans Glutamine increases postprandial energy expenditure and fat oxidation. When young, healthy volunteers were given 1.05 grams/1 kg body weight Glutamine in their meal, the energy expenditure after meal increased by 49% ($p < 0.05$), compared to the control group, which got an isocaloric mixture of Glycine, Alanine and Serine amino acids. Glutamine increased fat oxidation after meal by 42 kcal ($p < 0.05$), compared to the control group (Iwashita et.al. 2006).

When rats were given in their daily water and food 4% Glutamine, for 2 months, body weight ($p < 0.05$) and body fat% ($p < 0.5$) and RER (Respiratory Exchange Ratio) ($p < 0.05$) decreased significantly, but oxygen consumption ($p < 0.05$) increased significantly, compared to the control group (Prada et.al. 2007).

Glycemic Index GI

Glycemic Index GI is a measure, how quickly blood glucose levels rise after eating a particular type of food. It can be measured for each food item, relative to glucose, which has a GI value of 100. If the food has higher than 70 GI value, it is said to be high GI foodstuff. If the value is between 50 and 70, then it is said to be medium GI foodstuff. If it is lower than 50, it is said to be low GI foodstuff. The GI is affected by various food properties: Acidity, type of carbohydrate, amount of fat and protein, cooking, fiber content, water content etc. The higher the GI value, the faster the rise of blood glucose and the higher the blood Insulin content is, in normal persons.

Low glycemic index food has body weight and body fat mass decreasing properties.

When obese volunteers were on a 2000 kcal daily diet for 24 weeks, but the average GI value of food was either 86 (high GI value) or 53 (low GI value), body weight decreased by 10.0 kg in low GI value (GI = 53) group, which was significantly ($p = 0.047$) higher, than the 6.3 kg weight reduction in the high GI value (GI = 86) group. There were 32 volunteers in this experiment (Pittas et.al. 2005).

The body weight and body fat mass decreasing properties of low GI food has been verified in many human experiments (Fajcsak et.al. 2008; Maki et.al. 2007; Costa et.al. 2012).

Here are some examples of the GI values of different food items.

Foodstuff	GI value
Glucose	100
Fructose	15
Sugar	65
Honey	61
White wheat bread	75
White rice, boiled	73
Brown rice, boiled	68
Barley	28
Sweet corn	52
Spaghetti, white	49
Cornflakes	81
Muesli	57
Apple	36
Orange	43
Banana	51
Pineapple	59
Mango	51
Watermelon	76
Potato, boiled	78
Potato, mashed	87
Potato, French fries	63
Sweet potato, boiled	63
Milk, full fat	39
Milk, skim	37
Soy milk	34
Chickpeas	28
Kidney beans	24
Lentils	32
Soya beans	16

Glycine

Glycine is a natural amino acid, which exist both in food and living cells. It is an essential precursor for the strong antioxidant, Glutathione (GSH) in living cells. Glycine is known to give better sleep quality.

Glycine has body weight and fat mass decreasing properties.

When obese mice were given high fat diet and either water or Glycine (20% strong Glycine in water, 0.45 ml) daily, for 12 days, body weight in test group was 7.7% ($p < 0.01$) lower, compared to control group. Total fat mass was 26.1% ($p < 0.01$) in test group, compared to control group (Jing et.al. 2005).

In experiments with rats, Glycine decreases fat mass, fat cell size and serum triglycerides (Hafidi et.al. 2004).

The body weight decreasing properties of Glycine in experimental animals has been known since 1969 (Takeuchi et.al. 1969).

Glycine strongly decreases total cholesterol in experimental animals (Sugiyama et.al. 1989).

Goji berry

(Lycium Barbarum, Lycium Chinensis)

Goji is the Japanese name for the berry of Lycium Barbarum or Lycium Chinensis. Goji has been used thousands of years in Asia as a functional food and medicine. It contains large amounts of Betaine and Zeaxanthin.

Goji has body weight and waist circumference decreasing properties.

When 15 volunteers were given Goji juice 1.2 dl daily, for 14 days, waist circumference decreased by 5.5 cm ($p < 0.01$), being significantly more and the 0.9 cm decrease in the 14 person control group. Also each bolus of Goji juice increased the resting energy consumption by 10% ($p < 0.05$), within 1 hour of intake (Amagase et.al. 2011). This was a double blind experiment.

In China obesity is treated by giving 30 grams Goji berry with hot water both in the morning and evening (Qingfu et.al. 1993).

When obese rats were given Goji berry polysaccharides 10 mg/kg BW daily, for 3 weeks, body weight decreased in the test group by 6.8% ($p < 0.05$), compared to the control group. Also triglycerides and total cholesterol decreased significantly in the test group, compared to the control group (Zhao et.al. 2005).

The body weight, triglycerides and total cholesterol decreasing properties of Goji berry has been verified in other experiments too (Zhang et.al. 2002; Cui et.al. 2011). Also Lycium leaf extract decreases body weight, triglycerides and total cholesterol in rats (Kang et.al. 2010).

Golden Cane Palm

(Dypsis Lutescens)

Golden Cane Palm is very common in tropical and sub-tropical countries. Its cultivation is very easy.

Golden Cane Palm leaves have body weight and fat mass decreasing properties.

When obese mice were given high fat diet and 3% of Golden Cane Palm leaf methanol extract daily, for 11 weeks, body weight in test group was 18.1% (p < 0.05) lower, compared to control group. Total fat mass was 51.4% (p < 0.01) lower in test group, compared to control group. Also triglycerides were 10.8%, total cholesterol was 27.6% (p < 0.05) and serum glucose was 19.1% (p < 0.05) lower in test group, compared to control group (Koyama et.al. 2012).

Grape seeds

(Vitis Vinifera, Vitis Sp.)

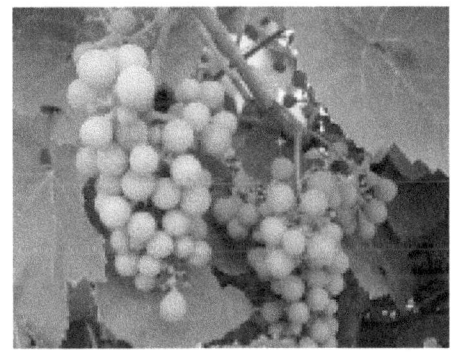

Grape seeds and grape seed water-ethanol extracts contain large amount of polyphenols, so called procyanides, which have many health effects, by decreasing high cholesterol and hypertension etc. These extracts have short name GSE (Grape Seed Extract).

Grape seed and GSE have body weight and body fat mass decreasing properties.

When mice were given high fat diet together with 250 mg/kg BW GSE daily, for 12 weeks, body weight was 20.3% (p < 0.05) and body fat mass was 33.3% (p < 0.05) lower in test group, compared to control group. Also triglycerides were 15.8% (p < 0.05) and total cholesterol was 11.8% (p < 0.05) lower, but HDL-cholesterol was 44.6% (p < 0.05) higher in test group, compared to control group (Park et.al. 2008).

The body weight, body fat mass, Leptin, triglycerides and total cholesterol decreasing but HDL-cholesterol and Adiponectin increasing properties of GSE and grape seeds has been verified in great many animal experiments (Decorde et.al. 2009; Arora et.al. 2011; Montagut et.al. 2010; Suwannaphet et.al. 2010; Charradi et.al. 2011; Terra et.al. 2011; Nakamura et.al. 2002; Caimari et.al. 2012; Ohyama et.al. 2011; Arora et.al. 2011; Moreno et.al. 2003; Baiges et.al. 2010; Choi et.al. 2010).

In human volunteers, GSE decreases up to 4% the daily energy intake (Vogels et.al. 2004).

Green Coffee Extract

(GCE)

The extract from green, raw coffee beans contains large amounts of Chlorogenic acid, which is a very strong antioxidant, and decreases high cholesterol levels and high blood pressure. GCE also contains large amounts of Caffeine.

GCE has body weight reducing effect.

When 16 volunteers were given 1050 mg GCE extract daily, for 6 weeks, body weight decreased by 8.04 kg or 10.5% (76.69 kg → 68.85 kg; $p < 0.0001$), BMI decreased by 2.92 or 10.3% (28.22 → 25.5; $p < 0.0001$) and body fat mass by 4.44 kg (28.13% → 23.69%; $p < 0.0001$), compared to the control group (Vinson et.al. 2012). Also heart rate decreased by 2.56 beats/minute (77.44 → 74.88; $p < 0.005$). This was a double blind experiment.

Both Chlorogenic acid and Caffeine in GCE extract decrease body weight, stimulate fatty acid beta-oxidation and inhibits fatty acid synthase (FAS) in animal experiments (Cho et.al. 2010).

In a meta-analysis of 3 other double blind experiments with human volunteers, the average body weight decrease was 2.47 kg ($p = 0.006$) with GCE extract, compared to the control groups. The daily use of GCE extract was 180 – 200 mg, and the duration of the experiments were between 4 – 12 weeks (Onakpoya et.al. 2011).

Also in animal experiments GCE strongly reduces body weight, compared to control groups (Shimoda et.al. 2006; Tanaka et.al. 2009).

Green tea

(Camellia Sinensis)

Green tea is one of the oldest refreshing drinks in the World. It has been used in China for at least 5000 years. It contains extremely large amounts of healthy polyphenols, called Catechins. The most important Catechins are Epigallocatechin, Catechin and EGCG (=Epigallocatechin-3-O-Gallate). Green tea has many medicinal uses. It decreases high cholesterol and high blood pressure, it is antiviral and it has anti-inflammatory properties.

Green tea has body weight and body fat mass decreasing properties.

When volunteers were given acutely 270 mg EGCG catechin, 24 hours energy expenditure increased by 4% ($p < 0.01$), respiratory quotient RQ decreased from 0.88 to 0.85 ($p < 0.05$), fatty acid oxidation increased by 35% ($p < 0.05$) and urinary Norepinephrine excretion increased by 40% ($p < 0.05$), compared to placebo group (Dulloo et.al. 1999).

When 50 obese volunteers were given green tea extract 300 mg daily, for 90 days, body weight decreased in test group by 9.24 kg ($p < 0.001$), compared to 50 person control group. Waist circumference decreased by 7 cm (p < 0.001) in test group, compared to control group. Also triglycerides decreased by 13% (p < 0.01), total cholesterol decreased by 15% (p < 0.001) and LDL-cholesterol decreased by 11% (p < 0.001), but HDL-cholesterol, increased by 11.4% (p < 0.001) in test group, compared to control group. Also Leptin decreased by 37.6% (p < 0.05), Insulin decreased by 20.0% (p < 0.001) and Cortisol decreased by 10.35% (p < 0.05), but growth hormone GH increased by 301% (p < 0.001) and IGF-1 increased by 9.5% (p < 0.01) in test group, compared to control group. This was a double blind experiment (Pierro et.al. 2009).

The body weight and body fat mass decreasing properties of green tea extract has been verified in many experiments with obese volunteers (Chantre et.al. 2002; He et.al. 2009; Suliburska et.al. 2012; Auvichayapat et.al. 2008; Nagao et.al. 2005; Nagao et.al. 2007; Harada et.al. 2005).

The body weight and body fat mass decreasing properties of green tea has been verified also in great many animal experiments (Han et.al. 1999; Murase et.al. 2006; Shimotoyodome et.al. 2005; Murase et.al. 2006; Sae-Tan et.al. 2011).

Growth hormone GH

(Somatotropin)

GH is a 191 amino acid protein, polypeptide, which is secreted by pituitary gland. GH is absolutely essential to the normal growth and development of human body. Both GH deficiency and GH overproduction (Agromegaly) has several serious side effects. The GH concentration in human plasma decreases dramatically with aging.

In an experiment with 106 adults with GH deficiency, aged 53 years, it was noticed, that in men the body weight was 7.5 kg (p < 0.001) and body fat mass was 6.6 kg (p < 0.001) higher, compared to healthy control group of the same height. In females the body weight was 3.6 kg higher, and body fat mass was 6.0 kg (p < 0.001) higher, compared to control female group of the same height. Females also lost about 2.4 kg (p < 0.001) of extracellular water (Rosen et.al. 1993).

When 32 adults with GH deficiency were given 10 micrograms/kg BW GH daily, for 18 months, body fat-% decreased from 31.9% to 28.3% (p < 0.001) and lean body mass increased from 59.0 kg to 61.5 kg (p < 0.001) (Baum et.al. 1996).

Some natural GH stimulators are:
- Deep sleep
- Hypoglycemia
- Niacin (B vitamin)
- High intensity exercise
- Lactate
- L-Arginine
- Glycine
- Tryptophan
- 5-Hydroxytryptophan
- Melatonin
- Sauna, hot bath, high body temperature

- Glutamine
- GABA
- High protein diet

Some natural GH inhibitors are:
- Hyperglycemia
- High serum triglycerides concentration
- Alcohol
- High fat diet
- High sugar diet

Guar Gum

Guar Gum is soluble fiber from the Cyamopsis Tetragonoloba beans (Cluster Beans). It is known to decrease cholesterol.

Guar Gum has body weight decreasing properties.

When hypercholesterolemic females were given daily 15 grams Guar Gum, Body weight decreased in test group significantly (62.9 kg → 60.4 kg; $p < 0.005$), compared to the control, group (Tuomilehto et.al. 1980). This was a double blind experiment.

When 9 obese volunteers were given Guar Gum 20 grams daily, for 8 weeks, body weight (95.6 kg → 91.3 kg; $p < 0.01$) and fat mass (46.1 kg → 43.6 kg; $p < 0.01$) decreased significantly in the test group, compared to the control group (Krotkiewski et.al. 1984).

In animal experiments Guar Gum decreases both body weight and body fat mass significantly (Pande et.al. 2012; Deshaies et.al. 1990; Asp et.al. 1981).

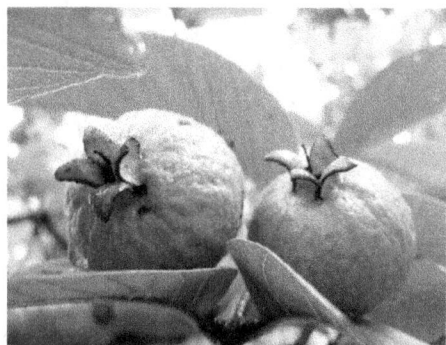

Guava

(Psidium Guajava)

Guava is a very popular tropical fruit. Guave contains large amounts of Lycopene, vitamin C and Polyphenols. Guava is known to decrease cholesterol, triglycerides and blood pressure.

Guava has body weight decreasing properties.

When obese rats were given daily Guava puree at doses of 500 mg/kg or 2000 mg/kg body weight, for 6 weeks, body weight decreased by 6.0% ($p < 0.05$) and 11.5% ($p < 0.05$), compared to the control group (Norazmir et.al. 2010).

Guduchi

(Tinospora Cordifolia)

Guduchi is a famous, climbing vine, which has been used medicinally in India for thousands of years. It has memory enhancing, antistress, antidepressant, antiallergic, cholesterol decreasing and blood sugar decreasing properties.

Guduchi stems have body weight decreasing properties.

When rats were given high fat diet and 50 mg/kg BW petroleum ether extract of Guduchi stems, body weight in test group was 30% ($p < 0.001$) lower, compared to control group. Also triglycerides were 85.0% ($p < 0.001$), total cholesterol was 59.7% ($p < 0.001$) and blood sugar was 31.9% ($p < 0.001$) lower, but HDL-cholesterol was 81.1% ($p < 0.001$) higher in test group, compared to control group (Dinesh et.al. 2011).

Guggulu

(Commiphora Mukul)

Guggulu is the oleoresin of Commiphora Mukul tree. Guggulu has been used as a medicine in India for hundreds of years. It is known to decrease cholesterol and blood pressure. The effective compouns are Guggulsterones.

Guggulu has body weight decreasing properties.

When 16 volunteers were given daily 414 mg Guggulu, for 3 months, body weight decreased by 8.2 kg ($p < 0.01$) in test group, compared to the 2.4 kg decrease in control group. Also waist circumference decreased in test group by 8.2 cm ($p < 0.01$), when it decreased only by 4.2 cm in the control group (Paranjpe et.al. 1990). This was a double blind experiment. The daily dose included also totally 336 mg dried fruits of Terminalia Chebula, Terminalia Bellerica, Emblica Officinalis and Piper Longum.

When 6 volunteers were given 750 mg Guggulsterones and 1650 mg Phosphate daily, for 6 weeks, body weight decreased in test group by 3.2% ($p < 0.05$), when it decreased only by 0.3% in the control group. Also body fat mass decreased by 20.6% (20.9 kg $\rightarrow$ 16.6 kg; $p < 0.01$), when it decreased only by 8.6% in the control group (Antonio et.al. 1999). This was a double blind experiment.

Also in other experiments with human volunteers, Guggulu dereases body weight significantly (Mehra et.al. 2009; Sidhu et.al. 1976; Bhatt et.al. 1995).

Guinea pepper

(Xylopia Aethiopica)

Guinea pepper is a medium size tree cultivated in Africa. The dried fruits are used as spice and medicine.

Guinea pepper has body weight decreasing properties.

When obese rats were fed Guinea pepper 250 mg/kg, 5 days a week, for 8 weeks, body weight decreased by 60% ($p < 0.01$), compared to the obese control rat group, which did not get Guinea pepper (Nwozo et.al. 2011). Also total cholesterol ($p < 0.05$) and LDL-cholesterol ($p < 0.05$) decreased significantly, compared to the control group.

In a study of anti-lipase effect of 19 Cameroonian spices, Guinea pepper most strongly inhibited the activity of Lipase enzyme (Etoundi et.al. 2010). This means, that Guinea pepper has anti-obesity properties.

In experiment with rats, Guinea pepper strongly decreased total cholesterol, LDL-cholesterol and triglycerides, compared to the control group (Johnkennedy et.al. 2011).

Gukhru

(Pedalium Murex)

Gukhru is a small plant, which is used in India as aphrodisiac to increase sexuality and libido. The English name is Land Caltrops. Gukhru increases testosterone and libido in animal experiments (Sharma et.al. 2012).

Gukhru fruits have body weight decreasing properties.

When rats were given high fat diet and either 200 mg/kg BW or 400 mg/kg BW Gukhru fruit ethanol extract daily, for 30 days, body weight in test groups were 31.9% ($p < 0.01$) and 43.9% ($p < 0.01$) lower, compared to control group. Also total cholesterol, LDL-cholesterol, VLDL-cholesterol and triglycerides were significantly ($p < 0.01$) lower in test groups, compared to cotrol groups (Balasubramanian et.al. 2008).

Gymnema

(Gymnema Sylvestre)

Gymnema is a climbing plant, which has been used in India for hundreds of years against diabetes.

Gymnema has body weight and fat mass decreasing properties.

When obese mice were given daily Gymnema leaf extract 250 mg/kg BW, for 45 days, body weight was 22.3% ($p < 0.001$) lower in test group, compared to the control group. Also triglycerides ($p < 0.001$), LDL-cholesterol ($p < 0.001$) and total cholesterol ($p < 0.001$) were significantly lower, but HDL-cholesterol ($p < 0.001$) was significantly higher in test group, compared to the control group (Manish et.al. 2011).

When 12 volunteers were given daily Gymnema capsules, together with chitosan, fenugreek and glucomannan, for 6 weeks, body weight decreased by 2.3 kg ($p < 0.01$), fat mass by 2.0 kg ($p < 0.01$) and waist circumference by 4.1 cm ($p < 0.05$) in test group, compared to the control group (Woodgate et.al. 2003). This was a double blind experiment.

The body weight and fat mass decreasing property of Gymnema has been verified in many animal experiments (Shigematsu et.al. 2001; Luo et.al. 2007; Reddy et.al. 2012).

5-Hydroxytryptohan

(5-HTP)

The human body makes 5-Hydroxytryptophan (5-HTP) from the essential amino acid Tryptophan from food. 5-HTP is again converted to Melatonin, which is the famous "Sleep" hormone. 5-HTP can be bought from markets as a supplement.

5-HTP has body weight decreasing properties.

When 10 obese volunteers were given 900 mg 5-HTP daily, for 6 weeks, body weight in test group decreased by 5.0 kg (99.7 kg → 94.7 kg; $p < 0.02$), when it did not change ($p > 0.05$) in the 10 person control group (Cangiano et.al. 1992). This was a double blind experiment.

117

Hawthorn berries and leaves

(Crataegus Oxyacantha, Crataegus Pinnatifida)

Hawthorn is an old medicinal plant, which leaves are used against hypertension. In China Hawthorn berries are also used to lower high cholesterol levels. Hawthorn has many Flavonoids and Polyphenols, such as Quercetin, Rutin, Isoquercetin, Chlorogenic acid, Hyperoside etc. Hawthorn berry is edible but almost tasteless.

Hawthorn berries and leaves have body weight and fat mass decreasing properties.

When obese hamsters were given daily high fat diet, together with Hawthorn 250 mg/kg, for 7 days, body weight was 10.3% ($p < 0.001$) lower in test group, than in the control group. Also body fat mass was 24.6% ($p < 0.001$) lower in test group, than in the control group. Also triglycerides, LDL-cholesterol and total cholesterol were significantly ($p < 0.001$) lower, but HDL-cholesterol significantly ($p < 0.001$) higher in the test group, than in the control group (Kuo et.al. 2009).

The body weight decreasing properties of Hawthorn has been verified also in many other experiments with mice and rats (Niu et.al. 2011; Kanyonga et.al. 2011; Kausar et.al. 2012).

HCA

(Hydroxy citric acid)

HCA or Hydroxy citric acid is a natural compound, which exists in large quantities in the fruit rinds on Malabar Tamarind, Garcinia Cambogia and other Garcinia species, such as Garcinia Indica and Garcinia Atroviridis. These trees grow naturally in South-Asia. The content of HCA in dried fruit rinds of these species can be between 10-30%. The rinds have been used for hundreds of years in food making, as a spice and color. HCA inhibits fatty acid synthesis, by inhibiting the critical enzyme, ATP citrate lyase.

HCA and fruit rinds of Garcinia species have body weight and body fat mass decreasing properties.

When rats were given high carbohydrate diet and 1.6% HCA in their daily diet, for 8 weeks, body weight decreased by 11.1% ($p < 0.05$) and body fat mass decreased by 19.0% ($p < 0.05$) in test group, compared to control group (Hong et.al. 2009).

The body weight and body fat mass decreasing properties of HCA has been verified in many experiments with rats and mice (Shara et.al. 2003; Park et.al. 2005; Kim et.al. 2008; Ishihara et.al. 2000).

HCA increases fatty acid oxidation both in untrained females (Lim et.al. 2003), untrained males (Tomita et.al. 2003) and in athletes (Lim et.al. 2002).

When 23 obese volunteers were given 3.45 grams dried rind powder of Garcinia Atrovidis fruit daily, for 8 weeks, body weight was 1.4 kg ($p < 0.05$) and body fat mass was 3.4 kg ($p < 0.05$)

lower in test group, compared to 19 person control group. This was a double blind experiment (Roongpisuthipong et.al. 2007).

The body weight and body fat mass decreasing properties of HCA has been verified in many double blind experiment with human volunteers (Preuss et.al. 2004; Hayamizu et.al. 2001; Anno et.al. 2004; Hayamizu et.al. 2003).

Hibiscus tea

(Hibiscus Sabdariffa)

Hibiscus tea is a very popular refreshing drink, which is known to Decrease blood pressure and cholesterol.

Hibiscus tea has body weight decreasing properties.

When obese mice were fed Hibiscus tea extract 120 mg/kg BW daily, for 60 days, body weight was 8.33% ($p < 0.05$) lower in test group, compared to the control group (Alarcon-Aguilar et.al. 2007).

The body weight decreasing property of Hibiscus tea has been verified in many experiments with rats and cells (Carvajal-Zarrabal et.al. 2005; Kim et.al. 2003; Yang et.al. 2010; Carvajal-Zabarral et.al. 2009; Iyare et.al. 2011; Iyare et.al. 2010; Kim et.al. 2007)

Himematsutake

(Agaricus Blazei, syn. Agaricus Brasiliensis)

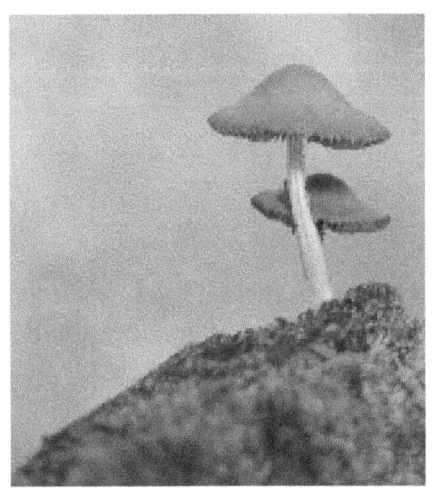

Himematsutake is an edible mushroom, which inhibits cancer cell growth and has immunostimulant properties. It is much cultivated in Asia and South America.

Himematsutake has body weight and fat mass decreasing properties.

Himematsutake decreased significantly both body weight and fat mass in obese rats, compared to control rats (Vincent et.al. 2012).

When human volunteers were given 3.0 grams Himematsutake water extract daily, for 3 months, both body weight ($p < 0.01$) and fat mass ($p < 0.01$) decreased significantly, compared to control group (Liu et.al. 2008).

HMB

(beta-Hydroxy-beta-Methylbutyrate)

HMB is a metabolite of the essentail amino acid Leucine. HMB has long time been a very popular sports supplement, because it reduces body fat mass and increases both body lean muscle mass and strength.

HMB has body fat reducing properties.

In a meta-analysis with 5 different experiments, HMB decreased the body fat mass by an average of 66 grams/week, compared to the control groups. The daily amount used was 3.0 grams on average, the duration of experiments was 4 weeks on average (Nissen et.al. 1997).

When 31 elderly volunteers were given HMB 3.0 grams daily, for 8 weeks, the body fat-% decreased by 1.1% (25.9% → 24.8%; $p < 0.05$), compared to the control group (Vukovich et.al. 2001). This was a double blind experiment.

When 75 volunteers were given 3.0 grams HMB daily, for 4 weeks, the lean body mass increased by 1.4 kg ($p = 0.08$) and fat-% decreased by 1.1% ($p = 0.08$). The changes in control group without HMB were 0.9 kg and 0.5% (Panton et.al. 2000).

When female Judo athletes were given 3.0 grams HMB daily, only 3 days, body weight decreased by 0.48 kg ($p < 0.05$) and body fat-% decreased by 1.05% ($p < 0.05$), compared to the control group without HMB (Hung et.al. 2010).

In experiments with cells, HMB increased fatt acid beta-oxidation by 30% ($p < 0.01$), compared to controls (Cheng et.al. 1998).

Honey

Honey is an ancient food item and it is also used in many medicinal purposes. Honey contains large amounts of functionally healthy Polyphenols and Flavonoids. The darker the honey is, the more Polyphenols it contains.

Honey has body weight and fat mass decreasing properties.

The energy content of honey is 330 kcal/100 g, whereas the energy content of common sugar is 405 kcal/100 g. So from 100 grams of honey we get 18.5% less kilocalories than from sugar.

When 38 volunteers were given either sugar or honey 70 grams daily, for 30 days honey decreased body weight by 1.3% and fat mass by 1.1%. In the sugar group, body weight increased by 0.6 kg and fat mass increased by 2.8% (Yaghoobi et.al. 2008). Also triglycerides decreased in the honey group by 11%, but only 0.6% in the sugar group.

When 48 type 2 diabetes patients were given daily hony, for 8 weeks, both body weight (p < 0.001) and triglycerides (p < 0.001) decreased significantly, compared to the control group (Bahmari et.al. 2009).

When rats were fed with 20% of their daily food either as sugar or honey, for 33 days, body weight decreased by 14.7% (p < 0.05) in honey group, compared to the sugar group. Also body fat mass decreased by 20.1% (p < 0.05) in honey group, compared to the sugar group. Triglycerides decreased by 29.6% (p < 0.05) in the honey group, compared to the sugar group (Nemoseck et.al. 2011).

In many other experiments with rats, the body weight and fat mass decreasing properties of honey, compared to the control groups, have been verified (Chepulis 2007; Chepulis et.al. 2008; Zaid et.al. 2010).

Obese persons with high triglyceride levels should always replace ordinary sugar by honey.

Hops

(Humulus Lupulus)

Hops have been used for hundreds of years in beer making and also as a medicine, to induce sleep. Hops contain many estrogenic compounds, like Isohumulone and Xanthohumol.

Hops, Isohumulone and Xanthohumol have body weight and fat mass decreasing properties.

When 21 volunteers were given 48 mg Isohumulone daily, for 12 weeks, body weight decreased in test group by 1.3 kg, being significantly (p < 0.01) more than the 0.3 kg decrease in control group. Fat mass decreased significantly (p < 0.001) in test group, compared to control group (Obara et.al. 2009).

When mice were given high fat diet together with 2% Hops extract daily, for 20 weeks, body weight decreased in the test group by 28.0% (p < 0.05), compared to the control group. Fat mass decreased in test group by 58.8% (p < 0.05), compared to control group (Sumiyoshi et.al. 2012).

The body weight and fat mass decreasing properties of Hops compounds has been verified in other experiments with mice and rats (Legette et.al. 2012; Yajima et.al. 2005).

Horse gram

(Dolichos Biflorus)

Horse gram is a bean, which is widely cultivated in India and Nepal for food. It is a close relative of the more familiar edible bean, Dolichos Lablab, or Hyasinth bean. Horse gram has been used in India for hundreds of years to decrease obesity. It is known to decrease cholesterol and triglycerides in animal experiments (Muthu et.al. 2005).

Horse gram has body weight decreasing properties.

When rabbits were given high fat diet, and 400 mg/kg BW methanol extract of whole Horse gram plant daily, for 11 weeks, body weight increased in test group by 14.05%, which was significantly (p < 0.01) less, than the 19.76% body weight increase in control group (Muthu et.al. 2006).

When 25 volunteers were given 900 mg Horse gram bean extract and Betel (Piper Betle) leaf extract mixture daily, for 8 weeks, body weight decreased in test group by 4.26 kg, which was significantly (p < 0.05) more, than the 1.77 kg body weight decrease in the 25 person control group. Leptin decreased by 17.3% (p < 0.05) in the test group, compared to the control group (Chatterjee et.al. 2010). This was a double blind experiment.

Hypocaloric protein diet

In hypocaloric protein diet people eat a lot of protein containing food, like meat, fish, chicken, beans etc., and only very small amounts of carbohydrates and fat, so as to minimize the daily amount of calories.

Hypocaloric protein diet has body weight decreasing properties.

When 83 diabetic volunteers were 16 weeks on protein diet or protein diet plus 3 aerobic exercise weekly, body weight decreased by an average of 11.4 kg, compared to the control values (Wycherley et.al. 2010).

When 32 volunteers were 8 weeks on a protein diet, and they ate 4 times weekly different beans, 160 – 320 grams at a time, body weight decreased by an average of 7.8%, which was significantly (p = 0.024) more, than in the control group with the same calorific value in their diet (Hemsdorff et.al. 2011).

When 100 volunteers were 12 weeks on protein diet, they lost body weight by an average of 7.3 kg. The control group was given carbohydrates (Noakes et.al. 2005).

When 215 volunteers were 12 weeks on protein diet, they lost body weight by an average of 6.8 kg. Triglycerides decreased by an average of 0.47 mmol/L, which was significantly (p < 0.001) more, than the 0.27 mmol/L in the control group (Clifton et.al. 2009).

When volunteers were 12 weeks on a protein diet, or protein diet plus 3 physical exercise weekly, body weight decreased in the protein group by 4.6 kg and in the exercised protein group by 7.0 kg. The control group lost 2.1 kg of body weight (Meckling et.al. 2007).

When on hypocaloric protein diet, volunteers can easily decrease body weight at least 6 kg in 3 months.

Ichang papeda, fruit peel

(Citrus Ichangensis)

Ichang papeda is a citrus fruit, which grows in south-western and west-central China. It is extremely cold hardy.

Ichang papeda fruit peel has body weight and body fat mass decreasing properties.

When obese mice were given high fat diet and 1% of Ichang papeda fruit peel 95% ethanol extract daily, for 8 weeks, body weight in test group was 13.8% ($p < 0.01$) lower, compared to control group. Also fat cell sizes were 56% ($p < 0.01$) lower in test group, compared to control group (Ding et.al. 2012).

Indian Coral Tree, leaves and seeds

(Erythrina Variegata)

Indian Coral Tree is a fast growing tree with ornamental, red flowers. Its leaves are edible, and they are used as vegetable salad in India. The leaves contain large amounts of protein and flavonoids. The leaves have many medicinal properties. They are used against obesity, diabetes, eye diseases etc.

Indian Coral Tree leaves and seeds have body weight decreasing properties.

When rats were given high fat diet and 400 mg/kg BW Indian Coral Tree seeds methanol extract daily, for 90 days, body weight was 17.8% ($p < 0.001$) lower in test group, compared to control group. Also triglycerides were 19.2% ($p < 0.001$), total cholesterol was 29.5% ($p < 0.001$), LDL-cholesterol was 30.3% ($p < 0.001$) and VLDL-cholesterol was 19.2% ($p < 0.001$) lower in test group, compared to control group (Balamurugan et.al. 2010).

The body weight, triglycerides and total cholesterol decreasing, but HDL-cholesterol increasing properties of Indian Coral Tree leaves have been verified in 2 other experiments (Balakhrishna et.al. 2009; Balakhrishna et.al. 2011).

Indole-3-Carbinol, I3C

Indole-3-Carbinol is an organic natural compound, which exists in large quantities in the common foods Broccoli, Kale, Cauliflower and Cabbage. It is also sold as a supplement.

Indole-3-Carbinol has body weight and total fat mass decreasing properties.

When obese mice were fed high fat diet and 0.1% Indole-3-Carbinol in their daily diet, for 10 weeks, body weight was 36% (p < 0.05) and body fat mass was 49% (p < 0.05) lower in test group, compared to control group. Also triglycerides were 72% (p < 0.05) and total cholesterol was 52% (p < 0.05) lower in test group, compared to control group (Choi et.al. 2012).

The body weight and body fat mass decreasing properties of Indole-3-Carbinol has been verified also in other experiments with mice (Chang et.al. 2011; Chang et.al. 2011).

Cabbage diet has a long time been a popular weight reduction diet. Besides the low calorific content of Cabbage, I-3-C may be the main reason to the weight loss of Cabbage diet.

Inositol

Inositol is a natural compound, which exists in many plants. It is especially abundant in soy lecithin.

Inositol has body weight and fat mass decreasing properties.

When female volunteers were given 2.0 grams Inositol daily, for 14 weeks, body mass index BMI decreased significantly in test group (35.0 → 34.4; p = 0.03), when it increased in control group (35.2 → 35.5; p = 0.04). Those volunteers with BMI lower than 37, BMI decreased even more: 29.2 → 28.3 (p = 0.01). Also HDL-cholesterol increased in test group by 5.1% (p = 0.009), compared to control group (Gerli et.al. 2007). This was a double blind experiment with 92 volunteers.

When mice were given Inositol 1.2 mg/g BW daily, for 15 days, both fat mass decreased by 33% (p = 0.009), compared to control group (Croze et.al. 2012).

Intellect tree, seeds

(Celastrus Paniculatus)

Intellect tree is a vine like plant, which grows in India and Sri Lanka. The seeds have been used hundreds of years as a medicine to improve memory, and against asthma, rheumatism, inflammation etc. The Indian name is Malkangani.

Intellect tree seeds have body weight decreasing properties.

When rats were given high fat diet and 65 mg/kg BW Intellect tree seeds methanol extract daily, for 6 weeks, body weight was 25.0% (p < 0.05) lower in test group, compared to control group. Also triglycerides, total cholesterol, LDL-cholesterol and VLDL-cholesterol were significantly (p < 0.05) lower in test group, compared to control group (Patel et.al. 2010).

Inulin and Frukto-oligosaccharides

Inulin and frukto-oligosaccharides are so called fructans, which are complex carbohydrates. They exist in many plants, such as chicory, garlic, Yacon root and Jerusalem artichoke. The normal dietary intake is between 1 – 11 grams/day. Fructans do not increase blood sugar, so they are well fitted to diabetes nutrition. They increase the bioavailability of Calcium, Magnesium, Zinc and Iron, and increase also the content of lactic acid bacteria.

Inulin and fructo-oligosaccharides have body weight and body fat mass decreasing properties.

When rats were given first 35 days normal diet or normal diet and 10% fructo-oligosaccharides, and then 15 days high fat diet or high fat diet and 10% fructo-oligosaccharides, body weight gain was 47.3% ($p < 0.05$) lower in test group, compared to control group (Cani et.al. 2005).

Also in other experiments with rats and mice Inulin (Jamieson et.al. 2008) and fructo-oligosaccharides (Nakamura et.al. 2011) decreased body weight and body fat mass, compared to control groups.

When obese volunteers were given 7 grams Inulin daily, for 4 weeks, total cholesterol decreased by 21.8% ($p = 0.028$), LDL-cholesterol decreased by 16.9% ($p = 0.028$), VLDL-cholesterol decreased by 31.1% ($p = 0.046$) and triglycerides decreased by 27.3% ($p = 0.046$) in test group, compared to control group (Balcazar-Munoz et.al. 2003). This was a double blind experiment.

When 40 obese volunteers were given daily 0.14 grams/kg BW fructo-oligosaccharides, for 6 months, body weight decreased in test group by 15.0 kg (91.2 kg → 76.2 kg; $p < 0.05$), when it increased 1.5 kg (90.7 kg → 92.3 kg) in the 15 person control group. Waist circumference decreased by 9.9 cm (105.1 cm → 95.2 cm; $p < 0.05$) in test group, but it increased by 0.4 cm in control group. LDL-cholesterol decreased by 28.8% ($p < 0.05$) in test group, but it did not change in control group (Genta et.al. 2009). This was a double blind experiment.

The body weight, body fat mass and hunger feeling decreasing effect of inulin and fructo-oligosaccharides has been verified in many double blind experiments with human volunteers (Antal et.al. 2008; Abrams et.al. 2007; Whelan et.al. 2006; Cani et.al. 2006).

Iodine

Iodine is an essential trace mineral in human nutrition. Thyroid gland makes 2 different Iodine containing thyroid hormones: Thyroxine (T4) and Triiodothyronine (T3). The recommended daily intake of Iodine for adults is typically 150 micrograms per day. Excellent sources of dietary Iodine are: Sea fish, Iodine containing salt, seaweeds and kelp. The daily intake of Iodine in Japanese diet is many times more, than in Europe or America, because large amounts of seaweeds and kelp used in daily diet.

Iodine deficiency may have body weight increasing properties.

When obese volunteers were given a daily 320 kcal diet and 60 micrograms Triiodothyronine T3 daily, for 12 weeks, body weight in test group decreased significantly ($p < 0.05$), compared to control group. This was a double blind experiment (Moore et.al. 1980).

The body weight decreasing property of Triiodothyronine T3 in obese volunteers has been verified also in other experiments (Moore et.al. 1981; Koppeschaar et.al. 1983). The used amounts of T3 were between 60 – 150 micrograms daily.

Ivy Gourd, fruit

(Coccinia Indica)

Ivy Gourd is a cucumber like vine, which is cultivated all over the World, especially in India. The green, raw fruits are eaten as vegetable and the red, ripened fruits are eaten as such. Ivy Gourd is famous for its blood glucose decreasing properties.

Ivy Gourd fruit has body weight and fat mass decreasing properties.

When rats were given high fat diet and 400 mg/kg BW Ivy Gourd fruit water extract daily, for 40 days, body weight was 8.97% ($p < 0.01$) and body fat mass was 23.7% ($p < 0.05$) lower in test group, compared to control group. Also blood sugar, tirglycerides, LDL-cholesterol and total cholesterol were significantly lower, but HDL-cholesterol was significantly higher in test group, compared to control group ($p < 0.01$ in all parameters) (Ahmed et.al. 2012).

Iwayomogi Mugwort

(Artemisia Iwayomogi)

Iwayomogi Mugwort is used in Korea and China as a vegetable and a medicinal plant against liver diseases. It is a close relative to our common Tarragon, Artemisia Dacunculus, which is used as a spice and vegetable.

Iwayomogi Mugwort has body weight and body fat mass decreasing properties.

When obese mice were given normal diet and 200 mg/kg BW Iwayomogi Mugwort ethanol extract daily, for 8 weeks, body weight was 16.7% ($p < 0.05$) and body fat mass was 28.5% ($p < 0.05$) lower in test group, compared to control group (Cho et.al. 2012).

When in another experiment rats were given high fat diet and Iwayomogi Mugworth oligosaccharide extract daily, for 4 weeks, body weight was 16.6% ($p < 0.05$) and body fat mass was 39.2% ($p < 0.05$) lower in test group, compared to control group (Jang et.al. 2003).

Japanese Catnip

(Schizonepeta Tenuifolia, Syn. Nepeta Spica)

Japanese Catnip is a very important medicinal plant in China, Korea and Japan. It is used in bronchitis, viral diseases, insomnia etc., and also as a food additive and herbal tea.

Japanese Catnip has body weight decreasing properties.

When mice were given high fat diet and 200 mg/kg BW Japanese Catnip water extract daily, for 15 weeks, body weight in test group was 13.9% ($p < 0.05$) lower, compared to control group (Roh et.al. 2012).

Japanese Ginseng

(Panax Japonicus)

Japanese Ginseng is an endemic Ginseng species in Japan, here its root are used against hypertension, diabetes and hyperlipidemia.

Japanese Ginseng root has body weight and body fat mass decreasing properties.

When obese mice were given high fat diet and 1% Saponins from Japanese Ginseng root daily, for 9 weeks, body weight was 15.7% ($p < 0.05$) and body fat mass was 45.2% ($p < 0.05$) lower in test group, compared to control group (Kim et.al. 2005).

Japanese Honeysuckle, flower buds

(Lonicera Japonica)

The dried flower buds of Japanese Honeysuckle has been used in China, Korea and Japan 3000 years as a medicine against bacterial and viral infections, high blood pressure etc. Its Chinese name is Jin Yin Hua.

Japanese Honeysuckle flower buds have body weight and body fat mass decreasing properties.

When rats were given normal diet and 5% dried Japanese Honeysuckle flower buds in daily diet, for 8 weeks, body weight decreased by 10% ($p < 0.05$) and body fat mass decreased by 25.8% ($p < 0.05$) in test group, compared to control group. Also alpha-Amylase was strongly inhibited by the methanol extract of flower buds (Kwon et.al. 2004).

Japanese red pine, needles

(Pinus Densiflora)

The needles of Japanese red pine have been used as a medicine for a long time in East-Asia. They contain large amounts of polyphenols, terpenes and tannins.

Japanese red pine needles have body weight and body fat mass decreasing properties.

When rats were given high fat diet together with 1% Japanese red pine needle hot water extract in their daily diet, for 6 weeks, body weight in test group was 12.0% ($p < 0.05$) lower, compared to control group. Body fat mass was 25.0% ($p < 0.05$) lower in test group, compared to control group. Also triglycerides ($p < 0.05$), total cholesterol ($p < 0.05$) and Leptin ($p < 0.05$) were significantly lower in test group, compared to control group (Jeon et.al. 2006).

Japanese Teasel, root

(Dipsacus Asperoides)

Japanese Teasel is a very old and famous Chinese medicinal plant. It is used against broken bones and osteoporosis and uterine bleeding. The part used is root, Radix Dipsaci. The Chinese name is XU DUAN.

Japanese Teasel root has body weight decreasing properties.

When obese OVX rats were given either 300 mg/kg BW or 500 mg/kg BW Japanese Teasel root ethanol extract daily, for 16 weeks, body weight in test groups were 6.0% ($p < 0.05$) and 10.1% ($p < 0.01$) lower, compared to control group (Liu et.al. 2009).

Jasonia

(Jasonia Montana)

Jasonia is a strongy aromatic plant, which occurs around the Mediterranian area and Sinai Peninsula. It is one of the most often used medicinal plant. It is non-toxic, and used against diabetes. It contains large amouts of flavonoids and polyphenols.

Jasonia has body weight decreasing properties.

When obese rats were given high fat diet together either 150 mg/kg BW or 300 mg/kg BW Jasonia ethanol extract daily, for 8 weeks, body weight decreased in test groups by 8.2% ($p < 0.05$) and 12.9% ($p < 0.05$), compared to control group. Also blood sugar, triglycerides, total cholesterol, LDL-cholesterol and VLDL-cholesterol decreased significantly ($p < 0.05$ in all parameters), but HDL-cholesterol increased significantly in test groups, compared to control group (Hussein et.al. 2011).

Java tea

(Orthosiphon Stamineus)

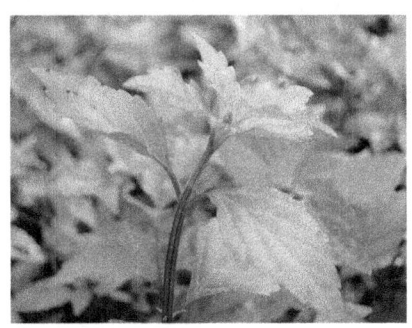

Java tea is made from the Orthosiphon Stamineus plant. It is very popular daily tea in Asia, especially Thailand, Vietnam, Myanmar and Indonesia. Java tea is known to decrease blood pressure and blood sugar.

Java tea has body weight and fat mass decreasing properties.

When normal rats were given 450 mg/kg BW dried Java tea daily, for 2 weeks, body weight decreased by 7.6% ($p < 0.05$) in test group, compared to control group. Body fat mass decreased by 36.9% ($p < 0.05$) in test group, compared to control group (Son et.al. 2011). Also in obese rats Java tea decreaseased significantly ($p < 0.05$) both body weight and body fat mass, when given daily for 7 days.

The blood pressure decreasing property of Java tea has been verified in many animal experiments (Matsubara et.al. 1999; Ohashi et.al. 2000; Azizan et.al. 2012). Also the triglycerides decreasing but HDL-cholesterol increasing properties of Java tea has been verified in experiments with rats (Sriplang et.al. 2007).

Javanese long pepper, fruits

(Piper Retrofractum, syn. Piper Chaba)

Javanese long pepper grows in Indonesia, where its fruits are used as a spice and also as a medicine in diarrhea, bronchitis and fungal infections. It is a close relative of the common Long pepper, Piper Longum, and Black pepper, Piper Nigrum. The fruits contain alkaloids Piperine, Pipernonaline, and Dehydropipernonaline. In experiments with men, Javanese long pepper fruit extract increases testosterone.

Javanese long pepper fruits have body weight and body fat mass decreasing properties.

When obese mice were given high fat diet and 50 mg/kg BW Javanese long pepper alkaloid mixture from the ethanol fraction, daily for 8 weeks, body weight was 19.5% ($p < 0.05$) and body fat mass was 18.0% ($p < 0.05$) lower in test group, compared to control group (Kim et.al. 2012).

Jerusalem Artichoke

(Helianthum Tuberosum)

Jerusalem Artichoke is a common root vegetable. It contains large amounts of Inulin. Oligofructose are sugars, which are produced by degradation of Inulin. Both Inulin and Oligofructose are knwon to decrease triglycerides in plasma. The energy content of Jerusalem Artichoke is only 38 kcal/100 grams. The cultivation of Jerusalem Artichoke is extremely easy, and the harvest yield is large.

Jerusalem Artichoke has body weight and body fat decreasing properties.

When 33 obese volunteers were given 14 grams of Jerusalem Artichoke Oligofructose daily, for 12 weeks, both body mass index BMI ($p < 0.05$) and body fat-% ($p < 0.05$) decreased significantly, compared to the control group (Antal et.al. 2008). Also triglycerides and sensation of hunger decreased significantly.

When given to obese rats, Jerusalem Artichoke decreases significantly both body weight ($p < 0.05$) and body fat-% ($p < 0.05$), compared to the control groups (Rendon-Huerta et.al. 2012; Cho et.al. 2010).

Jiaogulan

(Gynostemma Pentaphyllum)

Jiaogulan is a famous, small size herb, which originates from China. It has been used thousands of years as food and medicine against different diseases, such as diabetes. The Chinese name Xiancao means "Herb of Immortality". Jiaogulan is a strong adaptogen, which increases swimming endurance in animal experiments. It also decreases high blood pressure, cholesterol and blood sugar. The active compounds are Gypenosides.

Jiaogulan has body weight and body fat mass decreasing properties.

Jiaogulan inhibits strongly the Lipase enzyme (Shimura et.al. 1993).

Jiaogulan decreases strongly triglycerides, total cholesterol, LDL-cholesterol and blood sugar in experiments with rats on high fat diet (Megalli et.al. 2006; Megalli et.al. 2005).

When rats were given high fat diet and 200 mg/kg BW Gypenosides daily, for 4 weeks, body weight decreased by 7.5% ($p < 0.05$) and body fat mass decreased by 41.4% ($p < 0.01$), compared to control group (Tan et.al. 2011).

In experiments with obese mice, Jiaogulan decreases significantly body weight and total cholesterol and increases fatty acid oxidation (Gauhar et.al. 2012).

When mice were given 100 mg/kg BW Gypenosides daily, for 4 weeks, swimming endurance increased by 133% (23 min → 55 min; $p < 0.05$) in test group, compared to control group. Also serum lactate was lower, and glucose was higher, which means a higher rate of fatty acid oxidation in test group (Ding et.al. 2010).

Jicama

(Pachyrhizus Erosus)

Jicama originates from Mexico, but is nowadays cultivated all over the World for its edible tubers. The tubers can grow up to 20 kg in weight, and the flavor is sweet and much like apples.

Jicama tubers have body weight decreasing properties.

When rats were given Jicama tuber ethyl acetate extract 200 mg/kg BW daily, for 4 weeks, body weight in test group was 36.3% (p < 0.01) lower, compared to control group (Nurrochmad et.al. 2010).

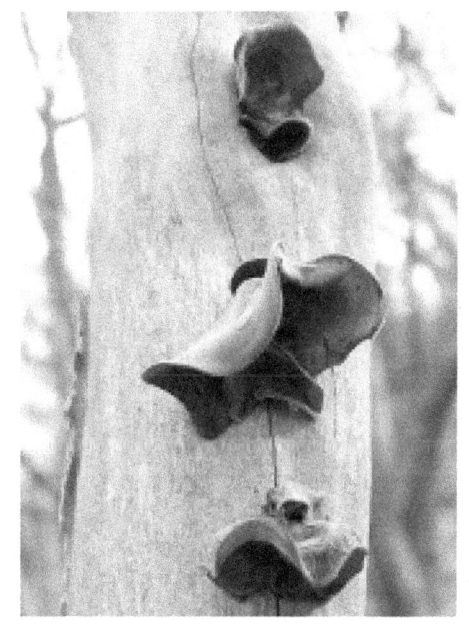

Judas ear mushroom

(Auricularia Auricula-judae)

Judas ear mushroom is a delicious, edible mushroom, which has been used as a food and medicine for a long time in China, Korea and Japan. It is known to decrease high cholesterol and it is also anti-carcinogenic.

Judas ear mushroom has body weight decreasing properties.

In experiments with cells, Judas ear mushroom water extracts inhibits triglyceride accumulation into 3T3-L1 fat cells (Yamagashi et.al. 2007).

When rats were given high fat diet and Judas ear mushroom water-ethanol extract 100 mg/kg BW daily, for 6 weeks, body weight in test group was 14.1% (p < 0.05) lower, compared to control group. Also triglycerides were 24.3% (p < 0.05), total cholesterol was 28.5% (p < 0.05) and LDL-cholesterol was 36.4% (p < 0.05) lower, but HDL-cholesterol was 9% higher in test group, compared to countrol group (Jeong et.al. 2007).

The body weight decreasing property of Judas ear mushroom has been verified also in another experiemnt with mice (Yuan et.al. 1998).

Jute mallow, leaves

(Corchorus Olitorius)

Jute is an annual plant, which can grow up to 3.5 meters high in wet places. It is known as a fiber plant, but the leaves are eaten as vegetable in Africa and Asia. The leaves contain very large amounts of flavonoids and polyphenols: Chlorogenic acid 7.5 mg/100g, Isorhamnetin 51.1 mg/100g, Quercetin 59.6 mg/100g, Caffeic acid 58.1 mg/100g and Hyperoside. These all are known to have body weight and body lipids decreasing properties.

Jute mallow leaves have body weight and fat mass decreasing properties.

When mice were given high fat diet and 1% of Jute Mallow leaves 60% ethanol extract daily, for 8 weeks, body weight was 6.6% ($p = 0.003$), body fat mass was 16.6% and triglycerides were 22.1% ($p = 0.009$) lower in test group, compared to control group (Wang et.al. 2011).

Kaempferol

Kaempferol is a flavonoid, which exist in many plants and edible food items. It is a very strong antioxidant.

Kaempferol has body weight and fat mass decreasing properties.

When rats on high fat diet were given Kaempferol, body weight and fat mass were significantly lower in test group, compared to control group (Chang et.al. 2011).

Kaempferol stimulates lipolysis and inhibits adipogenesis in experiments with 3T3-L1 cells (Park et.al. 2012).

In experiments with cells, Kaempferol increases up to 30% oxygen consumption, by increasing several fold cyclic AMP (cAMP). It also increases the thyroid hormone T3 (Da-Sailva et.al 2007).

The following plants are good sources of Kaempferol.

Kaempferol content mg/100g

Green tea	151.9
Garden cress	13.0
Capers	135.5
Komatsuna	9.7
Mizuna	8.7
Green Chili	3.9
Welsh onion leaves	83.2
Eggplant	8.0
Lemon grass	17.8

Kelp

(Laminaria Japonica)

Kelp has been used as food and medicine in China, Japan and Korea for thousands of years. Kelp is known to decrease high blood pressure and cholesterol. Kelp contains a carotenoid called Fucoxanthin, which is known to decrease body weight in animal experiments.

Kelph has body weight decreasing properties.

When obese mice on high fat diet were given in their daily diet 3% Kelp, for 63 days, body weight decreased in the test group by 16.2% ($p < 0.05$), compared to the control group. Triglycerides decreased by 16.0% ($p < 0.05$) in the test group, compared to the control group (Miyata et.al. 2009).

When obese rats were given high fat diet and 200 mg/kg BW Kelp daily, for 6 weeks, body weight decreased in the test group by 13.9% ($p < 0.05$), compared to the control group. Also triglycerides and total choleterol decreased significantly in the test group, compared to the control group (Lee et.al. 2011).

Kencur

(Kaempferia Galanga)

Kencur or aromatic ginger is a very popular vegetable in East-Asian countries. Normally the roots are used, but leaves can also be used. It is similar to the more familiar Galangal root, Alpinia Galangal.

Kencur has body weight decreasing properties.

When rats were given high fat diet and 20 mg Kencur 70% ethanol extract daily, for 4 weeks, body weight in test group was 21.3% ($p < 0.05$) lower, compared to control group. Total cholesterol was 48.0% ($p < 0.01$) and triglycerides were 76.4% ($p < 0.01$) lower, but HDL-cholesterol was 52.5% ($p < 0.01$) higher in test group, compared to control group (Achuthan et.al. 1997).

Ketogenic Diet

Ketogenic diet containst a lot of protein from fish, meat and chicken, and only very small amount of carbohydrates and fat, but a lot of fresh vegetables, and fruits. Olive oil or Sesame oil is used as cooking and salad oil. Red wine can be used as drink. Daily calorific value is unlimited.

Ketogenic diet is extremely effective to reduce body weight, and also very effective to reduce high blood pressure and high cholesterol values.

Ketogenic diet has body weight lowering properties.

When 31 obese volunteers were on Ketogenic diet for 12 weeks, body weight decreased significantly by 14.14 kg ($p < 0.0001$; 108.52 kg → 94.48 kg) and BMI decreased significantly by 4.7 kg/m2 ($p < 0.0001$; 36.46 → 31.76) (Perez-Guisado et.al. 2008).

When 106 volunteers were on Ketogenic diet for 6 weeks, body weight decreased significantly ($p < 0.001$; 86.15 kg → 79.43 kg) (Paoli et.al. 2011). BMI decreased from 31.45 kg/m2 to 29.01 kg/m2 ($p < 0.0001$).

When obese children, age between 12 – 15 and average weight 147.8 kg, were on Ketogenic diet for 8 weeks, body weight decreased b 15.4 kg (Willi et.al. 1998). BMI decreased by 5.6 kg/m2 and body fat-% decreased from 51.1% to 44.2%.

When 102 obese volunteers were on ketogenic diet for 12 weeks, body weight decreased by 13.3 kg (99.2 kg → 85.9 kg; $p < 0.0001$) and BMI decreased by 4.4 kg/m2 (37.4 → 33.0; $p < 0.0001$) (Dashti et.al. 2003).

When 17 obese volunteers were on ketogenic diet for 4 weeks, body weight decrerased by 6.3 kg (108.0 kg → 101.7 kg; $p = 0.006$) and body fat mass decreased by 5.13 kg (38.53 kg → 33.39 kg; $p = 0.083$) (Johnstone et.al. 2008).

Ketogenic diet decreases body weight ($p < 0.001$), BMI ($p < 0.001$), blood sugar ($p < 0.001$) and high cholesterol values ($p < 0.001$) also in diabetic volunteers and volunteers with high cholesterol levels (Dashti et.al. 2007; Dashti et.al. 2006).

Typically the body weight decreases in Ketogenic diet, where daily calorific value is not limited, by an average of 1.0 – 2.0 kg per week, depending on the initial weight.

Khuzestanian Savory

(Satureja Khuzestanica)

Khuzestanian Savory is a close relative to the common edible spice, Winter Savory, Satureja Montana. Khuzestanian Savory is endemic to south-Iran, where it has a long history as a medicinal plant.

Khuzestanian Savory has body weight decreasing properties.

When rats were given daily 150 mg/kg BW Khuzestanian Savory water extract, for 2 weeks, body weight in test group was 9.24% ($p < 0.001$) lower, compared to control group (Nazari et.al. 2006).

When 11 volunteers were given dried Khuzestanian Savory 250 mg daily, for 60 days, total cholesterol decreased by 23.0% (202.8 mg/dl → 156.2 mg/dl; $p = 0.008$), LDL-cholesterol decreased by 14.1% (120 mg/dl → 103 mg/dl; $p = 0.03$), but HDL-cholesterol increased by 10.3% (45.3 mg/dl → 50 mg/dl; $p = 0.03$), but in the 10 person control group there were no changes in any lipid parameters (Vosough-Ghanbari et.al. 2010). This was a double blind experiment.

King Oyster mushroom

(Pleurotus Eryngii)

King Oyster mushroom is a close relative of the common oyster mushroom, Pleurotus Ostreatus. King Oyster mushroom grows wild from Europe to Asia, and it is cultivated in China, Korea, Japan, USA and Italy as a delicious edible mushroom. It is the largest of all Oyster mushroom species.

King Oyster mushroom has body weight decreasing properties.

When rats were given high fat diet and 3% of King Oyster mushroom in their daily diet, for 10 weeks, body weight in test group was 5.9% ($p < 0.05$) lower, compared to control group (Koh et.al. 2005).

Korean black raspberry

(Rubus Koreanus)

Korean black raspberry originates from Korea, China and Japan. The delicious fruit is much used as a food and medicine. The raw fruits are used against impotence and as a diuretic.

Korean black raspberry has body weight decreasing properties.

When obese rats were given high fat food and 2% Korean black raspberry daily, for 4 weeks, body weight in test group was 6.48% ($p < 0.05$) lower, compared to control group (Cho et.al. 2004).

Also in cell experiments Korean black raspberry reduces significantly lipid accumulation in 3T3-L1 adipocytes, suggesting strong anti-obesity activity (Roh et.al. 2011).

In many swimming tests with mice, Korean black raspberry increases swimming endurance, which means mice are burning more fat during exercise, compared to control mice (Lee et.al. 2011; Jung et.al. 2007).

Kratom, leaves

(Mitragyna Speciosa)

Kratom is an evergreen tree. The young leaves are used in Thailand against pain, coughing, diarrhea and diabetes.

Kratom leaves have body weight decreasing properties.

When rats were given 40 mg/kg BW Kratom leaves methanol extract daily, for 60 days, body weight in test group was 17.6% ($p < 0.01$) lower, compared to control group (Kumarnsit et.al. 2006).

Kuding tea

(Ilex Kudingcha)

Kuding tea is made from the leaves of Ilex Kudingcha tree, which grows naturally in Southern China. Kuding tea has been used in China over 2000 years as a health tea. It decreases high blood pressure, high cholesterol and body fat.

Kuding tea has body weight and body fat mass decreasing properties.

When mice were given high fat diet and 0.05% Kuding tea ethanol extract in their daily diet, for 5 weeks, body weight was 13.9% ($p < 0.05$) lower in test group, compared to control group. Also adipocyte size, triglycerides, total cholesterol and LDL-cholesterol were significantly lower in test group (Fan et.al. 2012).

Kudzu, flowers

(Pueraria Lobata, syn. Pueraria Thomsonii)

Kudzu is a very old food and medicinal plant, which is much used in China, Korea and Japan. The root is edible. The flower contains large amounts, about 20%, different isoflavonoids.

Kudzu flower has body weight and fat mass decreasing properties.

When mice were given high fat diet and 5% Kudzu flower extract in their daily diet, body weight was 12.6% ($p < 0.05$) and body fat mass was 44.9% ($p < 0.05$) lower in test group, compared to control group (Kamiya et.al. 2012).

Also in another experiment with mice, Kudzu flower extract decreased both body weight and body fat mass in test group, compared to control group (Kamiya et.al. 2012).

When volunteers were given 300 mg Kudzu flower extract daily, for 8 weeks, body weight ($p < 0.05$) and body fat mass ($p < 0.05$) decreased significantly in test group, compared to control group (Kamiya et.al. 2011; Kamiya et.al. 2012). These were double blind experiments.

Kudzu, root

(Pueraria Lobata)

Kudzu root is extremely important herb in Chinese medicine. Kudzu root contains large amounts of Isoflavonoids, especially Puerarin, Genistein, Daidzein and Formonetin. The root is also an edible vegetable. Cultivation is extremely easy.

Kudzu root has body weight and body fat decreasing properties.

When obese rats were given 80 mg/kg BW Kudzu root 80% ethanol extract daily, for 49 days, body weight decreased in test group by 18% ($p < 0.05$), when it increased in control group by 8% ($p < 0.05$). Also fat mass decreased significantly ($p < 0.05$) in test group, compared to control group (Saunier et.al. 2011).

Also the main Isoflavonoid, Puerarin, decreased body weight in experiments with rats (Zhang et.al. 2010).

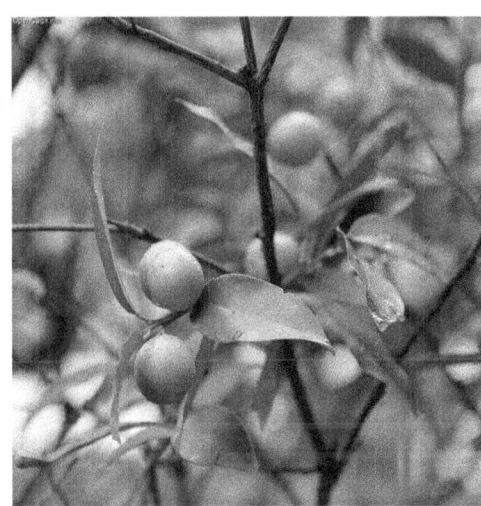

Kumquat

(Fortunella Japonica)

Kumquat is a small citrus fruit, which is cultivated all around the World. Kumquat is always eaten together with peel. Kumquat contains large amount of Flavonoids.

Kumquat has body weight decreasing properties.

When obese mice were fed daily 800 mg/kg Kumquat peel ethyl acetate extract, chloroform extract or ethanol extract, for 8 days, body weight decreased by 9.2% ($p < 0.05$), 8.2% ($p < 0.05$) and 4.7% ($p < 0.05$), compared to the control group, which was given water (Lien et.al. 2010). Also Kumquat decreased significantly both triglycerides and total cholesterol.

Also in other experiments it has been verified, that Kumquat decreases triglycerides and total cholesterol (Li et.al. 2008).

Kuthu

(Clerodendrum Glandulosum , syn. Clerodendrum Colebrookianum)

and Arni, leaves

(Clerodendrum Phlomidis)

Kuthu and Arni are famous medicinal plants in India. They are small size trees. The leaves are commonly used against obesity, diabetes and hypertension in North-India. The English common names for these trees are Glorybower or Bagflower.

Kuthu and Arni leaves have body weight and fat mass decreasing properties.

When obese mice were given high fat diet and 1% Kuthu leaves water extract daily, for 20 weeks, body weight was 23.6% (p < 0.001), body fat mass was 43.0% (p < 0.05), triglycerides were 72.7% (p < 0.05) and Leptin was 53.8% (p < 0.05) lower in test group, compared to control group (Jadeja et.al. 2011).

The same kind of body weight, body fat mass, triglycerides, total cholesterol and LDL-cholesterol decreasing properties has been verified also with Arni leaf extracts in animal experiments (Chidrawar et.al. 2012; Chidrawar et.al. 2011).

The blood pressure decreasing properties of both Kuthu and Arni is well documented (Lokesh et.al. 2012; Jadeja et.al. 2010).

L-Arginine

L-Arginine is an amino acid, which exists both in food and living cells. It plays a very important role in producing nitrogen oxide NO, and thus controlling blood pressure. It stimulates growth hormone synthesis, and it plays an important role in penile and clitoris erection. Good sources of L-arginine are nuts, garlic, sunflower seeds and beans.

L-Arginine has body weight and fat mass decreasing properties.

When obese diabetic rats were given normal food and 1.25% L-Arginine in drinking water daily, for 10 weeks, body weight was 16.4% (p < 0.01), fat mass was 33.2% (p < 0.05), triglycerides were 23% (p < 0.05), blood sugar was 25% (p < 0.05) and Leptin was 32% (p < 0.05) lower in test group, compared to control group (Fu et.al. 2005).

The body weight and body fat mass decreasing properties of L-Arginine has been verified in many animal experiments (Jobgen et.al. 2009; Tan et.al. 2011; Tan et.al. 2009; McKnight et.al. 2010; Clemmensen et.al. 2012).

When 15 obese volunteers were given 1000 mg L-Arginine daily, for 3 months, body weight decreased by 1.2 kg (77.7 kg → 76.5 kg; p < 0.05), fat-% by 3.0% (29.6% → 26.4%; p < 0.05), waist circumference by 1.4 cm (p < 0.05), systolic blood pressure by 7.2 mmHg (126.8 mmHg → 119.6 mmHg; p < 0.05), diastolic blood pressure by 5.0 mmHg (82.1 mmHg → 77.1 mmHg; p < 0.05), triglycerides by 20.9% (164.2 mg/dl → 129.8 mg/dl; p < 0.05) and LDL-cholesterol by 5.6% (p < 0.05), but Adinopectin increased by 13.1% (p < 0.05) (Watanabe et.al. 2009).

Also in other experiments with human volunteers, L-Arginine decreases fat mass, waist circumference and both systolic – and diastolic blood pressure (Alizadeh et.al. 2012; Lucotti et.al. 2006; Alizadeh et.al. 2010).

L-Carnitine

L-Carnitine is an essential, vitamin like natural compound, which exists in large quantities in muscle. It is made in human body from the amino acids Methionine and Lysine. L-Carnitine exists also in food, especially in meat products. L-Carnitine has a very important role in fatty acid oxidation, by transporting fatty acids into mitochondria. It is also sold as nutritional supplement. L-Carnitine is known to decrease high blood pressure and cholesterol, and it increases aerobic endurance. The normal dose is between 1 – 6 grams daily.

L-Carnitine has body weight and fat mass decreasing properties.

L-Carnitine stimulates lipolysis (Lee et.al. 2006), and it stimulates fatty acid oxidation and decreases RQ (Respiratory Quotient) value (Center et.al. 2012).

When mice were given high fat diet and 0.5% L-Carnitine in their daily food, for 12 weeks, body weight was 14.0% (p < 0.05), body fat mass was 24.5% (p < 0.05) and Leptin was 32.2% (p < 0.05) lower in test group, compared to control group (Mun et.al. 2007).

The body weight, body fat mass, triglycerides and total cholesterol decreasing properties of L-Carnitine has been verified in great many experiments with rats and mice (Iwami et.al. 2006; Park et.al. 2006; Bernard et.al. 2008; Gaafar et.al. 2010; Kim et.al. 2007; Mishra et.al. 2010; Amin et.al. 2009).

In a double blind experiment with human volunteers, 2 grams L-Carnitine daily for 24 weeks decreased muscle glycogen use by 55% and it activated PDC (Pyryvate Dehydrogenase Complex) 31% less at 50% VO2max level exercise, compared to control group (Wall et.al. 2011). This means that muscles used more fat and less carbohydrates as fuel during exercise.

With human volunteers 2 grams L-Carnitine daily increased significantly (p =0.021) fatty acid oxidation, compared to control group (Wutzke et.al. 2004).

When volunteers were given 4 grams L-Carnitine daily, for 2 weeks, running endurance increased by 10.77% (9.0 min: 83.5 min → 92.5 min; p < 0.05), compared to control group (Lee et.al. 2003). This means more fatty acid oxidation in test group, compared to control group.

The aerobic endurance and max VO2 increasing, but RQ value decreasing properties of L-Carnitine has been verified in many experiments with human volunteers (Arenas et.al. 1994; Wyss et.al. 1990; Cha et.al. 2001).

The body weight and body fat mass decreasing properties of L-Carnitine has been verified in many experiments with human volunteers (Malaguarnera et.al. 2007; Lurz et.al. 1998; Gwak et.al. 2007; Cha et.al. 2003).

L-Histidine

L-Histidine is a natural amino acid in human cells and food. It is needed in the L-Carnosine biosynthesis. Good dietary sources are Tuna, Soy products, Sesame seeds and Egg whites.

L-Histidine has body weight and body fat mass decreasing properties.

When rats were given either 20% Casein or 20% Casein and either 1%, 2.5% or 5% L-Histidine daily, for 8 days, body weight gain was 3.33%, 15.00% and 46.66% ($p < 0.05$ in all groups) lower in test groups, compared to the control group. Also body fat mass was significantly ($p < 0.01$) lower in test groups, compared to the control group. Also Insulin and Leptin levels were significantly lower in test groups (Kasaoka et.al. 2004).

When 9 volunteers were given 25 mg/kg L-Histidine daily, for 10 days, body weight decreased by 1.4% ($p = 0.009$) compared to the control group. Also blood Glucose decreased by 11% ($p = 0.04$) compared to the control group (Rajashekar et.al. 2008).

When 18 volunteers were given 25 mg/kg L-Histidine daily, for 8 weeks, body weight decreased by 0.7 kg ($p = 0.003$) compared to the control group (Rajashekar et.al. 2008).

The body weight, body fat mass and FAS enzyme decreasing, but lipolysis increasing properties of L-Histidine has been verified in many experiments with rats and mice (Walczewska et.al. 1993; Yoshimatsu et.al. 2002; Mong et.al. 2011).

Lactoferrin

Lactoferrin is a natural protein, which exist in milk, and especially in breast milk, colostrum and whey protein. It is antibacterial and antiviral.

Lactoferrin has body weight and fat mass decreasing properties.

When obese mice were given Lactoferrin, corresponding to 18% of daily energy need, for 50 days, body weight was 10.8% ($p < 0.001$) and body fat mass was 46.7% ($p < 0.001$) lower in test group, compared to whey protein control group, which got equivalent amount of whey protein daily (Pilvi et.al. 2009).

The body weight and fat mass decreasing properties of Lactoferrin has been verified in other experiments with rats and mice (Shi et.al. 2012; Ono et.al. 2011).

When 13 volunteers were given 300 mg Lactoferrin daily, for 8 weeks, body weight was 2.5 kg (p = 0.013), waist circumference was 3.5 cm (p = 0.073), hip circumference was 2.4 cm (p = 0.032), and heart rate was 3.6 beats/minute lower in test group, compared to the 13 volunteers control group (Ono et.al. 2010). This was a double blind experiment.

Lemon, peel

(Citrus Limon)

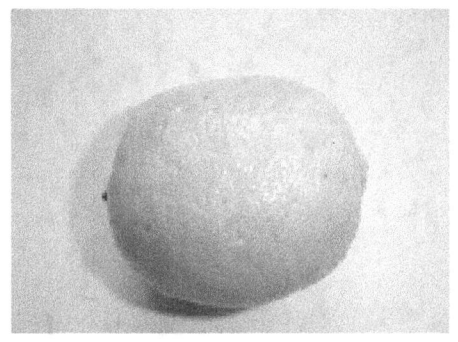

Lemon is a familiar fruit to everybody. The peel is normally used as a spice. It contains many times more the healthy flavonoids, than the fruit pulp. The following flavonoids exist in the peel: Eriocitrin, Hesperidin, Narirutin and Diosmin.

Lemon peel has body weight and body fat mass decreasing properties.

When mice were fed high fat diet and 0.5% Lemon peel flavonoids extract daily, for 12 weeks, body weight was 14.9% (p < 0.05) and fat mass was 36.0% (p < 0.05) lower in test group, compared to control group. Also Leptin was 43.1% (p < 0.05), triglycerides were 18.1% (p < 0.05), total cholesterol was 26.1% (p < 0.05), serum sugar was 65.8% (p < 0.05) and Insulin was 26.1% (p < 0.05) lower in test group, compared to control group (Fukuchi et.al. 2008).

When rats were given high fat diet and 5% Lemon peel daily, for 8 weeks, body weight gain was 61.2% (p < 0.05), total cholesterol ws 55.5% (p < 0.05), LDL-cholesterol was 82.7% (p < 0.05), VLDL-cholesterol was 53.4% (p < 0.05) and triglycerides were 53.5% (p < 0.05) lower, but HDL-cholesterol was 21.8% (p < 0.05) higher, compared to control group (Abdelbaky et.al. 2009).

Lemongrass

(Cymbopogon Citratus)

Lemongrass is a very popular spice all around the World. Its cultivation is easy, and it is known to decrease high blood pressure and high cholesterol levels.

Lemongrass has body weight decreasing properties.

When obese rats with high cholesterol levels were given Lemongrass ethanol extract 200 mg/kg BW daily, for 7 days, body weight decreased in test group by 22.6% (132.5 g → 102.5 g; p < 0.05), when it did not change in the control group (155.0 g → 152.5 g; p < 0.05). Total cholesterol decreased by 48.7% (p < 0.05) in test group, compared to control group (Agbafor et.al. 2007).

In another experiment with rats Lemongrass decreased significantly body weight, total cholesterol, LDL-cholesterol and VLDL-cholesterol, but increased significantly HDL-cholesterol (p < 0.05 in all Properties) (Adeneye et.al. 2007).

Also in experiments with chickens lemongrass decreased significantly body weight, compared to control group (Thayalini et.al. 2011).

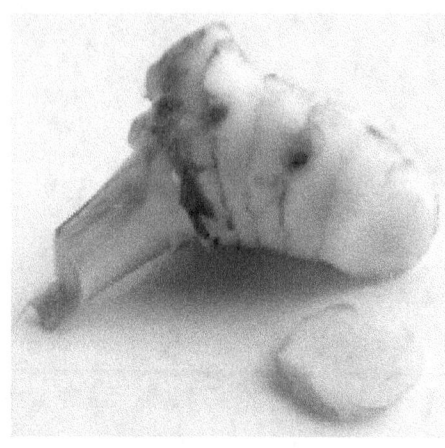

Lesser Galangal, root

(Alpinia Officinarum)

Lesser Galangal is a close relative to our familiar Ginger. It is used in Asia in the same way as a spice and food, as Ginger. It has also many medicinal properties in rheumatic pain, stomach problems etc.

Lesser Galangal root has body weight decreasing properties.

When chicken were given in their daily food either 2% or 5% Lesser Galangal root, for 4 weeks, body weight in test group were 5.5% (p < 0.05) and 12.0% (p < 0.05) lower, compared to control group. Also total cholesterol was significantly (p < 0.05) lower in test group, compared to control group (Seddeag et.al. 2010).

The body weight, triglycerides, total cholesterol and LDL-cholesterol decreasing but HDL-cholesterol increasing properties of Lesser Galangal root has been verified in many experiments with mice and rats (Shin et.al. 2003; Xia et.al. 2010; Beattie et.al. 2011).

Leucine

Leucine is an essential amino acid, which stimulates protein synthesis and decreases protein catabolism. In can be purchased as a pure amino acid powder from markets.

Leucine has body weight and body fat mass decreasing properties.

When 10 obese volunteers were given Leucine 2.25 grams daily, for 4 weeks, there was a 33.6 gram (p < 0.04) extra fatty acid oxidation per day in the experimental group, compared to the control group. Also RER-value decreased from 0.88 to 0.87, which means more fatty acid oxidation, compared to carbohydrate oxidation. Also Leucine decreased FAS synthesis (FAS = Fatty Acid Synthase) (Zemel et.al. 2012).

When mice were given 100% more Leucine in their daily diet, compared to the control group, for 14 weeks, the weight gain was 32% (p < 0.05) less, and adiposity was 25% (p < 0.01) less, than in the control group. Also total cholesterol decreased by 27% (p < 0.001) and LDL-cholesterol decreased by 53% (p < 0.001), compared to the control group (Zhang et.al. 2007).

In many other experiments with mice and rats, it has been verified, that Leucine decreases body weight and body fat mass, compared to the control groups (Freudenberg et.al. 2012; Vianna et.al. 2012; Torres-Leal et.al. 2011; Donato et.al. 2006; Freudenberg et.al. 2012).

Licorice

(Glycyrrhiza Glabra, G. Uralensis, G. Inflata)

There exists several different Licorice species in the World, but the common Licorice, Glycyrrhiza Glabra, is the most often used. Licorice has been used over 4000 years as a medicine and food component and component in drinks and sweeties. Licorice is antiviral, antibacterial, antifungal, anti-inflammatory, and it is used in bronchitis, asthma and hepatitis. It contains large amounts of flavonoids, especially Glabridin, and also Glycyrrhizic acid. Glycyrrhizic acid is hypertensive, but it is easily removed from Licorice extract by 95% ethanol extraction.

Licorice has body weight and body fat mass decreasing properties.

When obese mice were given high fat diet and 5 times weekly 80 mg Licorice 80% ethanol extract, for 49 days, body weight in test group was 18% ($p < 0.05$) lower, compared to control group. Also fat mass was significantly ($p < 0.05$) lower in test group, compared to control group (Saunier et.al. 2011).

The body weight and body fat mass decreasing properties of Licorice has been verified in great many experiments with mice, rats and chickens (Nakagawa et.al. 2004; Malik et.al. 2011; Mae et.al. 2003; Birari et.al. 2011; Aoki et.al. 2007; Sedghi et.al. 2010).

When obese volunteers were given daily 300 mg MCT oil, which has 1% Glabridin content, for 12 weeks, body weight gain in test group was 1.5 kg ($p < 0.05$) lower, compared to control group. This was a double blind experiment, with 103 volunteers (Tominaga et.al. 2006). Already very small amount of Licorice extract decreases body weight in obese persons.

The Licorice extract body weight and body fat mass decreasing properties has been verified also in other experiments with human volunteers (Tominaga et.al. 2009; Armanini et.al. 2003).

When volunteers with high cholesterol levels were given 100 mg/day, for 4 weeks, Licorice Glycyrrhizic acid free extract, total cholesterol decreased by 5% ($p < 0.05$), LDL-cholesterol decreased by 9% ($p < 0.05$), triglycerides decreased by 14% ($p < 0.05$) and systolic blood pressure decreased by 10% ($p < 0.05$) (Fuhrman et.al. 2002). The same kind of results has been obtained also in animal experiments (Mae et.al. 2003; Malik et.al. 2011; Birari et.al. 2011).

Lime fruit

(Citrus Aurantifolia)

Lime fruit is the familiar small, round and green colored healthy Citrus fruit, which has a sharp taste like Lemon. Lime fruit contains large amounts of flavonoids. The oil extracted from Lime fruit contains large amounts of a terpene called D-Limonene.

Lime fruit has body weight decreasing properties.

When rats with an average weight of 170 grams were given Lime fruit juice 1 ml daily, for 7 days, body weight decreased in test group by 13.8% (174 g → 150 g; $p < 0.05$), when it increased in control group by 7.5% (164.2 g → 177.6 g) (Bakare et.al. 2012). This would corresponds to 4 dl of daily Lime juice intake, when a person weights 70 kg.

In experiments with mice, oil extracted from Lime fruit decreased significantly body weight, compared to control group, when fed for 45 days (Asnaashari et.al. 2010).

D-Limonene from Lime fruit oil decreased significantly body weight, triglycerides, total cholesterol and systolic blood pressure, when given for 4 weeks, compared to control group (Santiago et.al. 2010).

Lipoic acid

Lipoic acid is a natural, Sulphur containing, vitamin-like compound, which exist in every living cell. It has a very important role in the cell energy production. Lipoic acid is also a very strong antioxidant. In animal experiments and experiments with cells it increases lifetime.

Lipoic acid has body weight decreasing properties.

When 82 volunteers were given daily 1800 mg Lipoic acid, for 20 weeks, body weight decreased significantly ($p < 0.05$), compared to the control group. The average body weight decrease was 2.76 kg (Koh et.al. 2011). This was a double blind experiment. About 22% of the volunteers lost more than 5% of their body weight. Totally there were 360 volunteers.

When 1127 volunteers were given daily 800 mg Lipoic acid, for 4 months, body weight decreased by 8% ($p < 0.001$) and BMI decreased by 2.0 units in the mildly obese group. In the clearly obese volunteer group, body weight decreased by 9% ($p < 0.001$) and BMI decreased by 3.5 units, compared to the control group (Carbonelli et.al. 2010). Abdominal circumference decreased in men by 9 cm and in women by 11 cm. Also blood pressure decreased.

Also in experiments with rats and mice, Lipoic acid decreases significantly both body weight and body fat mass, compared to the control groups (Kim et.al. 2004; Kim et.al. 2011; Shen et.al. 2005; Wang et.al. 2010; Prieto-Honoria et.al. 2009; Prieto-Honoria 2012; Valdecantos et.al. 2012; Thabet 2009).

Loquat, leaves

(Eriobotrya Japonica)

Loquat tree is known for its delicious fruits. The leaves are also used medicinally, especially in lung diseases. The leaves contain large amounts of Corosolic acid, which is known to decrease body weight and fat mass.

Loquat leaves have body weight and fat mass decreasing properties.

When obese mice were given daily 400 mg/kg BW Loquat leaves 50% ethanol extract, for 12 weeks, body weight was 7% ($p < 0.05$) lower in test group, compared to control group. Also triglycerides were significantly ($p < 0.05$) lower but Adinopectin was significantly ($p < 0.05$) higher in test group, compared to control group (Oh et.al. 2011).

The body weight, fat mass and triglycerides decreasing properties of Loquat leaves has been verified also in other experiments with mice and rats (Shih et.al. 2010; Tanaka et.al. 2010).

Lotus leaf and root

(Nelumbo Nucifera)

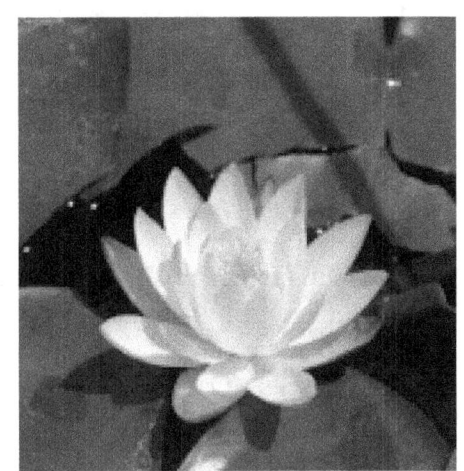

Lotus roots and seeds are used generally as a food in China, Korea and Japan. Lotus leaves are diuretic and they have for a long time been used against obesity.

Lotus leaf and root have body weight decreasing properties.

The body weight decreasing properties of lotus leaves have been documented in great many experiments.

When obese rats were given high calorific diet and Lotus leaf extract daily, for 6 weeks, body weight decreased by 15% ($p < 0.05$), compared to the control group, which was given high calorific diet. Also triglycerides ($p < 0.05$), total cholesterol ($p < 0.05$) and LDL-cholesterol ($p < 0.05$) decreased significantly in the Lotus group, compared to the control group (Du et.al. 2010).

When obese rats were given daily Lotus root Polyphenol extract, 0.5% of their daily diet, for 3 weeks, body weight gains was 43% lower in Lotus group, compared to the control group (Tsuruta et.al. 2011).

The body weight decreasing properties of Lotus leaf has been documented in many experiments (Okhoshi et.al. 2007; Wu et.al. 2010; Ono et.al. 2006; Siegner et.al. 2010).

Luffa

(Luffa Aegyptica, Luffa Cylindrica)

Luffa is a vegetable, which is cultivated all around the World. Its cultivation is very easy. Luffa decreases cholesterol and triglycerides.

Luffa has body weight decreasing properties.

When obese rabbits were given high fat diet together with 300 mg/kg BW Luffa methanol extract daily, for 8 weeks, body weight was 15.5% (p < 0.01) lower in test group, compared to the control group. Totally weight gain was 69.2% (p < 0.01) lower in test group. Total cholesterol decreased by 29%, triglycerides decreased by 52% and LDL-cholesterol decreased by 22%, but HDL-cholesterol increased by 38% (p < 0.01 in all parameters) in test group, compared to the control group (Thayyil et.al. 2011).

Also in other experiments with rats Luffa decreases body weight, total cholesterol and triglycerides, but increases HDL-cholesterol, compared to control group (Li et.al. 2004).

Luo Han Guo, fruit

(Siraitia Grosvenorii)

Luo Han Guo is a vine like plant, which is called either Buddha fruit or Monk fruit in English. The edible, delicious fruit is round and 5-7 cm in diameter, green colored. The fruit extract is 300 times sweeter than sugar. The plant is cultivated in South-China, in Guangxi, Guangdong, Guizhou, Hunan and Jiangxi provinces. The fruit contains Triterpene Glycosides, which are called Mongrosides.

Luo Han Guo fruit has body weight and fat mass decreasing properties.

When mice were given high fat diet and 2% Mongrosides daily, extracted from Luo Han Guo fruit, for 11 weeks, body weight in test group was 12.4% (p < 0.05) lower, compared to control group. Total fat mass was 36.6% (p < 0.05) lower in test group, compared to control group (Sun et.al. 2012).

The triglycerides, total cholesterol and blood sugar decreasing but HDL-cholesterol increasing properties of Luo Han Guo has been verified in many experiments (Qi et.al. 2008; Lin et.al. 2007).

Madagascar periwinkle, leaves

(Catharanthus Roseus)

Madagascar periwinkle is a famous medicinal plant, which originates from Madagascar, but is now cultivated all around the World. It is used especially against diabetes, but it is also anti-carcinogenic, and it decreases strongly high blood pressure, high cholesterol and high triglyceride levels.

Madagascar periwinkle leaves have body weight decreasing properties.

When hypertensive rats were given 200 mg/kg BW Madagascar periwinkle leaves ethanol extract daily, for 8 days, body weight decreased in test group by 7.7% (p < 0.0001), compared to control group. Also blood pressure decreased significantly in test group (Ara et.al. 2009).

When rats were given high fructose diet and 100 mg/kg BW Madagascar periwinkle dried leaves daily, for 60 days, body weight was 24% (p < 0.05) lower in test group, compared to control group. Also blood sugar, total cholesterol, triglycerides, LDL-cholesterol and VLDL-cholesterol were significantly (p < 0.05 in all parameters) lower in test group, compared to control group (Rasineni et.al. 2011).

Madras pea pumpkin

(Melothria Maderaspatana)

Madras pea pumpkin is an annual, climbing plant from India, which is a close relative to the more familiar Melothria Scabra from Mexico, which has edible small cucumber like fruits. The leaf tea of Madras pea pumpkin is used against high blood pressure and other illness.

Madras pea pumpkin leaf has body weight decreasing properties.

When 25 hypertensive patients were given Madras pea pumpkin leaf tea, 4 grams daily, for 45 days, body weight decreased by 5.02 kg (66.20 kg → 61.16 kg; p < 0.001). Systolic blood pressure decreased by 23.8 mmHg (159.4 mmHg → 135.6 mmHg; p < 0.001), Diastolic blood pressure decreased by 15.5 mmHg (101.0 mmHg → 85.5 mmHg; p < 0.001), heart rate decreased by 9.0 beats/minute (81.0/min → 72.0/min; p < 0.05), total cholesterol decreased by 16.33 mg/dl (201.99 mg/dl → 185.66 mg/dl; p < 0.001), LDL-cholesterol decreased by 12.8 mg/dl (131.46 mg/dl → 118.66 mg/dl; p < 0.001), VLDL-cholesterol by 5.71 mg/dl (34.49 mg/dl → 28.78 mg/dl; p < 0.05), triglycerides decreased by 28.51 mg/dl (172.41 mg/dl → 143.90 mg/dl; p < 0.001), but HDL-cholesterol increased by 2.8 mg/dl (36.04 mg/dl → 38.22 mg/l; p < 0.05) (Raja et.al. 2007).

Also in experiments with rats Madras pea pumpkin decreased significantly body weight, total cholesterol, LDL-cholesterol and triglycerides (Pandey et.al. 2010).

Maitake

(Grifola Frondosa)

Maitake is a famous, eatable mushroom, which decrease blood pressure and cholesterol.

Maitake has body weight and fat mass decreasing properties.

When obese mice were fed high fat diet and 20% Maitake mushroom in their daily diet, for 25 days, body weight was 14.7% (p < 0.01) lower in test group, compared to the control group. Fat mass in Maitake group was 37.1% (p < 0.01) lower, than in the control group. Maitake also significantly decreased triglycerides and total cholesterol, but increased HDL-cholesterol (Kubo et.al. 1997).

Mangiferin and Honeybush tea

(Cyclopia Sp.)

Mangiferin is a natural organic compound, which exist in many plant species, especially in Mango tree (Mangifera Indica) leaves, and in Honeybush tea from South-Africa. Mangiferin is anti-viral.

Mangiferin has body weight and fat mass decreasing properties.

The triglycerides, total cholesterol and LDL-cholesterol decreasing, but HDL-cholesterol increasing properties of Mangiferin has been verified in many animal experiments (Miura et.al. 2001; Muruganandan et.al. 2005).

Mangiferin is strongly lipolytic (Yoshikawa et.al. 2002).

When hamsters were fed high fat diet together with either 50 mg/kg BW or 150 mg/kg BW Mangiferin daily, body weight ($p < 0.05$), fat mass ($p < 0.05$) and triglycerides ($p < 0.05$) decreased significantly in test group, compared to control group (Guo et.al. 2011).

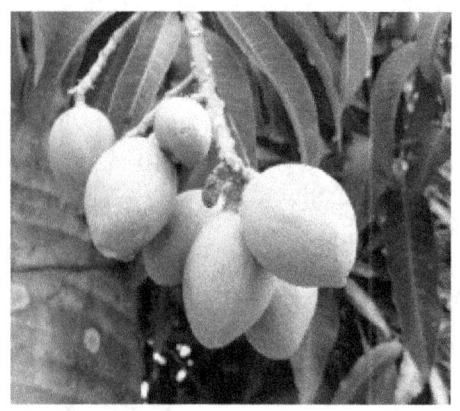

Mango

(Mangifera Indica)

Mango is a delicious tropical fruit and normally available all around the year in markets.

Mango has fat mass decreasing properties.

When mice were given high fat diet and 1% Mango daily, for 8 weeks, fat mass decreased by 36.9% ($p < 0.05$) in test group, compared to the control group. Also total cholesterol decreased by 14.2% ($p < 0.05$), blood sugar decreased by 32.2% ($p < 0.05$) and Leptin decreased by 80% ($p < 0.05$) in test group, compared to the control group (Lucas et.al. 2011).

Also in cell experiments Mango decreases fat mass (Taing et.al. 2012).

Mango tree, leaves

(Mangifera Indica)

Mango fruit is the familiar, delicious tropical fruit. But Mango tree leaves contain much higher amounts of flavonoids and polyphenols, than the fruit. Mango tree leaves are used in Asia, especially in India against diabetes, viral infections, bacterial infections, high blood pressure etc. The leaves and bark contain large amounts of Mangiferin, which is known to decrease body weight.

Mango tree leaves have body weight decreasing properties.

When diabetic rats were given daily either 30 mg, 50 mg or 70 mg Mango tree leaves water extract, for 42 days, body weight in test groups were 8.78% (p < 0.05), 10.6% (p < 0.05) and 14.88% (p < 0.05) lower, compared to control group. Also triglycerides were significantly (p < 0.05) lower in each test group, compared to control group (Morsi et.al. 2010).

The body weight, triglycerides, total cholesterol, LDL-cholesterol and VLDL-cholesterol decreasing, but HDL-cholesterol increasing properties of Mango tree leaves has been verified also in other experiments (Moreno et.al. 2006; Shah et.al. 2010).

Mangosteen

(Garcinia Mangostana)

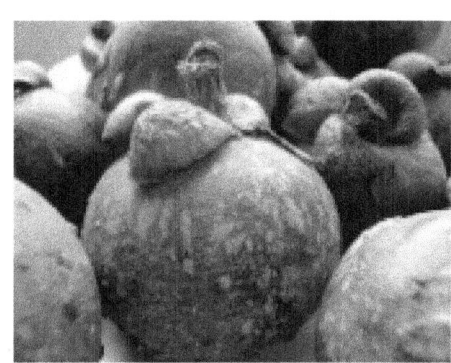

Mangosteen is a delicious tropical fruit. In Asia it has long time been used in obesity treatment. It contains large amounts of biologically active anti-inflammatory compounds.

Mangosteen has body weight decreasing properties.

When 11 volunteers were given 1.7 dl Mangosteen juice daily, for 8 weeks, the BMI decreased significantly by an average of 2.0 units (34 → 32; p = 0.006), compared to the 8 volunteer control group, where BMI increased by an average of 1.0 units (34 → 35) (Udani et.al. 2009). This was a double blind experiment.

Mashparni

(Teramnus Labialis)

Mashparni or Blue Swiss is an edible medicinal plant, which grows in Asia, Africa and South-America. The edible seeds contain 22.8% protein. The whole plant is aphrodisiac and used also against tuberculosis, rheumatism and catarrhs.

When rats were given high fat diet and either 250 mg/kg BW or 500 mg/kg BW Mashparni methanol extract daily, for 9 weeks, body weight was 14.7% (p < 0.05) and 29.6% (p < 0.05) lower in test groups, compared to control group. Also total cholesterol, LDL-cholesterol, VLDL-cholesterol and triglycerides were significantly (p < 0.05 in all parameters) lower, but HDL-cholesterol was significantly (p < 0.05) higher in test groups, compared to control group (Alagumanivasagam et.al. 2011).

Mate tea

(Ilex Paraguariensis)

Mate tree is a small tree, which originates from South-America. The tea made from its leaves is called Yerba Mate in Spanish. The tea is commonly drank in Chile, Argentina, Uruguay, Paraguay and Brazil as a stimulating and healthy drink. Mate tea contains large amounts of Caffeine, Theobromine, Chlorogenic acid, Saponins and Polyphenols.

Mate tea has body weight decreasing properties.

When 60 obese volunteers were given 3.0 grams Mate extract daily, for 6 weeks, the body fat-% decreased by 0.9% ($p = 0.04$) and the body fat mass decreased by 0.7 kg ($p = 0.04$), compared to the control group (Kim et.al. 2012). This was a double blind experiment.

When 48 volunteers were given YGD extract, which contains Mate, Guarana and Damiana extracts, 3 pills before each meal, for 45 days, body weight decreased by 5.1 kg ($p < 0.05$), compared to the control group (Andersen et.al. 2001). This was a double blind experiment.

When diabetic mice were given Mate tea water extract 100 mg/kg daily, for 7 days, body weight increased by 7.2%, being significantly ($p < 0.05$) lower, than the 16.3% increase in the control group (Hussein et.al. 2011).

When mice were given Mate tea water extract 100 mg/kg daily, for 3 weeks, body weight increased by 3.5%, being significantly ($p < 0.05$) lower than the 5.8% increase in the control group (Hussein et.al. 2011).

When hyperlipidemic mice were given Mate tea 1.0 g/kg daily, for 8 weeks, body weight was 7.4% ($p < 0.05$) lower, than in the control group, after this 8 weeks test period (Arcari et.al. 2009).

The body weight ($p < 0.01$) decreasing properties of Mate tea has been verified also in experiments with rats (Przygodda et.al. 2010; Kan et.al. 2012).

MCT oils

MCT short name comes from Medium Chain Triglycerides, which are C6-C12 carbon number fatty acid esters of glycerol. The best sources of MCT oils are coconut oil and palm kernel oil, which can contain over 60% of MCT oils. The fatty acids in these oils are Caproic acid (C6), Caprylic acid (C8), Capric acid (C10) and Lauric acid (C12). MCT oils are popularly used among sportsmen and also in hospitals, when treating patients with malnutrition. The ordinary vegetable oils are so called LCT (Long Chain Triglyceride) oils. MCT oils diffuse passively into the portal system, and they do not need bile acids or energy for absorption.

MCT oils have body weight and body fat mass decreasing properties.

When 73 volunteers were given daily either 5 grams MCT oil or 5 grams LCT oils (from rapeseed oil and soybean oil), for 12 weeks, body weight decreased by 5.7% (4.2 kg: 70.5 kg → 66.3 kg; $p < 0.05$), fat mass decreased by 3.8 kg (21.5%: 18.6 kg → 14.8 kg; $p < 0.05$) and waist circumference decreased by 5.1 cm (5.7%: 88.1 cm → 83.0 cm; $p < 0.05$) in test group. The changes in control group were 4.1% (2.9 kg: 67.6 kg → 64.7 kg), 2.3 kg (12.6%: 17.8 kg → 15.5 kg) and 3.3 cm (3.7%: 87.8 cm → 84.4 cm). The changes were significantly ($p < 0.05$) more in test group, compared to control group (Nosdaka et.al. 2003).

The body weight and body fat mass decreasing properties of MCT oils has been verified in great number of double blind experiments with human volunteers (Tsuji et.al. 2001; Kasai et.al. 2003; Han et.al. 2007; St-Onge et.al. 2008; Xue et.al. 2009; Zhang et.al. 2010; Xue et.al. 2009; Zhang et.al. 2009; Liu et.al. 2009; Takeuchi et.al. 2008; Costa et.al. 2012).

Melatonin

Melatonin is the famous sleep hormone, which is made in the body especially at night time, when there is little light. Melatonin is made from the amino acid Tryptophan in food. Melatonin is a strong antioxidant, and it strongly stimulates all the natural antioxidants in human body, such as SOD (Superoxide dismutase), GSH (Reduced Glutathione), Catalase, GR (Glutathione Reductase) etc. Melatonin is essential for good sleep quality. Alcohol use inhibits Melatonin biosynthesis, and deteriorates sleep quality.

Melatonin has body weight and body fat mass decreasing properties.

When middle-aged rats were given ordinary food and 4 micrograms Melatonin/ml in drinking water daily, for 12 weeks, body weight was 7% ($p < 0.05$), fat mass was 4.4%, Leptin was 33% ($p < 0.05$) and Insulin was 25% ($p < 0.05$) lower in test group, compared to control group, which was given pure water (Wolden-Hansen et.al. 2000).

When type 2 diabetic rats were given 1.1 mg Melatonin daily, for 30 days, bodyweight was 8.3% ($p < 0.001$), triglycerides were 30% ($p < 0.05$), total cholesterol was 27% ($p < 0.001$), Leptin was 35% ($p < 0.01$) and Insulin was 33% ($p < 0.01$) lower in test group, compared to control group (Nishida et.al. 2002).

The body weight, fat mass, triglycerides, Leptin, blood sugar and Insulin decreasing properties of Melatonin has been verified in great many animal experiments with mice and rats (Markova et.al. 2004; Rio-Lugo et.al. 2010; Hussein et.al. 2007; Bojkova et.al. 2008; Sanchez-Mateos et.al. 2007; Rasmussen et.al. 1999; Ciortea et.al. 2011; Nduhirabandi et.al. 2011; Puchalski et.al. 2003; Prunet-Marcassus et.al. 2003).

Milk Vetch, root

(Astragalus Membranaceus)

Milk Vetch root is a very old and famous Chinese medicinal plant. Its Chinese name is HUANG QI. The root is immunostimulant, antiviral, hypotensive and decreases triglycerides and cholesterol.

Milk Vetch root has body weight and body fat mass decreasing properties.

When type 2 diabetic rats were given 400 mg/kg BW Milk Vetch root polysaccharides in their daily food, for 5 weeks, body weight in test group was 6.8% ($p < 0.05$) lower, compared to control group (Wu et.al. 2005).

The Milk Vetch root body weight, body fat mass, triglycerides and total cholesterol decreasing but Adinopectin increasing properties has been verified in great many animal experiments (Ryu et.al. 1998; Mao et.al. 2009; Li et.al. 2010; Mao et.al. 2009; Deng et.al. 2009; Zhang et.al. 2011; Jiangwei et.al. 2011; Xu et.al. 2009; Juan et.al. 2011).

Mioga, Japanese Ginger

(Zingiber Mioga)

Mioga or Japanese Ginger is a very popular vegetable in Japan and Korea. The delicious flower buds and flavorful shoots are normally used.

When mice, which weighted 21 grams, were given 50 mg dried Mioga daily, for 13 days, had 10.4% ($p < 0.01$) lower body weight, compared to control group. Also fat mass was 33.8% ($p < 0.01$) lower in test group, compared to control group (Iwashita et.al. 2001).

Monkey head mushroom

(Hericium Erinaceus)

Monkey head mushroom is a very popular edible mushroom in China, Japan and Korea. It is also used for medical purposes.

Monkey head mushroom has body weight and fat mass decreasing properties.

When obese mice were fed high fat diet together with 2% Ethanol extract of Monkey head mushroom daily, for 4 weeks, body weight in test group was 42.4% ($p < 0.01$) lower, compared to contol group. Also total fat mass was 16.0% ($p < 0.05$) lower in test group, compared to control group. Triglycerides were 27.1% ($p < 0.01$) lower in test group, compared to control group (Hiwatashi et.al. 2010).

Morolo

(Annona Crassiflora)

Morolo is a delicious fruit, which grows in Brazil and Paraguay. The fruit peel and seeds contain very large amounts of differet antioxidants, such as Rutin, Ferulic acid, Xanthoxylin, Caffeic acid, Malic acid etc.

Morolo seeds have body weight decreasing properties.

When rats were given Morolo seeds water extract daily, for 14 days, body weight gain was 28% ($p < 0.05$) lower in test group, compared to control group (Roesier et.al. 2011). The daily water extract dose corresponds to 50 mg GAE/kg BW (GAE = Gallic Acid Equivalent).

Mulberry tree leaves and fruits

(Morus Alba, Morus Sp.)

Mulberry tree leaves are the only food source of silkworms. The leaves contain large amount of antioxidants, such as Resveratrol, Quercetin, Rutin and GABA. Mulberry leaves are used as a medicine against high blood pressure, high cholesterol levels and high blood sugar values. Mulberry fruits are delicious to eat and they can be dried.

Mulberry tree leaves and fruits have body weight and body fat mass decreasing properties.

When obese rats were given high fat food and 5% Mulberry leaves water extract daily, for 6 weeks, body weight increased in test group by 4.6%, being significantly ($p < 0.05$) lower, than the 10.8% body weight increase in control group. Also, when obese rats were given a high sugar diet with 5% Mulberry leaves water extract daily, for 6 weeks, body weight increased in test group by 3.3%, being significantly ($p < 0.05$) lower, than the 8.35% body weight increase in control group (Kim et.al. 2011). Also body fat mass was significantly ($p < 0.05$) lower in test group, compared to contol group.

Also in other experiments with mice (Oh et.al. 2009) and fat cells (Naowaboot et.al. 2012) Mulberry leaves decrease body weigt and fat mass.

When 10 volunteers with serum triglyceride value higher than 200 mg/dl, were given Mulberry Leaves extract 36 mg daily, for 12 weeks, body weight decreased by 2.1 kg (79.2 kg → 77.1 kg), triglycerides decreased by 19.2% (352 mg/dl → 252 mg/dl; $p = 0.058$) and diastolic blood pressure decreased by 3 mmHg (84 mmHg → 81 mmHg) (Kojima et.al. 2010). Apidonectin decreased by 26.9% ($p = 0.001$) and Leptin decreased by 9.6% ($p = 0.001$) in test group.

When 14 type 2 diabetic volunteers were given Mulberry leaves extract 1000 mg daily, for 12 weeks, LDL-cholesterol decreased by 10.7% ($p < 0.05$) and triglycerides decreased by 26.5% ($p < 0.01$), compared to the 9 person control group (Yang et.al. 2006). This was a double blind experiment.

When rats were given Mulberry fruit ethanol extract 200 mg/BW daily, for 6 weeks, body weight was by average 9.6% lower in test group, compared to control group. Also total cholesterol ($p < 0.05$) and triglycerides ($p < 0.05$) were significantly lower, but HDL-cholesterol ($p < 0.05$) significantly higher in test group, compared to control group (Choi et.al. 2007).

The Mulberry fruit body weight, triglycerides and total cholesterol decreasing but HDL-cholesterol increasing properties has been verified also in other experiments with rats (Yang et.al. 2010; Ha et.al. 2011).

Mulberry fruit water extract reduced lipid accumulation, suppressed fatty acid synthesis and stimulated fatty acid oxidation in experiments with hepatic cells (Ou et.al. 2011).

Mundi

(Sphaeranthus Indicus)

Mundi is a very old, annual medicinal plant in India. It is used as aphrodisiac and against diabetes, epilepsy and bronchitis. The English name is East Indian Globe Thistle.

The flowering heads of Mundi have body weight decreasing properties.

When obese rats were given high fat diet and 500 mg/kg BW Mundi flowering heads water extract daily, for 8 days, body weight decreased by 17.34% (19.42 grams) in test group, but increased by 34.12% (38.35 grams) in control group. Also triglycerides, total cholesterol and LDL-cholesterol decreased significantly in test group, compared to control group (Pande et.al. 2009).

When 30 obese volunteers were given daily 800 mg combined Mundi flower and Mangostan fruit extract, for 8 weeks, body weight was 3.7 kg ($p < 0.05$) and waist circumference was 5 cm ($p < 0.05$) lower in test group, compared to 30 person control group (Lau et.al. 2011). This was a double blind experiment.

Mustak

(Cyperus Rotundus)

Coco-grass or Mustak, as it is called in India, is an ancient food- and medicinal plant. This grass like plant makes underground, 2 – 3 cm long edible tubers. These tubers are used in India against obesity. The cultivation of Mustak is extremely easy, and it will easily spread itself.

Mustak tubers have body weight and fat mass decreasing properties.

When obese rats were given in their daily food 4 grams/kg BW Mustak tubers, for 4 weeks, body weight gain was 27.3% ($p < 0.05$) lower in test group, compared to control group. Also triglycerides, total cholesterol and LDL-cholesterol were significantly ($p < 0.05$ in all parameters) lower, but HDL-cholesterol was significantly ($p < 0.05$) higher in test group, compared to control group (Al-Tellawy et.al. 2011).

In many experiments with rats it has been verified, that Mustak tubers decrease body weight and body fat mass, compared to control groups (Lemaure et.al. 2007; Bambhole et.al. 1993; Bambhole et.al. 1988).

Also in experiments with human volunteers, Mustak tubers decrease body weight, compared to control groups (Bambhole et.al. 1984; Karnick et.al. 1992; Mangal et.al. 2009).

Myricetin

Myricetin is a common flavonoid in many plants. Good dietary sources are peas, beans, cabbage, broccoli, cauliflower, spinach, eggplant, bell pepper, carrot, strawberry, apple, plum, apricot, guava and tea.

Myricetin has body weight and body fat mass decreasing properties.

When obese rats were given high fat diet and either 75 mg/kg BW, 150 mg/kg BW or 300 mg/kg BW Myricetin daily, for 8 weeks, body weight gain was 18.3% ($p < 0.05$), 39.4% ($p < 0.05$) and 53.4% ($p < 0.05$) lower in test group, compared to control group. Total fat mass was 7.0% ($p < 0.05$), 16.5% ($p < 0.05$) and 24.4% ($p < 0.05$) lower in test groups, compared to control group (Chang et.al. 2012).

NAC

(N-Acetyl-L-Cysteine)

NAC is the acetylated form of the sulfur containing amino acid, L-Cysteine. Both NAC and L-Cysteine exist in nature in different proteins. NAC is a very strong antioxidant, and it has a strong mucolytic effect. For this reason it is used in bronchitis and asthma. In experiments with cells, it increases the lifetime of cells. It also stimulates the biosynthesis of reduced Glutathione, GSH, which is a strong antioxidant in human cells.

NAC has body weight and body fat mass decreasing properties.

When mice were fed high fat diet and 1 grams/liter of NAC in their drinking water as a daily drink, for 4 weeks, body weight in test group was 15.0% ($p < 0.05$) lower, compared to control group. Also the activity of FAS enzyme was significantly ($p < 0.05$) reduced, as was the contents of triglycerides ($p < 0.05$) and total cholesterol ($p < 0.05$) in liver, compared to control group (Lin et.al. 2008).

The body weight, body fat mass, triglycerides and Leptin decreasing properties of NAC has been verified in great many experiments with mice and rats (Lin et.al. 2004; Diniz et.al. 2006; Elshorbagy et.al. 2012; Calzadilla et.al. 2011; Pechanova et.al. 2006; Kim et.al. 2006; Novelli et.al. 2009).

Narrowleaf Sida, leaves

(Sida Rhomboidea)

Narrowleaf Sida is a medicinal plant, which is used in India against obesity and diabetes.

Narrowleaf Sida leaves have body weight and fat mass decreasing properties.

When mice were given high fat diet and 1% Narrowleaf Sida leaves hot water extract daily, for 16 weeks, body weight was 25.6% ($p < 0.001$) and fat mass was 23.4% ($p < 0.001$) lower in test group, compared to control group. Also triglycerides and total cholesterol were significantly lower in test group, compared to control group (Thounaojam et.al. 2010).

The body weight and fat mass decreasing properties of Narrowleaf Sida leaves has been verified in many experimentes with mice and rats (Thounaojam et.al. 2011; Patel et.al. 2009; Thounaojam et.al. 2009; Thounaojam et.al. 2009).

Nobiletin

Nobiletin is a flavonoid, which exist in the peels and white matter of several Citrus species. Especially the following Citrus species raw peels contain large amounts of Nobiletin: Citrus Depressa, Citrus Sunki, Citrus Tachibana and Citrus Platymamma (Choi et.al. 2007).

Nobiletin has body weight and fat mass decreasing properties.

When rats were given high fat diet and 0.1% Nobiletin in their daily food, for 4 weeks, body weight was 3.3% ($p < 0.05$) and body fat mass was 32.6% ($p < 0.05$) in test group, compared to control group (Nagata et.al. 2010).

The same body weight and body fat mass decreasing results of Nobiletin has been achieved also in other experiments with mice (Lee et.al. 2012; Mulvihill et.al. 2011).

Nomame tea

(Cassia Mimosoides syn. Chamaecrista Nomame)

Nomame tea is made from the Feather-leaved cassia, Cassia Mimosoides, leaves. It is used as a healthy tea in Japan and China.

Nomame tea has body weight decreasing properties.

Nomame tea inhibits very strongly the Lipase enzyme (Shimura et.al. 1992).

When rats were given high fat diet and 2.5% Nomame tea ethanol extract in their daily food, for 8 weeks, body weight in test group was 15.2% (p < 0.01) lower, compared to control group (Yamamoto et.al. 2000).

Oleanolic acid

Oleanolic acid is a natural triterpenoid, which exists in many plants and fruits, especially in clove, grapes, pomegranate and olive leaves. The dietary wine pomace, which is the byproduct of winemaking, consisting of seeds, skins, pulp etc. residue of grapes, is especially rich Oleanolic acid source. It can contain up to 4 – 11 g/100 g Oleanolic acid (Yunoki et.al. 2008).

Oleanolic acid has body weight and fat mass decreasing properties.

When obese mice were given high fat diet and 10 mg/kg BW Oleanolic acid daily, for 15 weeks, body weight was 11.5% (p < 0.05) and body fat mass was 45% (p < 0.05) lower in test group, compared to control group (Melo et.al. 2010).

Also in another experiment with mice, Oleanolic acid decreased body weight in test group, compared to control group (Buus et.al. 2011).

Oleanolic acid decreases strongly plasme triglycerides and the expression of lipogenic genes in experiments with rats (Yunoki et.al. 2008).

Olive tree leaf

(Olea Europaea)

Olive tree grows all around the Mediterranian area. The Olive fruits and the Olive oil has been used as food for thousands of years. Olive tree leaf is widely used against high blood pressure and high cholesterol levels. Olive tree leaf contains, just like Extra Virgin Olive oil, large quantities of healthy polyphenols and triterpenes, such as Oleuropin, Hydroxytyrosol and Oleanolic acid. Oleuropin content of dried leaves is over 2 weight-%.

Olive tree leaf and its poyphenols and triterpenes have body weight and fat mass decreasing properties.

When pigs were given in their daily diet 5% Olive tree leaves, for 44 days, body weight in test group was 12.7% (p < 0.05) lower, compared to control group (Paiva-Martins et.al. 2009).

When rats were given corn starch and 3% Olive tree leaf ethanol extract daily, for 16 weeks, body weight decreased by 6.0% (p < 0.05) and body fat mass decreased by 48.6% (p < 0.0001) in test group, compared to control group (Poudyal et.al. 2010).

The body weight and body fat mass decreasing properties of Olive tree leaf and its polyphenols and triterpenes has been verified in many experiments with mice and rats (Al-Qarawi et.al. 2002; Onderoglu et.al. 1999; Melo et.al. 2010; Oi-Kano et.al. 2012; Ebaid et.al. 2010).

When 66 either overweight (BMI=28.5) or obese (BMI=32.1) volunteers were given dried Olive tree leaves 150 mg daily, for 3 months, body mass index BMI decreased by 4.0 units (28.5 → 24.5; $p < 0.05$) in overweight group, and by 4.6 units (32.1 → 27.5; $p < 0.05$) in obese groups (Said et.al. 2011). The food supplement, Weightlevel, contained also 180 mg dried leaves of Alchemilla Vulgaris, 60 mg of dried leaves of Mentha Longifolia and 75 mg of dried leaves of Cuminum Cyminum)

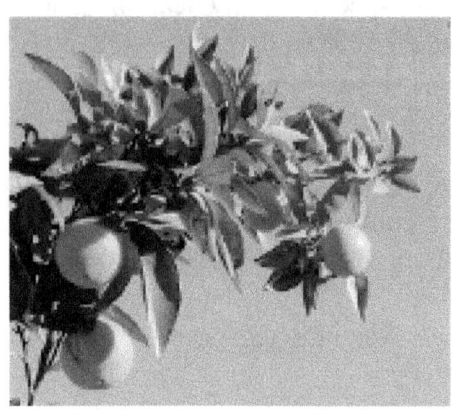

Orange, peel

(Citrus Sinensis)

Orange is a delicious fruit familiar to everybody. It can be purchased all around the year as a fresh fruit. Normally only the pulp is eaten, but orange peel contains many times more the healthy flavonoids, compared to pulp. Also the peel contains large amount of dietary fiber, pectin, which is known to have body weight and cholesterol decreasing properties.

Orange peel has body weight and body fat mass decreasing properties.

When mice were given high fat diet and 0.2% orange peel extract daily, for 10 weeks, body weight gain was 32% ($p < 0.05$) and body fat mass was 21% ($p < 0.05$) lower in test group, compared to control group (Huang et.al. 2009).

When chicken were fed ordinary maize and soybean meal together with 13.3% orange peel daily, for 35 days, body weight was 33.7% ($p < 0.05$) lower in test group, compared to control group (Oluremi et.al. 2010).

When obese rats were fed high fat diet and 5% orange peel daily, for 8 weeks, body weight gain in test group was 71.7% ($p < 0.05$) lower, compared to control group. Also triglycerides were 50.5% ($p < 0.05$), total cholesterol was 44.3% ($p < 0.05$) and LDL-cholesterol was 62.7% ($p < 0.05$) lower, but HDL-cholesterol was 31.9% ($p < 0.05$) higher in test group, compared to control group (Abdelbaky et.al. 2009).

Oyster mushroom

(Pleurotus Ostreatus, Pleurotus Sp.)

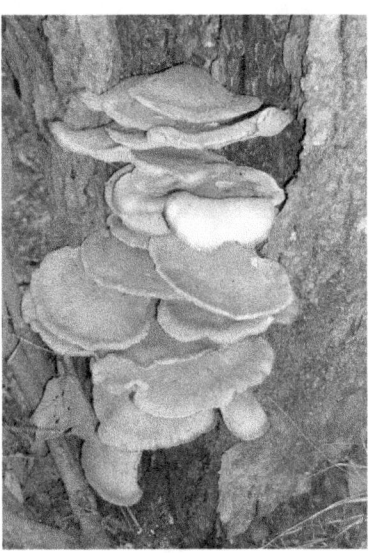

Oyster mushroom is a delicious edible mushroom, which is cultivated all over the World. It can be purchased both fresh and drid. It is known to decrease cholesterol and triglycerides.

Oyster mushroom has body weight decreasing properties.

When hypercholesterolemic rats were given 5% Oyster mushroom daily, for 42 days, body weight decreased by 16.89% ($p < 0.05$), total cholesterol decreased by 30.18% ($p < 0.05$), LDL-cholesterol decreased by 59.62% ($p < 0.05$) and triglycerides decreased by 52.75% ($p < 0.05$) in test group, compared to the control group (Alam et.al. 2011).

The body weight, total cholesterol, LDL-cholesterol and triglycerides decreasing properties of Oyster mushroom has been verified in a large number of experiments (Alam et.al. 2009; Yoon et.al. 2012; Refaie et.al. 2009; Ala et.al. 2011; Alam et.al. 2011).

Ox Knee, root

(Achyranthes Bidentata)

Ox Knee is a very old and famous Chinese medicinal plant. Root is the part used. It is used against broken bones, osteoporosis and in animal experiments it increases the swimming endurance. The Chinese name is NIU XI.

Ox Knee root has body weight decreasing properties.

When obese OVX rats were given either 25 mg/kg BW or 100 mg/kg BW Ox Knee root butanol extract daily, for 6 weeks, body weight in test groups were 7.1% ($p < 0.05$) and 14.2% ($p < 0.05$) lower, compared to control group (He et.al. 2010).

Pagoda tree, fruit

(Sophora Japonica)

Pagoda tree fruits are official medicine in Chinese and Korean Pharmacopeia.The fruits contain large amounts of flavonoids, Quercetin, Rutin, Kaempferol, Genistein etc.

Pagoda tree fruits have body weight and body fat mass decreasing properties.

When obese mice were given high fat diet and either 1% or 5% Pagoda tree fruit powder daily, for 4 weeks, body weight were 8.3% ($p < 0.05$) and 15.1% ($p < 0.05$), and body fat masses were 48% ($p < 0.05$) and 58% ($p < 0.05$) lower in test groups, compared to control group. Also blood sugar, triglycerides and total cholesterol were significantly ($p < 0.05$) lower in test groups, compared to control group (Park et.al. 2009).

Papaya, fruit

(Papaya Carica)

Papaya is a delicious tropical fruit, available all around the year as fresh, dried or canned product. It is known to decrease high cholesterol and high blood pressure.

Papaya fruit has body weight decreasing properties.

When rats were given high fat diet and either 200 mg/kg BW or 600 mg/kg BW Papaya fruit water extract daily, for 45 days, body weights in test groups were 17.4% ($p < 0.05$) and 23.9% ($p < 0.05$) lower, compared to control group. Also triglycerides were 20.8% and 41.9% ($p < 0.05$), total cholesterol was 7.0% and 39.8% ($p < 0.05$), LDL-cholesterol was 7.2% and 67.9% ($p < 0.05$) and VLDL-cholesterol was 16.5% and 41.9% ($p < 0.05$) lower, but HDL-cholesterol was 5.3% and 42.8% ($p < 0.05$) higher in test groups, compared to control group (Athesh et.al. 2012).

Parsley

(Petroselinum Crispum)

and Apigenin

Parsley is a familiar, extremely healthy vegetable. Its cultivation is very easy. It can be purchased as dry all around the year. Parsley is the best source of the Flavonoid Apigenin, which is a strong antioxidant, and has also anti-inflammatory, diuretic and testosterone stimulating properties.

Parsley and Apigenin have body weight decreasing properties.

When rats were given normal diet and 3 times weekly 10 mg/kg BW Apigenin, for 15 weeks, body weight in test group was 18.8% ($p < 0.0001$) lower, compared to control group (Park et.al. 2008).

Also in another experiment with mice Apigenin decreased body weight ($p < 0.05$) and food intake ($p < 0.05$) significantly, compared to control group, when given at a daily dose of 0.05%, for 4 weeks (Myoung et.al. 2010).

When obese rats were given high fat diet and either 10%, 15% or 20% Parsley in their daily diet, for 6 weeks, body weight gain in test groups were 28.33% ($p < 0.05$), 29.84% ($p < 0.05$) and 34.57% ($p < 0.05$) lower, compared to control group. Also triglycerides ($p < 0.05$), total cholesterol ($p < 0.05$), LDL-cholesterol ($p < 0.05$) and VLDL-cholesterol ($p < 0.05$) were significantly lower, but HDL-cholesterol (p < 0.05) was significantly higher in test groups, compared to control group (El-Kherbawy et.al. 2011).

Parwal

(Trichosanthes Dioica)

Parwal is a Cucumber like vegetable, which is widely cultivated in India as a food. It has large amounts of protein and vitamins. The English name is Pointed Gourd.

Parwal has body weight decreasing properties.

When rats were given Parwal water extract 50 mg/kg BW daily, for 15 days, body weight decreased by 13.5% (p < 0.001) in the test group, compared to the control group. Also triglycerides (p < 0.05) and total cholesterol (p < 0.05) decreased signifiantly in the Parwal group, compared to the control group (Sharmal et.al. 2007).

Passion fruit

(Passiflora Edulis, Passiflora Sp.)

Passion fruit is a delicious tropical fruit, and normally only the fruit pulp is used. But the fruit peel is eatable, and can be ground and dried and mixed to other foods. The peel is known to decrease blood pressure, total cholesterol, LDL-cholesterol and triglycerides, but it increases HDL-cholesterol in human experiments. It also decreases pain in knee arthritis and asthma symptoms in human experiments.

When 19 volunteers were given dried Passion fruit peel flour 30 grams daily, for 2 months, body weight decreased by 1.84 kg (73.76 kg → 71.92 kg; p < 0.0001), compared to control group. Also total cholesterol decreased by 18.2% (p < 0.0001) and LDL-cholesterol decreased by 20.6% (p = 0.0034), compared to the control group (Ramos et.al. 2007).

In another experiment with human volunteers, Passion fruit peel decreased significantly triglycerides, but increased HDL-cholesterol (Janebro et.al. 2008).

In experiments with rats, Passion fruit peel decreased significantly body weight, total cholesterol and triglycerides, but increases HDL-cholesterol (Barbalho et.al. 2012).

Pectin

Pectins are polysaccharides, contained in the walls of plant cells. Pectin is white or light brown in color, and it is prepared commercially from citrus fruit peels or apple molasses. Apples contain 0.5 – 1.5%, bananas contain 0.5 – 1.0%, carrots contain 0.6 – 1.0%, oranges contain 0.3 – 0.8% but citrus fruit peels contain up to 30% Pectin. Extraction of Pectin from citrus fruit peels is very simple. Pectin is known to have cholesterol decreasing properties.

Pectin has body weight and fat mass decreasing properties.

When rats were given high fat diet (20% fat) and Pectin 10% of daily food, for 9 weeks, body weight was 12.7% ($p < 0.05$) and body fat mass was 45% ($p < 0.05$) lower in test group, compared to control group. Also triglycerides decreased by 33.7% ($p < 0.05$), total cholesterol decreased by 10.6% ($p < 0.05$) and LDL-cholesterol decreased by 31.8% ($p < 0.05$) but HDL-cholesterol increased by 47.3% ($p < 0.05$) in test group, compared to control group. In experiments with 3T3-L1 fat cells, Pectin decreased Leptin by 85% ($p < 0.05$), compared to control value (Kwon et.al. 2005).

Also in another experiment with rats, Pectin decreased body weight, triglycerides and total cholesterol significantly, compared to control group (Sanchez et.al. 2008).

When 30 obese volunteers were given in their daily ordinary food noodles or noodles with 12% per weight of Pectin, for 30 days, body weight decreased by 3.05% (1.78 kg: 58.15 kg → 56.37 kg), waist circumference decreased by 5.41% and hip circumference decreased by 2.88% in test group, but in the 30 person control group body weight increased by 0.16% (0.9 kg: 58.33 kg → 58.42 kg), waist circumference decreased by 0.01% and hip circumference increased by 0.04% (Jitpukdeebodintra et.al. 2009).

When 14 obese volunteers were given daily 2.78 grams Pectin with their ordinary daily food, for 4 weeks, body weight decreased by 5.32 kg (5.84%: 88.07 kg → 82.75 kg), waist circumference decreased by 6.44 cm (7.20%: 90.95 cm → 84.51 cm), hip circumference decreased by 5.21 cm (4.43%: 116.59 cm → 11.38 cm), compared to original values (El-Shebni et.al. 1988).

Pepino

(Solanum Muricatum)

Pepino is a delicious fruit, which is grown in many countries. Pepino belongs to the same Solanum-group as Eggplant.

Pepino has body weight, body fat mass, triglycerides and total cholesterol decreasing properties.

When type 2 diabetic mice were given in their daily diet either 1%, 2% or 5% Pepino, for 8 weeks, body fat mass decreased by 29.4% ($p < 0.05$), 32.4% ($p < 0.05$) and 33.6% ($p < 0.05$), compared to the control group. Body weight decreased in all test groups by an average of 6.2%, compared to the control group. Triglycerides decreased by 19.5% ($p < 0.05$), 23.9% ($p < 0.05$) and 35.8% ($p < 0.05$), compared to the control group. Total cholesterol decreased by 5.3% (p < 0.05), 22.7% (p < 0.05) and 23.3% (p < 0.05) compared to the control group (Wang et.al. 2012).

Peppermint

(Mentha Piperita)

Peppermint is a very healthy vegetable, tea and spice, known to everybod. Its cultivation is very easy.

Peppermint has body weight decreasing properties.

When rats were given fructose containing diet and 250 mg/kg BW Peppermint water extract daily, for 3 weeks, body weight decreased by 18.2% (p < 0.05) in test group, compared to control group. Also total cholesterol decreased by 30.5% (p < 0.05), LDL-cholesterol decreased by 53.6% (p < 0.05), VLDL-cholesterol decreased by 45.6% (p < 0.05) and triglycerides decreased by 45.5% (p < 0.05), but HDL-cholesterol increased by 102.7% (p < 0.05), compared to control group (Badal et.al. 2011).

In another experiment with rats Peppermint decreased significantly body weight, total cholesterol, LDL-cholesterol and triglycerides, but increased HDL-cholesterol, compared to control group (Barbalho et.al. 2009).

When 25 volunteers were given 40 grams Peppermint daily, for 4 weeks, body mass index BMI decreased in 48.7% of volunteers. In the whole group LDL-cholesterol decreased by 20.7% (167.36 mg/dl → 132.6 mg/dl; p = 0.0163) and systolic blood pressure decreased by 7.4% (121.9 mmHg → 112.8 mmHg; p = 0.0101). Also total cholesterol decreased in 67% and triglycerides decreased in 58% of volunteers (Barbalho et.al. 2011).

Persimmon

(Diospyros Kaki)

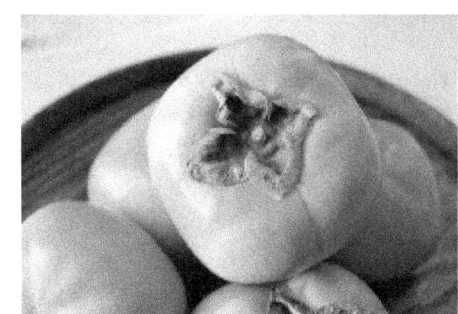

Persimmon or Sharon is a delicious fruit, which is known to decrease cholesterol and triglycerides.

Persimmon has body weight and fat mass decreasing properties.

When rats were given high fat diet together with 7% Persimmon daily, for 30 days, body weight decreased by 6.2% (p < 0.05) in test group, compared to the control group. Also total cholesterol, LDL-cholesterol and triglycerides decreased significantly (p < 0.05 in all parameters), compared to the control group (Al-Sayed et.al. 2009).

The body weight, fat mass, triglycerides and total cholesterol decreasing properties of Persimmon has been verified in other experiments with mice (Matsumoto et.al. 2008; Moon et.al. 2010).

Persimmon, leaves

(Diospyros Kaki)

Persimmon of Sharon is a delicious fruit. But the leaves of Persimmon tree are used as a functional healthy tea in Japan and Korea. This tea is known to decrease high blood pressure.

Persimmon tree leaves have body weight and fat mass decreasing properties.

When rats were given high fat diet together with 5% dried Persimmon leaves daily, for 6 weeks, body weight in test group was 8.4% ($p < 0.05$) lower, compared to control group. Total fat mass was 10.0% ($p < 0.05$) lower in test group, compared to control group. Triglycerides were 31.2% ($p < 0.05$) and total cholesterol was 50.1% ($p < 0.05$) lower in test group, compared to control group (Lee et.al. 2006).

Phellinus Linteus mushroom

Phellinus Linteus is a medicinal mushroom, which grows on mulberry trees. It is a very famous medicinal mushroom in China, Korea and Japan, due to its anticancer properties. Its English name is Black Hoof fungus, Japanese name is Meshimakobu, Chinese name is Song Gen and its Korean name is Sanghwang.

Phellinus Linteus mushroom has body weight decreasing properties.

When obese rats were fed high fat diet together with either 50 mg/kg BW or 100 mg/kg BW Phellinus Linteus mushroom water extract daily, body weight gain in test groups were 5.8% ($p < 0.05$) and 30.1% ($p < 0.05$) lower, compared to control group. The body weight gain in high fat control group was 154.98 grams, in 50 mg/kg BW group 145.92 grams in 100 mg/kg BW group 108.25 grams. Also triglycerides ($p < 0.05$), total cholesterol ($p < 0.05$) and LDL-cholesterol ($p < 0.05$) were significantly lower, but HDL-cholesterol ($p < 0.05$) was significantly higher in test groups, compared to control group (Song et.al. 2010).

Phosphorous

Phosphorous is an essential mineral in human nutrition. The bones and teeth especially contain large amounts of phosphorous. ATP and Creatine phosphate are phosphorous containing molecules, which have critical role as energy sources in cells. The recommended dietary allowance RDA of phosphorous is between 700 – 1200 mg daily. Excellent sources of phosphorous are: Rice bran (1677 mg/100g), pumpkin seeds (1172 mg/100g), watermelon seeds (815 mg/100g), sunflower seeds (1158 mg/100g), wheat germ (1146 mg/100g), Parmesan cheese (807 mg/100g), sesame seeds (774 mg/100g), flax seed (642 mg/100g).

When 30 obese females were on low-energy diet for 8 weeks, and were given phosphate (Redusan Kombi, Pharma AB, Sweden) daily for 4 weeks, resting metabolic rate (RMR) was $12 - 19\%$ ($p < 0.05$) higher in test group, compared to placebo group. Also triiodothyronine T3 level was increased in test group, compared to placebo group. This was a double blind experiment (Nazar et.al. 1996).

The same kind of results has been achieved also in another experiment with obese females (Kaciuba-Uscilko et.al. 1993).

When 6 obese volunteers were given 750 mg Guggulsterones and 1650 mg phosphates daily, for 6 weeks, body weight was 2.3 kg ($p < 0.05$), fat mass was 2.9 kg ($p < 0.01$) and body fat-% was 2.0% ($p < 0.01$) lower in test group, compared to 6 person control group. This was a double blind experiment (Antonio et.al. 1999).

In double blind experiments with elite athletes, phosphates at a daily dose between $3 - 4$ grams, increases significantly maximum oxygen uptake VO2 max, aerobic endurance and mean power output (Kridet et.al. 1990; Cade et.al. 1984; Stewart et.al. 1990; Kreidet et.al. 1992; Folland et.al. 2008; Brewer et.al. 2012).

Pineapple, fruit and leaves

(Ananas Comosus)

Pineapple is the familiar delicious fruit, which is available all around the year in markets. All parts, fruit, stem and leaves, contain an enzyme called Bromelain, which is used both medicinally in various diseases and to tender meat. Pineapple fruit is also used all around the World against obesity, and in India it is mentioned in the famous Ayurveda medicine as a fruit against obesity (Chandrasekaran et.al. 2012). Bromelain exists only in fresh fruit, in heated or canned fruits there is no Bromelain, because heat destroys this enzyme.

Pineapple fruit and leaves have body weight and body fat mass decreasing properties.

In experiments with fat cells, Bromelain inhibits adipogenesis and 3T3-L1 adipocyte differentiation and stimulates lipolysis (Dave et.al. 2012).

When obese rats were given high fat diet and either 400 mg/kg BW or 600 mg/kg BW Pineapple leaves water extract daily, for 4 weeks, body weights were 6.4% ($p < 0.001$) and 22.3% ($p < 0.001$) lower, and fat masses were 25.1% ($p < 0.05$) and 40.2% ($p < 0.05$) lower in test groups, compared to control group. Triglycerides, total cholesterol, LDL-cholesterol and VLDL-cholesterol were significantly ($p < 0.001$) lower, but HDL-cholesterol was significantly ($p < 0.001$) higher in test groups, compared to control group (Vuyyuru et.al. 2012).

The triglycerides, total cholesterol and LDL-cholesterol decreasing but HDL-cholesterol increasing properties of Pineapple leaves has been verified also in other animal experiments (Xie et.al. 2005; Xie et.al. 2007).

Pole Butterflybush, flowers

(Buddleja Officinalis)

Pole Butterflybush grows in Western and Southern China, in Sichuan and Yunnan provinces. Its Chinese name is Mi Meng Hua. The spring flowers have been used for thousands of years in China as a medicine in great many eye diseases. They contain large amounts of flavonoids, saponins and terpenoids.

Pole Butterflybush flowers have body weight and body fat mass decreasing properties.

When mice were given high fat diet and 200 mg/kg BW Pole Butterflybush flower water extract daily, for 15 weeks, body weight was 10% ($p < 0.05$) and body fat mass was 55% ($p < 0.01$) lower in test group, compared to control group (Roh et.al. 2012).

Pomelo, peel

(Citrus Grandis)

Pomelo is a large, green and delicious Citrus fruit, which has a very thick, white peel. Normally only the fruit flesh is used, but the peel contains large amounts of healthy flavonoids.

Pomelo peel has body weight decreasing properties.

When obese mice were given high fat diet and 1200 mg/kg BW Pomelo peel ethanol extract daily, for 3 weeks, body weight was 32.0% ($p < 0.05$) lower in test group, compared to cotrol group. Also total cholesterol, LDL-cholesterol and triglycerides were significantly ($p < 0.05$) lower in test group, compared to control group (Lien et.al. 2010).

When rats were given high fat diet together with 1% Pomelo peel daily, for 10 weeks, body weight gain in test group was 6.9% ($p < 0.05$) lower, compared to control group. Also triglycerides, LDL-cholesterol and total cholesterol were significantly ($p < 0.05$) lower in test group, compared to control group (Hong et.al. 2010).

Prickly pear, fruit and seeds

(Opuntia Ficus Indica)

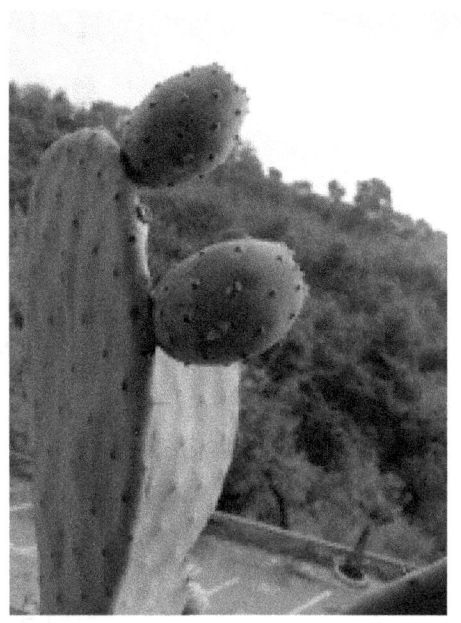

Prickly pear is a very healthy cactus fruit, which is cultivated all around the World. The fruit contains very strong antioxidants called Betalains.

Prickly pear fruit and seeds have body weight decreasing properties.

When 1/3 (33%) of ordinary food was replaced by Prickly pear seeds in rats daily food, for 63 days, body weight in test group was 18.0% (p < 0.05) lower, compared to control group (Ennouri et.al. 2006).

When rats were given Prickly pear fruit extract 240 mg/kg BW daily, for 7 days, body weight gain was significantly (p < 0.05) lower in test group, compared to control group. The fruit extract also significantly increased urine volune in test group (Bisson et.al. 2010).

When obese rats were given 5 mg NeOpuntia fiber from dried Prickly pear leaves, for 4 weeks, body weight in test group was 10.6% (p < 0.05) lower, compared to control group (Al-Tellawy et.al. 2011).

In diabetic rats Prickly pear fruit decreases significantly both blood glucose (p < 0.05) and total cholesterol (p < 0.05), but increases significantly (p < 0.05) HDL-cholesterol in test group, compared to control group (El-Razek et.al. 2011).

Propolis

Propolis is the wax, collected by honey bees, which contain large amount of different flavonoids and polyphenols. Propolis has many different health effects. It is antiviral, antibacterial, anti-inflammatory, and it decreases high blood pressure and high cholesterol levels.

Propolis has body weight and body fat mass decreasing properties.

When obese type 2 diabetic rats were given high fructose diet and 300 mg/kg BW Propolis daily, for 8 weeks, body weight in test group was 39.6% (p < 0.05) lower, compared to control group. Also Insulin and systolic blood pressure were significantly lower in test group, compared to control group (Zamami et.al. 2007).

The body weight and body fat mass decreasing properties of Propolis has been verified in many other experiments (Koya-Miyata et.al. 2009; Ichi et.al. 2009; Iio et.al. 2010).

Proso millet

(Panicum Miliaceum)

Proso millet has been cultivated for its grain over 7000 years. It is well adapted to many soil and climatic conditions. It needs very little water. It does not contain gluten.

Proso millet has body weight and fat mass decreasing properties.

When obese mice were given normal food and 1.0% Proso millet water extract daily, for 4 weeks, body weight was 8% ($p < 0.05$) and body fat mass was 22.2% ($p < 0.05$) lower in test group, compared to control group. Also triglycerides were 19.5% ($p < 0.05$) and total cholesterol was 16.2% ($p < 0.05$) lower, but HDL-cholesterol was 25.9% ($p < 0.05$) higher in test group, compared to control group (Park et.al. 2011).

The body weight and body fat mass decreasing properties of Proso millet has been verified also in another experiment with mice (Park et.al. 2012).

In experiments with cells, Proso millet inhibits strongly lipid accumulation into 3T3-L1 fat cells (Park et.al. 2011).

Pu-Erh tea

(Camellia Sinensis)

Pu-Erh tea is fermented green tea, which is produced especially in the Yunnan province, in southern China. The fermentation time can be over 10 years. Pu-Erh tea has many health properties. It is known to decrease high cholesterol and triglyceride levels. Pu-Erh tea contains extremely large amounts of polyphenols and flavonoids, up to 30% of dry weight.

Pu-Erh tea has body weight and body fat mass decreasing properties.

When rats were given normal diet and 1.5% Pu-Erh tea leaves daily, for 30 weeks, body weight in test group was 13.3% ($p < 0.001$) lower, compared to control group. Also triglycerides, total cholesterol and LDL-cholesterol were significantly ($p < 0.05$) lower in test group, compared to control group (Kuo et.al. 2005).

The body weight, body fat mass, triglycerides, total cholesterol, LDL-cholesterol, FAS enzyme activity and Leptin decreasing properties of Pu-Erh tea has been verified in great many experiments with mice and rats (Cao et.al. 2011; Huang et.al. 2012; Chiang et.al. 2005; Oi et.al. 2012; Gong et.al. 2010; Hou et.al. 2009).

When human volunteers were given 1.0 gram Pu-Erh tea leaves daily, for 3 months, body weight decreased by 1.2 kg ($p < 0.05$), total cholesterol decreased by 8.4% ($p < 0.01$), LDL-cholesterol decreased by 11.8% ($p < 0.01$) and triglycerides decreased by 8.4% ($p < 0.01$) in test group, being significantly more than in the control group (Fujita et.al. 2008). This was a double blind experiment with 47 volunteers.

Also in other experiments with human volunteers, Pu-Erh tea decreases significantly body weight, triglycerides, LDL-cholesterol and total cholesterol (Chu et.al. 2011; Fujita et.al. 2008).

Pumpkin, stem parts

(Cucurbita Moschata)

Pumpkin is a very popular vegetable all over the World. Its cultivation is very easy.

Pumpkin stem parts have body weight and body fat mass decreasing properties.

When mice were given high fat diet and 500 mg/kg BW Pumpkin stem parts water extract daily, for 8 weeks, body weight was 18% ($p < 0.05$) and body fat mass was 39.8% ($p < 0.05$) lower in test group, compared to control group (Choi et.al. 2007).

Purple Carrot

(Daucus Carota)

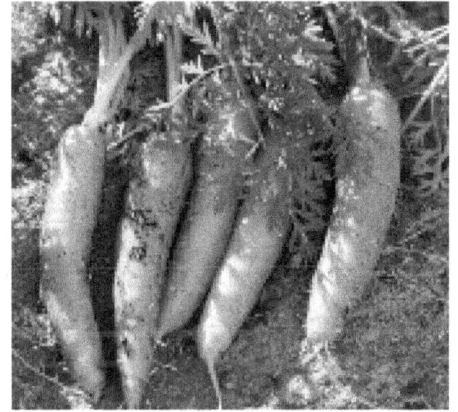

Purple carrot has, compared to ordinary carrot, very large amounts of Lycopene, Chlorogenic acid and Athocyanides, which are known to decrease body weight and body fat mass.

Purple carrot has body weight and fat mass decreasing properties.

When obese rats were fed high fat diet and purple carrot juice daily, for 8 weeks, body weight gain in test group was 10.6%, which was significantly ($p < 0.05$) less, than the 14.3% weight gain in control group. Also fat mass was 42.1% ($p < 0.05$) lower in test group, compared to control group (Poudyal et.al. 2010).

When rats were given maize starch diet and purple carrot juice daily, for 8 weeks, body weight gain in test group was 5.4%, which was significantly ($p < 0.05$) less, than the 10.8% weight gain in control group. Also fat mass was 34.1% ($p < 0.05$) lower in test group, compared to control group (Poudyal et.al. 2010).

Purple potato

(Solanum Tuberosum)

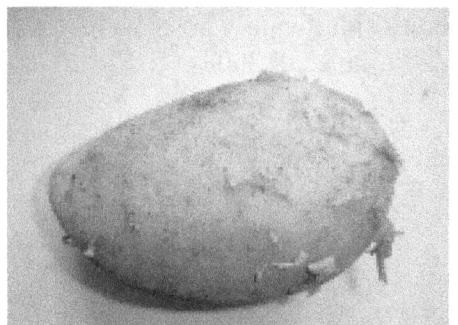

Except ordinary white potatoes, there exists also purple colored potatoes and dark blue or almost black potatoes. The color is caused by Anthocyanids, for example Cyanidin-3-Glucoside, which is known to decrease body weight. But ordinary French fries increase body weight and body fat mass.

Purple potato has body weight and fat mass decreasing properties.

When rats were given high fat diet and 200 mg/kg BW purple potato ethanol extract daily, for 4 weeks, body weight decreased in test group by 5.6% ($p < 0.05$), compared to control group. Also fat mass decreased in test group by 56% ($p < 0.05$), compared to control group (Yoon et.al. 2008).

Purple Sandsburry

(Spergularia Purpurea)

Purple Sandsburry is a small, red flowered medicinal plant, which is especially popular in North-Afric against high blood pressure and diabetes.

When rats were given Purple Sandsburry water extract 10 mg/kg BW daily, for 15 days, body weight decreased in test group by 13.5% ($p < 0.001$), compared to control group. Also total cholesterol ($p < 0.05$) and triglycerides ($p < 0.05$) decreased significantly in test group, compared to control group (Jouad et.al. 2003).

Purslane

(Portulaca Oleraceae)

Purslane is a popular vegetable, which contains large amounts of healthy Polyphenols, Anthocyanins, Melatonin, alpha-Linolenic acid and beta-Carotene. Its cultivation is very easy. Purslane is known to decrease cholesterol and triglycerides.

Purslane has body weight decreasing properties.

When obese rats were given daily Purslane ethanol extract at doses of 150 mg/kg, 300 mg/kg or 500 mg/kg body weight, for 8 weeks, body weight decreased significantly ($p < 0.01$) in all test groups, compared to the control group. The body weight of control group ws 206.9 grams, in the 150 mg/kg group it ws 200.7 grams, in the 300 mg/kg group it ws 187.1 grams and in the 500 mg/kg group it was 176.2 grams (Hussein 2010). Also triglycerides and total cholesterol decreased significantly in test groups.

When mice were fed Purslane water extract at different doses, the swimming endurance was significantly increased, as was serum Glucose, but triglycerides and Lactate were significantly decreased, compared to the control group (Lu et.al. 2009). This means Purslane increases the fatty acid beta-oxidation significantly.

Purslane, seed

(Portulaca Oleraceae)

Purslane is a very healthy vegetable, which contains large amounts of different nutrients. Purslane seeds contain even more of these nutrients, and also beta-Sitosterol, which decreases cholesterol.

Purslane seeds have body weight decreasing properties.

When 15 type 2 diabetes patients were given 10 grams Purslane seeds daily, for 8 weeks, body weight decreased in test group by 10.2 kg (83.26 kg → 73.06 kg; $p < 0.001$), compared to control group. Also triglycerides decreased by 19.7% ($p < 0.001$), total cholesterol decreased by 16.6% ($p < 0.001$) and LDL-cholesterol decreased by 11.3% ($p < 0.001$), but HDL-cholesterol increased by 19.5% ($p < 0.001$) in test group, compared to control group (El-Sayed 2011).

Purusharatna

(Hybanthus Enneaspermus, Synonymes: Ionodium Suffruticosum, Viola Enneasperma, Viola Suffruticosa)

Purasharatna is the Sankrit language name for this plant, which in English is called Spade Flower. The plant is a member of the Violacae family. It grows naturally from India to Australia. It is used in India as an aphrodisiac plant, which is known to increase testosterone levels in animal experiments (Narayanswamy et.al. 2007).

Purusharatna has body weight decreasing properties.

When rats were given high fat diet and 200 mg/kg BW Purusharatna Methanol extract daily, for 2 weeks, body weight in test group was 20.0% ($p < 0.001$) lower, compared to control group. Also triglycerides ($p < 0.001$), total cholesterol ($p < 0.001$), LDL-cholesterol ($p < 0.001$) and VLDL-cholesterol ($p < 0.001$) were significantly lower, but HDL-cholesterol ($p < 0.001$) was significantly higher in test group, compared to control group (Muthu et.al. 2012).

The body weight, triglycerides and cholesterol decreasing properties of Purasharatna has been verified also in another experiment with rats (Kumar et.al. 2012).

Psyllium

(Plantago Ovata)

Psyllium husk is a very popular dietary supplement, which is used in stomach problems, hypertension and high cholesterol levels.

Psyllium husk has body weight and body fat mass decreasing properties.

When 111 obese volunteers were given either 6 grams or 9 grams Psyllium husk daily, for 12 weeks, body weight decreased by an average of 4.56 kg in the test groups, compared to the 3.79 kg in control group. LDL-cholesterol decreased in the test groups by an average of 0.31 mmol/L, being significantly (p = 0.03) larger, than the 0.06 mmol/L decrease in control group (Salas-Salvado et.al. 2008). This was a double blind experiment.

When obese, hypertensive volunteers were given Psyllium husk 7 grams daily, for 6 months, the following parameters decreased significantly (p < 0.05 in all parameters): Body mass index BMI, triglycerides, LDL-cholesterol, systolic blood pressure and diastolic blood pressure. Totally there were 141 volunteers in this experiment (Cicero et.al. 2007).

When 18 obese volunteers were given Psyllium 12 grams daily, for 12 weeks, body weight decreased by 2.0 kg (p = 0.007) and body fat-% decreased by 2.0% (p = 0.002), compared to the 18 person control group. Also LDL-cholesterol decreased by 22% (p = 0.002) and total cholesterol decreased by 15% (p = 0.001) in the test group, compared to the control group (Pal et.al. 2011).

The body weight and cholesterol decreasing property of Psyllium husk has been verified also in other experiments (Frati-Munari et.al. 1983).

In animal experiments with rats Psyllium husk significantly decreases body weight, total cholesterol and blood pressure, compared to the control groups (Galisteo et.al. 2005; Galisteo et.al. 2010; Wang et.al. 2007).

Psyllium husk should be taken 10 – 15 grams daily, to be effective.

Pycnogenol, Flavangenol

(Pinus Pinaster)

The bark extract (Pycnogenol or Flavangenol) of French Maritime Pine (Pinus Pinaster) contains very strong antioxidants, Catechin oligomers, which have been used in humans against impotence, high blood pressure etc.

Pycnogenol and Flavangenol have body weight and fat mass decreasing properties.

When obese rats were given high fat food and Flavangenol in drinking water, at a dose of 3 micrograms/2 ml daily, for 15 days, body weight decreased in Flavangenol group by 8.0% (p < 0.05), compared to control group (Tanida et.al. 2009).

The body weight and also strong fat mass decreasing properties of Pycnogenol and Flavangenol has been verified in many experiments (Hasegawa et.al. 1999; Shimada et.al. 2011; Shimada et.al. 2012).

Pyruvate

Pyruvic acid in natural metabolite in every living cell. It has a very important role in the cell energy production. It can be purchased as Creatinepyruvate or Calciumpyruvate.

Pyruvate has body weight and body fat mass decreasing properties.

When 18 volunteers were given 6.0 grams Pyruvate daily, for 6 weeks, the body fat mass decreased by 2.1 kg (p = 0.005) and body fat-% decreased by 2.6% (21.0% → 18.4%; p = 0.005), compared to the control group (Kalman et.al. 1998). This was a double blind experiment.

When 12 volunteers were given Pyruvate 6.0 grams daily, for 6 weeks, body weight decreased by 1.2 kg (p < 0.001), body fat mass decreased by 2.5 kg (p < 0.001) and body fat-% decreased by 2.7% (23.0% → 20.3%; p < 0.001), compared to the control group (Kalman et.al. 1999). This was a double blind experiment.

The body weight and body fat mass reducing properties of Pyruvate has been verified also in many other experiments with humans (Koh-Banerjee et.al. 2005; Stanko et.al. 1994; Stanko et.al. 1992; Stanko et.al. 1992) and animal experiments with rats (Ivy et.al. 1994; Cortez et.al. 1994).

Pyruvate stimulates the beta-oxidation of fatty acids. In the Cortez experiments with rats, the RER-value (RER = Respiratory Exchange ratio) decreased from 0.87 to 0.81, which means, the cells use more fat compared to carbohydrate for energy production.

Quercetin

Quercetin is a flavonoid, which is a very strong antioxidant. It exists in many food plants, especially in red onion. Quercetin is antiviral, anti-inflammatory, antihypertensive and cholesterol decreasing flavonoid, which has many positive health effects. It can be also purchased from markets in pill form.

Quercetin has body weight and body fat mass decreasing properties.

When obese rats were given normal food and 10 mg/kg BW Quercetin daily, for 10 weeks, body weight was 5.3% ($p < 0.05$), triglycerides were 33.1% ($p < 0.05$), total cholesterol was 17.5% ($p < 0.05$) and Insulin was 75.5% ($p < 0.05$) lower in test group, compared to control group (Rivera et.al. 2008).

When rats were made obese by feeding MSG (Monosodium glutamate) and were given 75 mg/kg BW Quercetin daily, for 42 days, body weight was 23.0% ($p < 0.05$) lower in test group, compared to MSG control group. Also Leptin, triglycerides, total cholesterol, LDL-cholesterol and VLDL-cholesterol were significantly ($p < 0.05$) lower, but HDL-cholesterol was significantly ($p < 0.05$) higher in test group, compared to control group (Seiva et.al. 2012).

The body weight, body fat mass, triglycerides, total cholesterol and systolic blood pressure decreasing, but Adinopectin and HDL-cholesterol increasing properties of Quercetin has been verified in great many experiments with mice and rats (Panchal et.al. 2012; Jung et.al. 2012; Kobori et.al. 2010; Yamamoto et.al. 2006; Jeong et.al. 2012).

When volunteers were given 150 mg Quercetin daily, for 8 weeks, waist circumference ($p = 0.004$) and systolic blood pressure ($p = 0.044$) were significantly lower, but HDL-cholesterol ($p = 0.0235$) was significantly higher in test group, compared to control group. This was a double blind experiment with 49 healthy volunteers (Pfeuffer et.al. 2011).

When 49 smoking males were given 100 mg Quercetin daily, for 10 weeks, total cholesterol ($p < 0.05$), LDL-cholesterol ($p < 0.01$), systolic blood pressure ($p < 0.01$) and diastolic blood pressure ($p < 0.01$) were significantly lower, but HDL-cholesterol ($p < 0.05$) was significantly higher in test group, compared to the 49 person control group. This was a double blind experiment (Lee et.al. 2011).

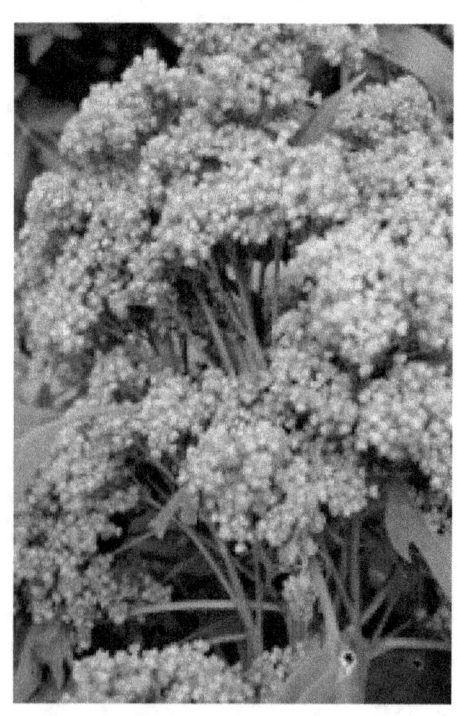

Quinoa

(Chenopodium Quinoa)

Quinoa originates from Peru. It is a high altitude growing edible seed, which has been cultivated in Peru for thousands of years. The seeds contain large amounts of protein, and also the compound 20-Hydroxyecdysone. Quinoa decreases total cholesterol, LDL-cholesterol and triglycerides.

Quinoa has body weight and fat mass decreasing properties.

When 22 volunteers were given 19.5 grams Quinoa daily, for 30 days, total cholesterol ($p = 0.0006$), LDL-cholesterol ($p = 0.0002$) and triglycerides ($p = 0.0471$) decreased significantly, compared to the baseline values. Also body weight decreased by 1.2 kg (71.9 kg → 70.7 kg; $p > 0.5$), but not significantly (Farinazzi-Machado et.al. 2012).

When mice were given Quinoa 20-Hydroxyecdysone at a dose of 10 mg/kg daily, for 13 weeks, weight gain in Quinoa group was 18% (p < 0.05) less than in the control group (Kizelsztein et.al. 2009). Body fat mass decreased by 41% (p < 0.05) in the Quinoa group, compared to the control group.

Also in other experiments with mice and rats, Quinoa decreases both body weight and fat mass (Foucault et.al. 2012; Seidlova-Wuttke et.al. 2010; Meneguetti et.al. 2011).

Radish leaves

(Raphanus Sativus)

Radish is a known root vegetable. Normally only the root is eaten, but radish leaves are used as a vegetable in Asia, especially in Korea. The leaves contain much higher levels of nutrients, than the root. It has Calcium 316 mg/100g, Iron 3.2 mg/100g and vitamin C 63 mg/100g.

Radish leaves have body weight decreasing properties.

When rats were fed high diet and 10% Radish leaves daily, for 6 weeks, body weight in test group was 5.76% (p < 0.05) lower, compared to control group (Rhee et.al. 2005).

When rats were given high fat diet and 10% enzyme-treated radish leaf powder daily, for 4 weeks, body weight in test group was 9.2% (p < 0.05) lower, compared to control group. Also total cholesterol, LDL-cholesterol and triglycerides were significantly lower, but HDL-cholesterol was significantly higher in test group, compared to control group (Kim et.al. 2011).

Radish seeds and sprouts

(Raphanus Sativus)

Radish sprouts have very high nutrient contents and they are very popular functional food, especially in Asia. Radish sprouts are known to decrease blood Glucose.

Radish seeds and sprouts have body weight and body fat mass decreasing properties. When obese rats were given high fat diet together with either 125 mg/kg BW, 250 mg/kg BW or 500 mg/kg BW Radish seed water extract daily, for 84 days, body weight in test groups decreased by 9.66% (p < 0.01), 22.52% (p < 0.01) and 25.02% (p < 0.01), compared to the control group. Also body fat mass (p < 0.01), triglycerides (p < 0.01), LDL-cholesterol (p < 0.01), total cholesterol (p < 0.01), Adiponectin level (p < 0.01) and Leptin level (p < 0.01) decreased significantly, but HDL-cholesterol (p < 0.01) increased (p < 0.01) significantly in test groups, compared to the control groups (Lee et.al. 2009).

The triglycerides, total cholesterol and blood Glucose decreasing but HDL-cholesterol increasing properties of Radish sprouts has been verified in other experiments with rats (Taniguchi et.al. 2006; Taniguchi et.al. 2007).

Red beet leaf

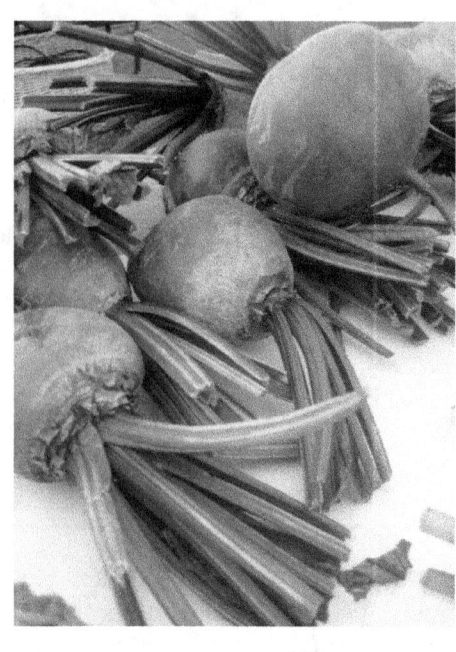

(Beta Vulgaris)

Red beet is a very common edible root vegetable, which decreases blood pressure. But red beet leaves contain very large amounts of Polyphenols, Flavonoids, Folic acid and Betalains.

Red beet leaves have body weight and body fat mass decreasing properties.

When mice were fed high fat and cholesterol, and also given in their daily food 8% of dried red beet leaves, for 4 weeks, body weight gain was significantly by 32.5% ($p < 0.05$) lower, than in the control group without red beet leave. Also body fat mass was significantly ($p < 0.05$) lower in test group, compared to the control group. Triglycerides were 13.5% ($p < 0.05$) lower in the test group, compared to the control group (Lee et.al. 2009).

Red Grapefruit and blood Orange

(Citrus Paradisi, Citrus Sinensis)

Red Grapefruit and blood Orange are delicious fruits, which contain large amounts of nutrients. Red Grapefruit has Flavonoids and Lycopene, blood Orange has Flavonoids and Cyanidin-3-Glucoside (C3G).

Red Grapefruit and blood Orange have body weight and body fat mass decreasing properties.

When obese volunteers were given daily 1.5 Grapefruit with normal diet, for 12 weeks, body weight decreased 1.6 kg ($p < 0.05$) in test group, compared to the control group. There were totally 91 volunteers in this experiment (Fujioka et.al. 2006).

When 42 obese volunteers were given 1.5 Grapefruit daily, with normal food, for 6 weeks, body weight decreased by 0.6 kg ($p = 0.097$), waist circumference decreased by 2.45 cm ($p = 0.0002$), systolic blood pressure decreased by 3.2 mmHg ($p = 0.03$), total cholesterol decreased by 6.0% ($p = 0.02$) and LDL-cholesterol decreased by 15.4% ($p < 0.001$) in test group, compared to the control group (Dow et.al. 2012).

When obese mice were given high fat diet together with Moro blood Orange juice daily, for 12 weeks, body weight decreased by 18.9% ($p < 0.05$) and fat mass decreased by 46.6% ($p < 0.05$) in test group, compared to the control group, which got water (Titta et.al. 2009).

Red mold rice

Red mold rice is rice, which is fermented by Monascus fungus (Monascus Purpureus, Monascus Pilosus etc.). Red mold rice is used in Asia as food and in other parts of the World to decrease high cholesterol and high blood pressure.

Red mold rice has body weight and fat mass decreasing properties.

When obese rats were given high fat diet together with 4% red mold rice daily, for 6 weeks, body weight gain in test group was 30.5% ($p < 0.05$) lower, than in the control group. Fat mass decreased in test group by 38.63% ($p < 0.001$), compared to the control group. Total cholesterol, LDL-cholesterol and triglycerides decreased also significantly in test group, compared to the control group (Chen et.al. 2008).

The body weight, fat mass, total cholesterol, LDL-cholesterol and triglycerides decreasing properties of red mold rice has been verified also in other experiments (Lee et.al. 2011; Kim et.al. 2010).

Red onion

(Allium Cepa)

Red onion has significantly more flavonoids, especially Quercetin and Rutin, than the ordinary yellow onion. These flavonoids are known to have body weight, triglycerides and cholesterol decreasing properties. Especially red onion peel contain up to several percent of Quercetin.

Red onion has body weight and fat mass decreasing properties.

When rats were given high fat diet and 5% onion powder in their daily diet, for 8 weeks, body weight was 7.0% lower in test group, compared to control group (Lee et.al. 2008).

When rats were given ordinary food and 5% onion peel powder in their daily food, for 3 months, body weight was 7.2% ($p < 0.05$), body fat mass was 16.9% ($p < 0.05$), triglycerides were 40.7% ($p < 0.05$) and total cholesterol was 11.0% ($p < 0.05$) lower, but HDL-cholesterol was 80.1% ($p < 0.05$) higher in test group, compared to control group (Kim et.al. 2004).

The body weight, body fat mass and triglycerides decreasing properties of onion has been verified also in other experiments with rats (Kim et.al. 2012; Yoshinari et.al. 2012; Choi et.al. 2008).

In human volunteers onion decreases significantly triglycerides ($p < 0.05$), total cholesterol ($p < 0.01$) and LDL-cholesterol ($p < 0.01$) (Lee et.al. 2010; Nam et.al. 2007).

Red raspberry

(Rubus Idaeus)

and Blackberry

(Rubus Fruticosus)

Red raspberry and Blackberry are very delicious berries. Red raspberry contains large amounts of healthy Ellagic acid, up to 150 mg/100g dry weight. The calorific value of Red raspberry is only 34 kcal/100g. Blackberry contains up to 550 mg/100g dry weight the Anthocyanin Cyanidin-3-Glucoside, which is known to have weight decreasing properties. It also contains Ellagic acid 24 mg/100g dry weight.

Red raspberry and Blackberry have body weight decreasing properties.

When obese OVX rats were given normal diet and 10% Blackberry daily, for 100 days, body weight in test group was 8.46% ($p < 0.05$) lower, compared to control group (Kaume et.al. 2012).

When hamsters with high cholesterol levels were given cholesterol rich diet and 5 ml Blackberry nectar daily, for 98 days, total cholesterol was 15.7%, LDL-cholesterol was 44.1% and triglycerides were 30.9% ($p < 0.05$ in all parameters) lower in test group, compared to control group (Ribeiro et.al. 2011).

Ellagic acid decreases body weight of rats on high fat diet (Panchal et.al. 2012).

Red raspberry inhibits Lipase activity (Slanc et.al. 2009).

In experiments with mice on high fat diet, Red raspberry ketone compound RK (=4-(4-hydroxyphenyl) butan-2-one) decreases significantly body weight in test group, compared to control group (Morimoto et.al. 2005).

Red raspberry is strongly diuretic (Zhang et.al. 2011).

The leaves of different raspberries and blackberries contain even 200 times more Ellagic acid than berries. The content of Ellagic acid can be up to 2.0 – 7.0% dry weight (Gudej et.al. 2004).

Red Wine

(Vitis Vinifera)

Red wine is a familiar drink to everybody. Red wine contains very large amounts of healthy polyphenols, between 1000 – 4000 mg/liter, which is 10 times more than in white wines. Red wine has many positive effects to cardiovascular system.

Red wine has body weight decreasing properties.

In experiments with 3T3-L1 fat cells, red wine inhibits the adipocyte differentiation (Choi et.al. 2005).

When rats were given normal food and either water or red wine daily, for 8 weeks, body weight gain was 28.4% ($p < 0.05$) lower in test group, compared to control group. Also the size of adipocytes was reduced by 15% ($p < 0.05$) in test group, compared to control group. The alcohol content of the used red wine was 13% (Monteiro et.al. 2009).

When hypertensive rats were given normal food and either water or water and 1.0% red wine polyphenols daily, for 8 weeks, body weight in test group was 7.1% ($p < 0.001$) lower, compared to control group (Mitzutani et.al. 1999).

Also in other experiments with rats, red wine lowers body weight compared to control group (Bargallo et.al. 2006).

Rehmannia, root

(Rehmannia Glutinosa)

Rehmannia root is a very old and famous medicinal plant in China, used against hypertension, loss of blood and to give physical strength. It is called DIHUANG in Chinese.

Rehmannia root has body weight decreasing properties.

When obese rats were given high fat food and either 1 gram/kg BW or 2 grams/kg BW Rehmannia root ethanol extract daily, for 10 weeks, body weight in test group were 6.7% and 11.9% ($p < 0.05$) lower, compared to control group (Jiang et.al. 2008).

Also in another experiment with obese OVX rats, body weight was 12.2% ($p < 0.05$) lower in test group treated by Rehmannia, compared to control group (Cho 2005).

Reishi

(Ganoderma Lucidum)

Reishi is a very famous medicinal mushroom, which has been used in China, Korea and Japan for thousands of years against hepatitis, asthma, bronchitis, insomnia, hypertension and gastric ulcers.

Reishi has body weight decreasing properties.

When obese rats were given high fat diet and 5% dried Reishi daily, for 4 weeks, body weight was 4.77% ($p < 0.05$) lower in test group, compared to control group (Amin et.al. 2012).

In a second experiment rats were given normal diet and 5% dried Reishi daily, for 4 weeks. Body weight was 6.6% lower in test group, compared to control group. Also total cholesterol was 20.6% ($p < 0.01$) lower in test group, compared to control group (Kabir et.al. 1988).

In experiments with fat cells, Reishi inhibits adipocyte differentation, and fatty acid synthase (FAS) enzyme (Thyagarajan-Sahu et.al. 2011).

Resveratrol

(3,5,4-trihydroxystilbene)

Resveratrol is a natural phenolic compound, Stilbene, which exists in the skin of grapes and especially in the root of Japanese Knotweed, Polygonum Cuspidatum. Resveratrol is under intense research due to its multitude health effects. It is hypotensive, decreases cholesterol, and it has anti-aging properties.

Resveratrol has body weight and body fat mass decreasing properties.

When obese type 2 diabetic rats were given high fat diet and 25 mg/kg BW Resveratrol daily, for 8 weeks, body weight was 14.5% ($p < 0.05$) lower in test group, compared to control group. Also triglycerides were 21.6% ($p < 0.05$), total cholesterol was 16.9% ($p < 0.05$), LDL-cholesterol was 23.3% ($p < 0.05$) and VLDL-cholesterol was 22.8% ($p < 0.05$) lower, but HDL-cholesterol was 51.9% ($p < 0.05$) higher in test group, compared to control group (Hussein et.al. 2013).

The body weight and body fat mass decreasing properties of Resveratrol has been verified in great many animal experiments (Kim et.al. 2010; Kim et.al. 2011; Shang et.al. 2008; Baile et.al. 2011; Franco et.al. 2012; Sun et.al. 2011; Macarulla et.al. 2009; Chen et.al. 2012; Rivera et.al. 2009; Cho et.al. 2012; Alberdi et.al. 2011).

Rocket Ligularia

(Ligularia Stenocephala)

Both Rocket Ligularia and Ligularia Fischeri are used as a vegetable in Korea. In other parts of Asia they are used as anti-viral and anti-bacterial medicine.

Rocket Ligularia has body weight and fat mass decreasing properties.

When obese rats were fed high fat diet and Butanol extract of Rocket Ligularia at a dose of 200 mg/kg BW daily, for 2 weeks, body weight was 11.6% ($p < 0.05$) lower in test group, compared to control group. Also fat mass was significantly lower in test group, compared to control group. Total cholesterol decreased by 16.6% ($p < 0.05$) and LDL-cholesterol decreased by 23.5% ($p < 0.05$) in test group, compared to control group (Nugroho et.al. 2010).

Rooibos tea

(Aspalathus Linearis)

Rooibos tea originates from South-Africa, and it contains large amounts of healthy flavonoids and polyphenols.

Rooibos tea has body weight decreasing properties.

When mice were given high fat diet together with Rooibos tea daily, for 14 weeks, weight gain in test group was 10%, which was significantly ($p < 0.05$) lower, than the 20% weight gain in control group, which was given water. The strength of Rooibos tea was 10 grams dried leaves in 1 liter water (Beltran-Debon et.al. 2009).

Rose hip

(Rosa Canina, Rosa Sp.)

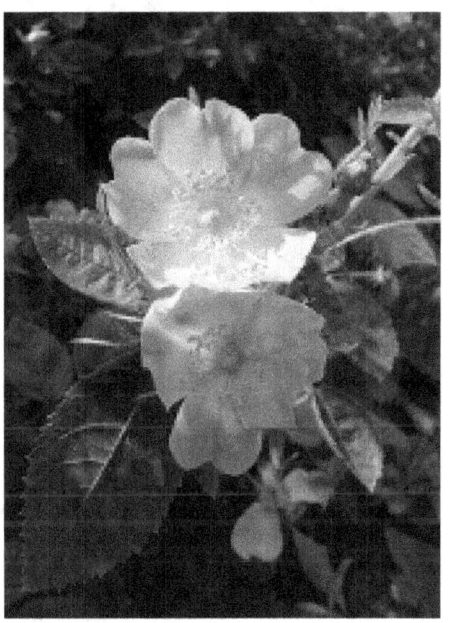

Rose hip is an edible berry, which contains large amounts of vitamin C and Lycopene. Also the Rose seeds can be used as a tea or in grounded form the seeds can be added to food.

Rose hip and Rose seeds have body weight and fat mass decreasing properties.

When obese mice were fed high fat diet together with 33% Rose hips daily, for 10 weeks, body weight decreased by 31.0% ($p < 0.001$) and body fat-% decreased by 24.9% (43.3% → 18.4%; $p < 0.001$), compared to the control group. Also total cholesterol decreased in the test group by 38% ($p < 0.01$), compared to the control group (Andersson et.al. 2011).

The body weight decreasing and body fat-% decreasing properties of Rose hip and Rose seeds has been verified in a number of experiments with mice (Hisashi et.al. 2006; Matsuda et.al. 2006; Ninomiya et.al. 2007; Goto et.al. 2012).

One of the effective compounds is trans-Tiliroside.

Rose root

(Rhodiola Rosea, Rhodiola Sachalinensis, Rhodiola Sp.)

There exists several tens of different Rhodiola species in the World. Rose roots are famous adaptogens, just like Ginseng root and Siberian Ginseng. In animal experiments, Rose root increases swimming endurance, which means better fat use in muscle cells. All Rose root species contain Salidroside and Tyrosol as active compounds.

Rose root has body weight and fat mass decreasing properties.

When obese rats were given 30 mg/kg BW Sachalin Rose root (Rhodiola Sachalinensis) root extract daily, for 8 weeks, body weight in test group was 6.4% ($p < 0.01$) lower, compared to control group. Also triglycerides were 42.7% ($p < 0.01$) lower in test group, compared to control group (Oh et.al. 2006).

Both Salidroside and Tyrosol inhibit fat accumulation and differentiation of 3T3-L1 fat cells (Lee et.al. 2011; Wang et.al. 2004).

In many animal experiments Rose root decreases significantly both triglycerides and total cholesterol (Shen et.al. 2008; Gao et.al. 2009; Li et.al. 2011).

Rosemary

(Rosmarinus Officinalis)

Rosemary is a very popular spice. It contains strong antioxidants, especially Carnosic acid, Carnosol and Rosmarinic acid.

Rosemary has body weight and fat mass decreasing properties.

When obese and lean rats were given Rosemary ethanol extract 0.5% in their daily diet, for 64 days, body weight decreased both in lean and fat rats 10% ($p < 0.01$), compared to the control groups. Triglycerides decreased by 57% ($p < 0.001$) and total cholesterol decreased by 25% ($p < 0.001$) in test groups, compared to the control groups (Vaquero et.al. 2012).

When mice were given high fat diet and Rosemary leaf extract 200 mg/kg BW daily, for 50 days, body weight gain was 64% ($p < 0.01$) and body fat mass gain was 57% ($p < 0.01$) lower in test group, compared to the control group (Harach et.al. 2010).

The body weight and fat mass decreasing properties of Rosemary has been verified also in other experiments with rats (Ibarra et.al. 2011; Wang et.al. 2011).

In experiment with mice, Rosemary significantly decreases triglycerides, total cholesterol and LDL-cholesterol, but increases HDL-cholesterol, compared to control group (Sheyab et.al. 2012).

Rucola or Rocket

(Eruca Sativa)

Rucola is a delicious salad plant, which grows wild around the Mediterranian countries. Also the seeds are edible and both Rucola salad and seeds are used as aphrodisiacs in Asian countries, in Jordania, Saudi Arabia etc.

Rucola has body weight decreasing properties.

When mice were fed daily 0.1 ml Rucola ethanol extract, for 30 days, body weight was 9.6% ($p < 0.01$) lower in test group, compared to control group. Also the size of testis were 39.6% higher in Rucola group, compared to control group (Homady et.al. 2000).

The Rucola seed oil decreases significantly total cholesterol, LDL-cholesterol and triglycerides in rats (El-Gengaihi et.al. 2004).

Rutin

Rutin is a flavonoid, which exist in many food plants. It is abundant in red onion and buckwheat, and especially abundant in tartary buckwheat, Fagopyrum Tataricum, and buckwheat sprouts. Rutin is a strong antioxidant, which has several positive health effects. Rutin is a very cheap supplement, which can be bought in markets as 500 mg pills.

Rutin has body weight and body fat mass decreasing properties.

In experiments with 3T3-L1 fat cell, Rutin strongly decreases fat accumulation into fat cells (Hsu et.al. 2007; Wu et.al. 2011).

When rats were given high fat and high carbohydrate diet and 0.16% Rutin in their daily diet, body weight decreased by 11.78% ($p < 0.001$), body fat mass decreased by 41.6% ($p < 0.001$), triglycerides decreased by 33.3% ($p < 0.01$), total cholesterol decreased by 20.0% ($p < 0.01$), blood sugar decreased by 26.9% ($p < 0.05$) and Insulin decreased by 24.3% ($p < 0.001$) in test group, compared to control group (Panchal et.al. 2011).

The body weight and body fat mass decreasing properties of Rutin has been verified in many other experiments with mice and rats (Hsu et.al. 2009; Choi et.al. 2006).

Sacred Lotus root

(Lotus Nucifera)

Sacred Lotus is cultivaed all over in Asia, especially in China, Korea, Japan and Taiwan. All parts, roots, leaves and seeds, are edible. The roots are very popular as a vegetable.

Sacred Lotus roots have body weight and body fat mass decreasing properties.

When rats were given Sacred Lotus root hot water extract 400 mg/kg BW daily, for 6 weeks, body weight in test group was 14.0% ($p < 0.05$) lower, compared to the control group. Total body fat mass was 45.4% ($p < 0.05$) lower in test group, compared to conrol group (Du et.al. 2010).

When obese, diabetic mice were given dried Sacred Lotus root 5% in their daily diet, for 3 weeks, body weight in test group was 8.9% lower, compared to control group. Serum adinopectin was significantly ($p < 0.05$) higher in test group, compared to control group. The FAS activity in liver was 58.6% ($p < 0.05$) lower in test group, compared to control group (Tsuruta et.al. 2012).

Safflower, flower

(Carthamus Tinctorius)

Safflower is commonly cultivated for the edible seeds and seed oil. The flowers are also edible. The flower tea is used in Thailand as a healthy tea, and in China it is a very old medicinal plant, which is used to increase blood circulation and blood volume. Its Chinese name is HONG HUA.

Safflower flower has body weight decreasing properties.

When rats, which were given normal diet and 2% cholesterol in their daily food, were given 250 mg/kg BW Safflower flower dichloromethane extract daily, for 4 weeks, body weight in test group was 11.1% ($p < 0.05$) lower, compared to control group (Arpornsuwan et.al. 2010).

Safflower oil

(Carthamus Tinctorius)

Safflower oil is popular cooking oil. It contains large amounts of unsaturated fatty acids. Safflower oil is one of the World's oldest cooking oils, it is known already from Egypt, 5000 years ago.

Safflower oil has body weight and body fat mass decreasing properties.

When obese rats were given 45% lard, and 5% Safflower oil daily, for 10 weeks, body weight in test group was 23.58% (p < 0.05) lower, compared to the 45% lard control group. Also total cholesterol was 23.3%, LDL-cholesterol was 18.2%´, triglycerides were 25.3% and Insulin was 59.7% (p < 0.05 in all parameters) lower in test group, compared to control group (Zhang et.al. 2010).

The body weight and body fat mass decreasing but aerobic swimming endurance increasing properties of Safflower oil has been verified in many experiments with rats and mice (Zhang et.al. 2011; Hsu et.al. 2006; Shimomura et.al. 1990).

When type 2 diabetic volunteers were given Safflower oil 8 grams daily, for 16 weeks, belly fat mass was 6.3% (p = 0.0422) lower, and also blood sugar (p = 0.0343) was lower, but Adiponectin increased by 20.3% (p = 0.0051), and also HDL-cholesterol (p = 0.0228) and fat free mass (p = 0.0432) increased significantly, compared to control groups. These were double blind experiments (Norris et.al. 2009; Michelle et.al. 2011).

Saffron

(Crocus Sativus)

and Gardenia fruit

(Gardenia Jasminoides)

Saffron and Gardenia fruit contain both large amounts of the carotenoid Crocin. Saffron also contains carotenoids Crocetin and Safranal, and Gardenia fruit contains the carotenoid Geniposide. Saffron is a very famous and expensive spice and Gardenia fruit is used in Asia medicinally, against high blood pressure etc.

Saffron, Gardenia fruit and Crocin have body weight and fat mass decreasing properties.

Crocin in Saffron and Gardenia fruit decreases both body weight (p < 0.05), fat mass (p < 0.05), triglycerides (p < 0.05), LDL-cholesterol (p < 0.05) and total cholesterol (p < 0.05) significantly in test mice, compared to control group (Lee et.al. 2005).

Geniposide in Gardenia fruit decreases significantly body weight (p < 0.05) and fat mass (p < 0.05) in test mice, compared to control group (Kojima et.al. 2011).

In human volunteers Saffron extract decreases both body weight (p < 0.05) and hunger (Gout et.al. 2010). This was a double blind experiment.

Also in other experiments Saffron, Crocin and Crocetin decrease fat mass, triglycerides, total cholesterol and LDL-cholesterol (Sheng et.al. 2006; Asdaq et.al. 2010; Xi et.al. 2007; Sheng et.al. 2008).

Sal tree, leaves

(Shorea Robusta)

Salt tree is a very old medicinal plant in India. In Ayurveda Sal tree has been used for hundreds of years against obesity, wounds, gonorrhea, dysentery and leprosy.

Sal tree leaves have body weight decreasing properties.

When obese rats were given fattening monosodium glutamate (MSG) and Sal tree leaves ethanol extract 200 mg/kg BW daily, for 48 days, body weight was 30.6% (p < 0.001) lower in test group, compared to control group. Also triglycerides were 21.5% (p < 0.001) and total cholesterol was 15.6% (p < 0.001) lower, but HDL-cholesterol was 22.4% (p < 0.001) higher in test group, compared to control group (Supriya et.al. 2012).

Salacia

(Salacia Reticulata)

Salacia, which is also called Kotala Himbutu, is a vine like medicinal plant, which has been used in Sri Lanka and South-India for thousands of years, against diabetes. Roots are the part which are used.

Salacia has body weight and fat mass decreasing properties.

When obese type 2 rats were given Salacia root water extract 0.2% of their daily diet, for 6 weeks, body weight decreased in the test group by 5.4% (p < 0.05), compared to the control group. Body fat mass decreased in the test group by 9.57% (p < 0.05), compared to the control group. And finally Insulin decreased in the test group by 51.3% (p < 0.05), compared to the control group (Kishino et.al. 2009).

The Salacia body weight and fat mass decreasing properties have been verified in a number of experiments with mice, rats and chicken (Akase et.al. 2011; Wang et.al. 2012; Im et.al. 2008; Shimada et.al. 2010; Yoshikawa et.al. 2002).

Salvia Hypoleuca

Salvia Hypoleuca is a close relative to the common Sage, Salvia Officinalis. There are several hundreds of different Sage species in the World. Common Sage is known to decrease cholesterol and high blood pressure. Salvia Hypoleuca is used as a traditional medicinal plant in Iran against diabetes.

Salvia Hypoleuca has body weight decreasing properties.

When obese rats were given high fat diet together with 200 mg/kg BW Salvia Hypoleuca ethanol extract daily, for 4 weeks, body weight decreased in test group by 45.3% ($p < 0.01$), compared to control group. Also triglycerides and LDL-cholesterol decreaased significantly ($p < 0.05$) in test group, compared to control group (Estakhr et.al. 2011).

Also in another experiment Salvia Hypoleuca at a dose of 50 mg/kg BW decreased body weight in rats, but only by 4%, at this low dose (Javdan et.al. 2011).

Sasabamboo

(Sasa Borealis, Sasa Sp.)

Bamboo has been used as a food and medicine in Asia for thousands of years. Sasabamboo leaves are used as a health tea in Korea and Japan, for example against diabetes.

Sasabamboo leaves have body weight and body fat mass decreasing properties.

When obese mice were given high fat diet together with 5% daily of Sasamboo leaves extract (70% ethanol extract), for 12 weeks, body weight was 7.7% ($p < 0.05$) and total fat mass was 18.9% ($p < 0.05$) lower in test group, compared to control group. Serum Glucose was 17.0% ($p < 0.05$) lower, insulin was 61.8% ($p < 0.05$) lower and Leptin was 24.5% ($p < 0.05$) lower in test group, compared to control group (Yang et.al. 2010).

The body weight and body fat mass decreasing properties of Sasamboo leaves has been verified in many animal experiments (Ryou et.al. 2012; Kang et.al. 2012; Kim et.al. 2007).

Satsuma Mandarin, peel and pulp

(Citrus Unshiu)

Satsuma mandarin is a very popular citrus fruit in the whole World. It contains large amounts of flavonoids, and especially large amount of the carotenoid beta-Cryptoxanthin, which is known to decrease body weight. The amount of beta-Cryptoxanthin in Satsuma mandarin pulp is typically 1.8 mg/100 g edible portion. The calorific value of Mandarin pulp is only 42 kcal/100 g, and with peel together only 33 kcal/100 g. Also mandarin juice contain typically 9.2 mg/100 g Synephrine (Dragull et.al. 2008), which is known to decrease body weight.

Satsuma mandarin peel and pulp have body weight and body fat decreasing properties.

When type 2 diabetic mice were given normal food and 2% of Mandarin peel 60% ethanol extract in their daily food, for 6 weeks, body weight was 5.8% ($p < 0.05$), fat mass was 11% ($p < 0.05$), triglycerides were 36.5% ($p < 0.05$) and total cholesterol was 10.8% ($p < 0.05$) lower in test group, compared to control group (Park et.al. 2012).

The body weight and body fat decreasing properties of Mandarin peel has been verified in many experiments with rats and mice (Takayanagi et.al. 2011; Yang et.al. 2008; Kim et.al. 2003).

Mandarin peel extract stimulates lipolysis (Tsujita et.al. 2007), and inhibits fat accumulation into 3T3-L1 fat cells (Jung et.al. 2011).

When female volunteers were given 4.7 mg beta-Cryptoxanthin daily, for 3 weeks, Adiponectin increased by 13.2% ($p = 0.009$), but triglycerides decreased by 13.8% ($p = 0.052$) and systolic blood pressure decreased by 4.4% ($p = 0.052$) (Iwamoto et.al. 2012).

In experiments with human volunteers, beta-Cryptoxanthin decreases significantly ($p < 0.01$) body fat mass, compared to control group (Tsuchida et.al. 2008). This was a double blind experiment.

Schisandra berry

(Shisandra Chinensis)

Schisandra berry is a very famous adaptogen, which has many positive effects on human health. It grows well in cold climates, and it is a very popular functional food and medicinal plant in Russia, China, Korea and Japan.

Schisandra berry has body weight and body fat mass decreasing properties.

When obese rats were given high fat diet with 200 mg/kg BW methanol extract of Schisandra berry daily, for 5 weeks, body weight in test group was 14.1% ($p < 0.05$) lower, compared to the control group. Also body fat-% ($p < 0.05$), triglycerides ($p < 0.05$), total cholesterol ($p < 0.05$) were significantly lower, but HDL-cholesterol ($p < 0.05$) was significantly higher in test group, compared to the control group (Park et.al. 2012).

The body weight, triglycerides, LDL-cholesterol and total cholesterol decreasing but HDL-cholesterol increasing property of Schisandra berry has been verified in 3 other experiments (Gao et.al. 2008; Kim et.al. 2011; Na et.al. 2010).

Seaweed and fatty fish combination

Seaweeds contain large amount of the anti-obesity carotenoid Fucoxanthin. Also fatty fish contains large amount of the anti-obesity polyunsaturated fatty acids DHA (Docosahexaenoic acid) and EPA (Eicosapentaenoic acid). Other good sources for Fucoxanthin are Wheatgrass, Chlorella and Spirulina. In Japan and Okinawa it is very common to eath both seaweed and fatty fish on the same meal.

Seaweed and fatty fish combination synergistically decreases body weight and body fat mass.

When rats were given either control food (group 1), control food and seaweed (group 2), control food and fish oil (group 3) or control food and seaweed and fish oil (group 4), fatty acid beta-oxidation in liver increased by 42% in group 2, by 154% in group 3 and by 381% in group 4, compared to control group 1. Also triglycerides in serum and liver were synergistically decreased by the combination of seaweed and fish oil (Murata et.al. 2002).

In another experiment it was shown, that Fucoxanthin in seaweeds increased the DHA content in liver (Tsukui et.al. 2007).

And lastly in 2 different experiments with mice it was shown, that seaweed and fish oil combination synergistically decreases body weight and body fat mass, compared to control group (Okada et.al. 2011; Maeda et.al. 2007).

Sesame oil, cold pressed

(Sesamum Indicum)

Sesame oil is popular food oil in many parts of the World. In Asia it is considered as health oil. Cold pressed sesame oil contains large amounts of healthy lignans, Sesamin and Sesamol, which stimulate fatty acid oxidation.

Cold pressed sesame oil has body weight decreasing properties.

When 50 hypertensive volunteers were given 35 grams sesame oil daily, for 45 days, body weight decreased by 5.8 kg (74.30 kg → 68.50 kg; $p < 0.001$) and body mass index BMI decreased by 2.32 units (29.40 → 27.08; $p < 0.001$), compared to control values. Also systolic blood pressure decreased by 19.37 mmHg (144.35 mmHg → 124.88 mmHg; $p < 0.001$) and diastolic blood pressure decreased by 14.1 mmHg (97.90 mmHg → 83.80 mmHg; $p < 0.001$), compared to control values (Sankar et.al. 2006).

Also in another experiment with human volunteers, sesame oil decreased body weight, BMI, systolic blood pressure and diastolic blood pressure, compared to control values (Sankar et.al. 2006).

Sesame, seeds

(Sesamum Indicum)

Sesame seeds is very nutrient rich, it contains large amounts of protein, Calcium and especially the healthy lignans, Sesamin and Sesamol.

Sesame seeds have body weight decreasing properties.

The Sesame lignans Sesamin and Sesamol inhibit strongly the activity of FAS enzyme and other lipogenic enzymes, but stimulate strongly the fatty acid oxidation enzymes (Ashakumary et.al. 1999; Sirato-Yasumoto et.al. 2001; Ide et.al. 2004; Ide et.al. 2012; Kushiro et.al. 2002; Ide et.al. 2009; Sharma et.al. 2012).

When type 2 diabetic rats were given high fructose diet together with 2 grams/kg BW defatted sesame seed cake, for 30 days, body weight decreased by 1.8% ($p < 0.01$) in test group, but increased by 18.5% in the control group. Also triglycerides, total cholesterol, and LDL-cholesterol decreased significantly, but HDL-cholesterol increased significantly in test group, compared to control group (Bigoniya et.al. 2012).

Also in another experiment with rats, sesame seeds decreased strongly body weight, compared to control group (Zyla et.al. 2005).

When 14 type 2 diabetic volunteers were given 30 grams defatted sesame seed flour daily, for 60 days, body weight decreased in test group by 2.0 kg, being significantly ($p < 0.05$) more than the 1.3 kg weight loss in the 14 volunteers control group (Figueiredo et.al. 2008).

Sesamol and germinated Sesame seeds

(Sesamum indicum)

Sesame seeds are very nutrient rich and they contain large amounts of antioxidative lignans, such as Sesamin and Sesamol. When Sesame seeds are germinated, the amount of Sesamol increases up to 475 mg/kg, after 4 days of germination (Hahm et.al. 2009).

When obese rats were given high fat food and Sesamol 8 mg/kg BW daily, for 30 days, body weight was 12.1% ($p < 0.01$) lower in test group, compared to the control group. Also total cholesterol decreased by 51.1% ($p < 0.001$), LDL-cholesterol decreased by 60.2% ($p < 0.001$) and triglycerides decreased by 47.0% ($p < 0.001$), but HDL-cholesterol increased by 23.6% ($p < 0.001$) in test group, compared to control group (Sharma et.al. 2012).

Shampoo Ginger

(Zingiber Zerumbet)

Shampoo Ginger is called Lempyang in Malaysia and Indonesia. It is a close relative to our familiar Ginger root, Zingiber Officinalis. Shampoo Ginger has been cultivated thousands of years in Malaysia, Indonesia and Taiwan as a spice and medicinal plant. The root is used like normal Ginger in food making. The roots have many medicinal applications, against swellings, sores, loss of appetite, muscular discomfort etc.

Shampoo Ginger has body weight and fat mass decreasing properties.

When obese rats were given high fat diet and 300 mg/kg BW Shampoo Ginger ethanol extract daily, for 8 weeks, body weight was 11.9% ($p < 0.01$) lower in test group, compared to control group. Total fat mass was 24.7% ($p < 0.05$) lower in test group, compared to control group. Also triglycerides, total cholesterol and LDL-cholesterol were significantly ($p < 0.05$ in all parameters) lower, but HDL-cholesterol was significantly ($p < 0.05$) higher in test group, compared to control group (Chang et.al. 2012).

Shiikuwasha, peel

(Citrus Depressa)

Shiikuwasha is a very popular, mandarin like citrus fruit, grown especially in Okinawa, Japan, for its delicious juice.

Shiikuwasha peel has body weight and fat mass decreasing properties.

Whe mice were given high fat diet and 1.5% Shiikuwasha peel methanol extract in their daily diet, for 5 weeks, body weight was 10.5% ($p < 0.05$), fat mass was 50.8% ($p < 0.05$), triglycerides were 29.9% ($p < 0.05$) and Leptin was 75.5% ($p < 0.05$) lower in test group, compared to control group (Lee et.al. 2011).

Shiitake

(Lentinus Edodes)

Shiitake is the very famous and delicious mushroom, which has been cultivated in Asia for hundreds of years as a food and medicine. Shiitake is known to decrease blood pressure and cholesterol.

Shiitake has body weight and body fat mass decreasing properties.

When rats with high cholesterol levels were given 5% Shiitake in their daily food, for 42 days, following properties decreased in test group, compared to the control group: Body weight by 13.51% (p < 0.05), total cholesterol by 34.33% (p < 0.05), triglycerides by 53.21% (p < 0.05) and LDL-cholesterol by 75.00% (p < 0.05) (Yoon et.al. 2011).

When obese rats were given high fat diet and 6% Shiitake in their daily diet, for 6 weeks, body weight was gain 28.68% (p = 0.077), body fat mass 35% (p < 0.05) and triglycerides 55% (p < 0.05) lower in test group, compared to the control group (Handayani et.al. 2011).

The body weight, body fat mass and triglycerides decreasing properties of Shiitake has been verified in 2 other experiments with rats (Handayani et.al. 2012; Yoshioka et.al. 2010).

Siberian Ginseng

(Eleutherococcus Senticosus)

Siberian Ginseng is a very famous adaptogenic plant from Siberia, China and Korea. It has been researched over 70 years very intensively. Both in experiments with animals and humans, it increases the resistance against physical and mental stress, and increases also immunity.

When obese mice were fed Siberian Ginseng water extract 2.5 mg daily, for 12 weeks, body weight was 21.3% (p < 0.05) lower in test group, compared to control group. Body fat mass was 48.4% (p < 0.05) lower in test group, compared to control group (Shin et.al. 2005). Also plasma triglycerids were significantly (p < 0.05) lower in test group, compared to control group.

The body weight, body fat mass and triglycerides decreasing properties of Siberian Ginseng has been verified in many experiments with mice and rats (Park et.al. 2010; Hong et.al. 2009; Cha et.al. 2004).

Siberian tea

(Bergenia Crassifolia)

Siberian tea is used as a health tea in Russia and Mongolia. The blackened, wintered leaves are used. The root is included in Russia Pharmacopoeia.

Siberian tea has body weight decreasing properties.

When mice were given Siberian tea 10% water extract at a dose of 9.0 ml/kg BW daily, for 7 days, body weight in test group was 16.5% (p < 0.05) lower by average, compared to control group (Shikov et.al. 2010).

Siberian tea decreased triglycerides by 45% (p < 0.05) and total cholesterol by 12.5% (p < 0.05) in experiments with rats, compared to control group (Shikov et.al. 2012).

Sibiraea

(Sibiraea Angustata)

Sibiraea is a small bush, which grows at the altitude between 3000 – 4000 meters in Tibet and Western-China. The local people regard it as a healthy tea, but they avoid of giving it to sheep feed, since it is known to cause weight loss.

Sibiraea aerial parts have body weight and fat mass decreasing properties.

When obese mice were given high fat diet together with 250 mg/kg BW Sibiskoside extracted from Sibiraea, daily for 42 days, body weight was 27% ($p < 0.05$) lower in test group, compared to control group. Also fat mass was significantly ($p < 0.01$) lower in test group, compared to control group (Yoshitaki et.al. 2009). Sibiskoside (=1-O-b-D-Glucopyranosyl-Geraniol-5.10-Olide) is non-toxic even at doses of 2500 mg/kg BW.

The body weight and fat mass decreasing properties of Sibiraea has been verified in many other experiments (Xiao et.a. 2010; Xia et.al. 2011; Jiabing et.al. 2010).

Sickle-leaved Hare's ear, root

(Bupleurum Falcatum, Bupleurum Chinense)

Sickle-leaved Hare's ear has been used in China, Korea and Japan over 2000 years as a medicinal plant in liver diseases, such as hepatitis and also in cardiovascular diseases, fatigue, virus infection, Malaria etc.. It is an official medicine in Chinese Pharmacopeia. Its Chinese name is Chai Chu.

Sickle-leaved Hare's ear root has body weight and body fat mass decreasing properties.

When obese rats were given high fat diet and 1000 mg/kg BW Sickle-leaved Hare's ear root water extract daily, for 12 weeks, body weight decreased by 13.2% ($p < 0.01$) and body fat mass decreased by 29.0% ($p < 0.01$) in test group, compared to control group. Also triglycerides, total cholesterol and LDL-cholesterol decreased significantly ($p < 0.01$), but HDL-cholesterol increased significantly ($p < 0.01$) in test group, compared to control group (Tzeng et.al. 2012).

SINETROL

SINETROL is a mixture of extracts of 4 Citrus fruit pulps, peels and seeds and Guarana. These are: Red Orange (Citrus Sinensis), sweet orange (Citrus Aurantium var. Sinensis), bitter orange (Citrus Aurantium var. Amara) and grapefruit (Citrus Paradisi). The composition is: Polyphenols 60%, flavonoids 16.7%, anthocyanins 2% and caffeine 3.6%.

SINETROL has body weight and body fat mass decreasing properties.

When 10 volunteers were given 1.4 grams SINETROL daily, for 12 weeks, body weight decreased by 5.2 kg ($p < 0.05$) and body fat mass decreased by 4.4% ($p < 0.05$), compared to the 10 person control group. The body weight decreased in test group from 70.5 kg to 64.9 kg, and body fat-% decreased from 30.7% to 25.9%. This was a double blind experiment (Dallas et.al. 2008).

Skim milk, fat free sour milk, fat free yoghurt

Milk products contain large amounts of Calcium, which is known to have body weight decreasing properties. They also contain good quality protein, part of which is Whey protein, which is known to decrease body weight. Fat free, non-sugar and lactobacillus fermented yoghurt is the best possible milk product for overweight persons, who want to decrease body weight.

Skim milk, fat free sour milk and fat free, non-sugar, lactobacillus fermented yoghurt have body weight and body fat mass decreasing properties.

When 22 obese (BMI = 38.27) volunteers were put on a reduced (-500 kcal/day) diet, and given 3 glasses skim milk daily, for 8 weeks, body weight in test group decreased by 4.43 kg, when it decreased in the 20 person (BMI = 38.25) control group only 2.87 kg. Also body fat mass decreased in test group by 3.82 kg, but only 2.77 kg in control group. Also waist circumference decreased in test group by 6.32 cm, but only 3.98 cm in control group (Faghih et.al. 2011).

When volunteers were given either 6 dl skim milk or 6 dl fruit juice at breakfast, the energy intake at lunch in milk group was significantly lower by 8.5% ($p = 0.04$: 2432 kcal in milk group, 2658 kcal min juice group), compared to the isocaloric fruit juice group (Dove et.al. 2009). So skim milk reduced both appetite and energy intake acutely.

When obese (BMI = 29.1) volunteers on a hypocaloric diet were training for 16 weeks, and given either yoghurt or sugar water before and after every training session, body weight decreased in yoghurt group by 2.6 kg, but only 1.2 kg in control group. Also fat mass decreased by 3.4 kg in yoghurt group, but only 2.3 kg in control group (Thomas et.al. 2011).

In animal experiments skim milk and especially fat free, lactobacillus fermented milk products and yoghurt decrease body weight and body fat significantly more than casein, soy protein or whey protein (Buonopane et.al. 1992; Eller et.al. 2010; Fried et.al. 2012; Sagwai et.al. 2010; Ramchandran et.al. 2011; Sato et.al. 2008; Xie et.al. 2011).

Sleeping Plant, leaves

(Phyllanthus Amarus)

There are many Phyllanthus species in the World. The Sleeping Plant, Phyllanthus Amarus, is an annual weed, which grows in Africa and Asia. It is used medicinally against many diseases, such as diabetes, anemia, hypertension, liver diseases, inflammation, skin ulcers etc.

Sleeping Plant, Phyllanthus Amarus, leaves have body weight decreasing properties.

When normal rats were given daily either 300 mg/kg BW or 600 mg/kg BW Sleeping Plant, Phyllanthus Amarus, leaf water extract, for 31 days, body weight in test group was 10.6% ($p < 0.05$) and 20.2% ($p < 0.001$) lower, compared to control group (Adeneye 2012).

The body weight decreasing property of Sleeping Plant, Phyllanthus Amarus, has been verified also in another experiment (Adeneye et.al. 2007).

Smoking

Smoking is known to have many serious side effects, such as lung cancer, emphysema and cardiovascular diseases. Generally smoking persons weight less than non-smoking persons. This has been verified in many different research studies (Chiolero et.al. 2008).

Smoking cessation has body weight increasing properties.

Nicotine increases energy expenditure by about 3%, and it will also decrease appetite (Chiolero et.al. 2008).

When analyzing data of current and past weight and smoking status of 5247 adults, smoking cessation increased body weight in men by an average of 4.4 kg and in females by an average of 5.0 kg, during the next 10 years after cessation of smoking (Flegal et.al. 1995).

Snap Ginger

(Alpinia Calcarata)

Snap Ginger is also called Indian Ginger and Kulanjan in Hindi language. It is cultivated in India, Sri Lanka and Malaysia for its roots. It is a close relative to our common Ginger root. The root is used against obesity, diabetes, rheumatism, stomachache, fever and respiratory problems. It is antibacterial and antifungal.

Snap Ginger root has body weight decreasing properties.

When diabetic rats were given 300 mg/kg BW Snap Ginger root ethanol extract daily, for 3 weeks, body weight was 12.1% (p < 0.001) lower in test group, compared to control group. Triglycerides were 33.6% (p < 0.001) and total cholesterol was 23.2% (p < 0.01) lower in test group, compared to control group. Also blood sugar was significantly (p < 0.001) lower in test group, compared to control group (Raj et.al. 2011).

The triglycerides, total cholesterol, LDL-cholesterol and VLDL-cholesterol decreasing but HDL-cholesterol increasing properties of Snap Ginger has been verified also in other rat experiments (Prabhu et.al. 2010).

Snowparsley, seeds and Osthole

(Cnidium Monnieri)

Snowparsley is also called Common Cnidium. It is a very important medicinal plant in China, Korea and Japan. The seeds contain Osthole as active compound. The seeds are used against impotence, asthma and fungal infections.

Snowparsley seeds and Osthole have body weight decreasing properties.

When obese rats were given high fat diet and 10 mg/kg BW Osthole daily, for 4 weeks, body weight was 7.1% (p < 0.05) lower in test group, compared to control group (Qi et.al. 2011).

The body weight decreasing properties of Osthole has been verified also in experiments with mice (Du et.al. 2011).

Soy bean

(Glycine Max)

Soy bean is one of the World's most cultivated crops. Soy contains large amounts of protein and the healthy lipolytic isoflavonoids Genistein and Daidzein. Fat free soy flour contains up to 50% protein, which is 2 times more than in lean meat. Soy is known to decrease high blood pressure, cholesterol and triglyceride values. In many meal replacement formulas soy is used as the protein source.

Soy has body weight and body fat mass decreasing properties.

When 37 obese volunteers were given 90 grams soy protein in their daily 1200 kcal diet, the body weight decreased in test group by 7.0 kg, being significantly (p < 0.001) more, than the 2.9 kg weight loss in the 50 person control group, which was also given a daily 1200 kcal diet. Body fat mass decreased in test group by 4.3 kg, which was significantly (p = 0.003) more than the 1.4 kg body fat mass reduction in control group. Waist circumference decreased in test group by 6.0 cm, which was significantly (p = 0.003) more than the 2.9 cm reduction in control group. Also total cholesterol (p = 0.013) and LDL-cholesterol (p < 0.009) decreased significantly more in test group, compared to control group (Allison et.al. 2003).

The body weight and body fat mass decreasing properties of soy has been verified in many experiments with human volunteers (Deibert et.al. 2004; Liao et.al. 2007; Roccisano et.al. 2012)

and experiments with mice and rats (Choi et.al. 2011; Grant et.al. 1995; Shinjo et.al. 1992; Davis et.al. 2005).

Soy protein isolate

(Glycine Max)

Soy protein isolate is extracted soy flour, where almost all carbohydrates and fat has been removed. As a result, the protein content of soy isolate is between 80 – 90% and the calorific value is between 385 – 390 kcal/100g. This isolate contains very large amounts of the following amino acids: L-Arginine 7.6g/100g, Glutamine 10.7g/100g, Histidine 2.6g/100g and branched chain BCAA amino acids 18.2g/100g. All these amino acids are known to decrease body weight and body fat mass.

Soy protein isolate has body weight and body fat mass decreasing properties.

When rats were given in their daily food either 20% casein or 20% soy protein isolate, for 44 days, body weight was 16.4% ($p < 0.05$) and body fat mass was 52.9% ($p < 0.05$) lower in test group, compared to control group (Simmen et.al. 2010).

When rats were given high fat diet and either casein or soy protein isolate daily, for 5 weeks, body weight, body fat mass and Leptin were significantly ($p < 0.05$) lower, but Adinopectin was significantly ($p < 0.05$) higher in soy protein isolate group, compared to casein reference group (Al-Dwairi et.al. 2012).

The body weight and fat mass decreasing properties of soy protein isolate has been verified in many other experiments (Aoyama et.al. 2000; Aoyama et.al. 2000).

Spice bush, bark

(Lindera Erythrocarpa, Lindera Obtusiloba)

The bark of different Spice bushes are used in China and Korea to increase blood circulation, to decrease inflammation and to protect liver.

Spice bush bark has body weight and body fat mass decreasing properties.

When rats were given high fat diet and Spice bush (Lindera Erythrocarpa) bark ethanol extract 250 mg/kg BW daily, for 56 days, body weight gain was 20.0% ($p < 0.05$) and body fat mass was 48.2% ($p < 0.05$) lower in test group, compared to control group (Ahn et.al. 2010).

In experiments with 3T3-L1 fat cells, Japanese Spice bush (Lindera Obtusiloba) reduced strongly intracellular lipid accumulation by 70% (Freise et.al. 2010).

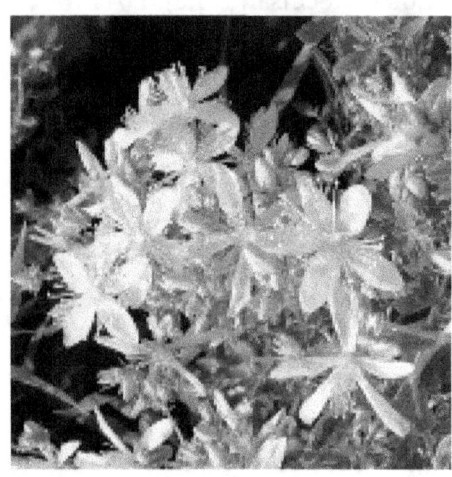

St. John's Wort

(Hypericum Perforatum)

St. John's Wort is a very old medicinal plant. The antidepressant properties were known in Europe over 500 years ago. The plant is also antiviral and antibacterial. It contains large amounts of flavonoids, especially Hyperforin and Hypericin.

St. John's Worth has body weight and fat mass decreasing properties.

When obese rats were given high fat diet and 100 mg/kg BW St. John's Wort 50% water-ethanol extract daily, for 15 days, body weight was 13.0% (p < 0.001) lower in test group, compared to control group. Also triglycerides, total cholesterol, LDL-cholesterol and blood sugar were significantly lower, but HDL-cholesterol was significantly higher in test group, compared to control group (p < 0.01 in all parameters) (Husain et.al. 2011).

When 9 volunteers were given Citrus Aurantium extract 900 mg, Caffeine 528 mg and St. John's Wort 900 mg daily, for 6 weeks, body weight decreased by 1.5 kg (p = 0.05), body fat-% decreased by 2.9% (p = 0.01) and fat mass decreased by 3.1 kg (13%; p = 0.01) in test group, the changes being significantly more than in the 7 person control group (Colker et.al. 1999). This was a double blind experiment.

Also in experiments with fat cells, St. John's Wort inhibits adipocyte differentiation (Amini et.al. 2009).

Stevia, herb

(Stevia Rebaudiana)

Stevia is a very famous plant. The active compound, Stevioside, is 300 times sweeter than sugar. Stevia originates from Paraguay, South-America, where it has been used as sweetener and medicine for hundreds of years. Stevia is known to decrease high blood pressure and heart rate.

Stevia herb has body weight and body fat mass decreasing properties.

When mice were given high fat diet and 1 ml/kg Stevia herb water extract daily, for 15 weeks, body weight gain was 13% (p < 0.05) lower in test group, compared to control group. Also body fat mass was significantly (p < 0.05) lower in test group, compared to control group (Park et.al. 2010).

When diabetic rats were given 250 mg/kg BW dried Stevia herb daily, for 3 weeks, body weight was 6.7% lower in test group, compared to control group (Sumon et.al. 2008).

Stoneage diet

The early human beings, who lived 2 million years – 100 000 years ago, lived in so called Paleolithic time period. They were hunters and also gathered plant foods. Their daily diet was mostly lean meat, fish, birds, eggs, roots, wild vegetables, berries, fruits, nuts and honey. They drank water. There was no salt, no grains, no bread, no butter, no vegetable oils, no red wine. The fat content of daily food was low, because wild animal fat content is very low. About 65% of daily calories came from animals and 35% from plants.

This kind of diet is called "Stoneage diet" or "Paleolithic diet". It is now heavily researched, because it seems to be more healthy, than the famous Mediterranean diet.

Stoneage diet has body weight decreasing properties.

When 13 diabetic volunteers were 3 months either on Stoneage diet or on the normal Diabetic diet, the following properties decreased significantly on the Stoneage diet, compared to the diabetic diet: body weight decreased by 3.0 kg ($p = 0.01$), Body Mass index BMI decreased by 1.0 kg/m2 ($p = 0.04$), and waist circumference decreased by 4.0 cm ($p = 0.02$) (Jönssön et.al. 2009).

When 10 Australian aboriginals in an experiment lived again 7 weeks in their original lands in Western Australia so, that they hunted and gathered all their food from nature, their body weight decreased by 8.0 kg (81.9 kg → 73.9 kg; 9.76% decrease). The total energy per day was 1200 kcal, and about 64% came from animal protein. Fat content of diet was only 13%, because wild animals contain very little fat (O'Dea 1984).

When pigs were on daily Stoneage diet for 13 months, body weight decreased 22% ($p = 0.0009$), compared to the control group, which got normal grain food (Jönssön et.al. 2006).

Sour Mandarin, peel

(Citrus Sunki, syn. Citrus Reticulata var. Austera)

The peel of Sour mandarin is used in Asia as a medicine in digestive problems and asthma.

Sour mandarin peel has body weight and fat mass decreasing properties.

When mice were given high fat diet and 150 mg/kg BW Sour mandarin peel 80% ethanol extract daily, for 70 days, body weight was 16.6% ($p < 0.05$), body fat mass was 36.3% ($p < 0.05$), triglycerides were 39.3% ($p < 0.05$) and total cholesterol was 17.6% ($p < 0.05$) lower in test group, compared to control group (Kang et.al. 2012).

Sudachi, fruit peel

(Citrus Sudachi)

Sudachi is a delicious citrus fruit, which has small, round and yellow fruits. It is cultivated especially in the Tokushima prefecture, in Japan. Both the pulp and peel are edible.

Sudachi fruit peel has body weight and body fat mass decreasing properties.

In experiments with 3T3-L1 fat cells, Sudachi stimulates very strongly lipolysis (Sakuramata et.al. 1998).

When 40 volunteers with metabolic syndrome were given 1.3 grams Sudachi dried peel powder daily, for 12 weeks, body weight decreased by 1.3 kg (76.9 kg → 75.6 kg; $p < 0.01$), waist circumference decreased by 1.8 cm (99.1 cm → 97.3 cm; $p < 0.01$) and diglycerides decreased by 23.8% (185 mg/dl → 141 mg/dl; $p < 0.01$) in test group, compared to control group. This was a double blind experiment (Akaike et.al. 2012).

Sugar

(Sucrose, fructose, glucose)

Sucrose and even fructose are added to almost every food nowadays, and they are widely used in making food and sweet drinks. Both sucrose and glucose increase blood glucose levels and thus also the blood Insulin levels increase. Insulin is a 51 amino acid peptide hormone made by pancreas, which has a critical role in regulation of carbohydrate and fat metabolism in the body. Insulin stores glucose in liver and muscle cells as glycogen and in fat cells as triglycerides. Insulin stops the use of fat as energy source by inhibiting the release of the hormone Glucagon. Thus Insulin is a fattening hormone. The Insulin level goes to basal value 2 hours after a meal. So if a person eats many times per day meals with high glycemic index GI foods, such as potatoes, white rice, white bread, sucrose containing drinks etc., the level of Insulin will stay high most of the day, in non-diabetic persons. So Insulin will store most of the day sugar as glycogen and as fat in the body, and he can still feel hunger.

Sucrose and fructose have body weight and body fat increasing properties.

For a long time it has been known from animal experiments, that even though the daily energy input does not change, the high fat- and sugar content of food increases body fat mass and body weight.

When rats were given either high sugar diet, or high fat diet or normal laboratory diet for 55 weeks, with the same total energy intake daily, body fat-% in sugar group was 45%, in fat group 46% but only 33% in the control group (Oscai et.al. 1987).

When studying 23 lean men (body weight 72.7 kg; fat-% 11.1%), 17 lean females (body weight 52.5 kg; fat-% 16.7%), 23 obese men (body weight 96.8 kg; fat-% 20.2%) and 15 obese females (body weight 90.0 kg; fat-% 42.7%), who all had the same total energy and total fat intake daily, it was noticed, that obese persons got more added sugar (men: 38.0% vs. 25.2%; females: 47.9% vs. 31.4%) from daily carbohydrates, compared to lean persons.

Also obese persons got less dietary fiber (men: 20.9 g vs. 27.0 g; females: 15.7 g vs. 22.7 g) from daily food, compared to lean persons (Miller et.al. 1994).

The body weight, body fat mass and triglycerides increasing but fat oxidation decreasing properties of sucrose and fructose has been verified in great many experiments with human volunteers (Vermunt et.al. 2003; Sartor et.al. 2012; Elliott et.al. 2002; Teff et.al. 2004; Teff et.al. 2009; Cox et.al. 2012; Le et.al. 2006; Le et.al. 2009; Stanhope et.al. 2009; Malik et.al. 2006).

Sweet Basil

(Ocimum Basilicum)

Sweet Basil is a very delicious vegetable and spice, which can be purchased fresh or dried all around the year. It is known to decrease cholesterol and triglycerides.

Sweet basil has body weight decreasing properties.

When rats were given high fat diet and 0.5 grams/kg BW Sweet Basil water extract daily, for 10 weeks, body weight in test group was 8.8% (p = 0.073) lower, compared to control group. Also triglycerides, total cholesterol and LDL-cholesterol were all significantly (p < 0.05) lower, but HDL-cholesterol was significantly (p < 0.05) higher in test group, compared to control group (Harnafi et.al. 2009).

When chicken were given 10% Sweet Basil in their daily diet, for 2 weeks, body weight gain was 52.0% (p < 0.05) lower in test group, compared to control group (Gadir et.al. 2006).

Sweet potato

(Ipomoea Batatas)

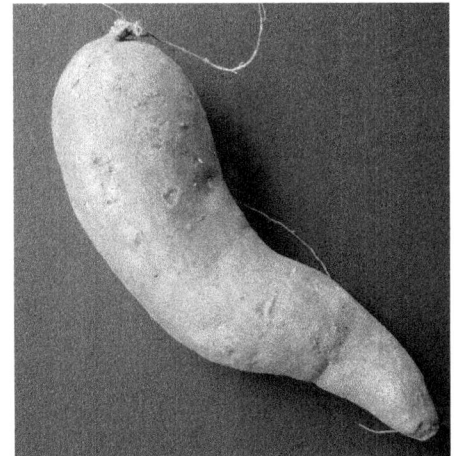

Sweet potato is the familiar vegetable root. Besides food, it is also used as a medicinal plant. In Japan Sweet potato (Caiapo) is used raw against diabetes and hypertension.

Sweet potato has body weight decreasing properties.

When 30 type 2 diabetes patients were given Sweet potato (Caiapo) 4 grams daily, for 12 weeks, body weight decreased in the test group by 3.7 kg (78.9 kg → 75.2 kg; p = 0.003), which was significantly more than the 1.0 kg (77.2 kg → 76.2 kg) in the control group. Also blood Glucose was significantly (p < 0.001) lower in test group, compared to the control group (Ludvig et.al. 2004). This was a double blind experiment.

When 24 type 2 diabetes patients were given Sweet potato (Caiapo) 4 grams daily, for 5 months, Adiponectin increased by 11.0% (5.97 mcg/ml → 6.63 mcg/ml; $p = 0.013$) and triglycerides decreased by 9.1% (2.32 mmol/L → 2.07 mmol/L; $p = 0.032$), compared to the control group (Ludvik et.al. 2008). This was a double blind experiment.

In other experiments Sweet potato and the close relatives Dioscorea Niopponica and Dioscorea Tokorinis decrease body weight and body fat mass, compared to the control groups (Ju et.al. 2011; Hwang et.al. 2011; Kusano et.al. 200; Cho et.al. 2010; Kwon et.al. 2003; Song et.al. 2009; Xuiong et.al. 2009).

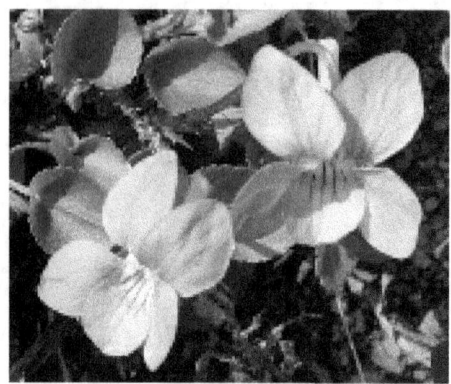

Sweet Violet

(Viola Odorata)

Sweet Violet is a very old medicinal plant. Its leaves and flowers can be eaten in salads. Hippocrates mentions it already 2400 years ago against liver diseases.

Sweet Violet has body weight decreasing properties.

When rats were given high fat diet and 300 mg/kg BW Sweet Violet methanol extract daily, for 6 weeks, body weight gain was 9.1% ($p < 0.05$) lower in test group, compared to control group. Also total cholesterol decreased by 28.2% ($p < 0.05$) and LDL-cholesterol decreased by 30.4% ($p < 0.05$) in test group, compared to control group (Siddiqi et.al. 2012).

Taiwan Galangal

(Alpinia Pricei)

Taiwan Galangal is endemic to Taiwan. It is a close relative to the familiar Ginger, and the root is used as a spice and in cooking the same way.

Taiwan Galangal root has body weight and body fat mass decreasing properties.

When obese mice were given high sugar diet and 5% Taiwan Galangal root ethanol extract daily, for 4 weeks, body weight in test group was 15% ($p < 0.05$) and total fat mass was 25% ($p < 0.05$) lower, compared to control group. Leptin was 56.6% ($p < 0.05$) lower, but Adiponectin was 37.4% ($p < 0.05$) higher in test group, compared to control group (Chou et.al. 2009).

Tamarind

(Tamarindus Indica)

Tamarind is a very popular sour fruit, which is used much in different foods in Asia. It is known to decrease blood pressure and cholesterol.

Tamarind fruit and seeds have body weight decreasing properties.

The body weight decreasing property of Tamarind has been verified in 5 different researchs.

When obese rat were fed high fat diet and either 5 mg/kg BW, 25 mg/kg BW, 50 mg/kg BW or 300 mg/kg BW Tamarind pulp water extract daily, for 10 weeks, body weight decreased in test groups by 3.2%, 11.3%, 12.1% and 12.3% ($p < 0.05$ in all groups), compared to the control group. Also triglycerides, LDL-cholesterol and total cholesterol decreased significantly, but HDL-cholesterol increased significantly in test groups, compaed to the control group (Khairunnuur et.al. 2010).

The body weight decreasing properties of Tamarind fruits and seeds has been verified also in other experiments (Azman et.al. 2012; Jindal et.al. 2011; Ukwuani et.al. 2008; Shahraki et.al. 2011).

Tart Cherry

(Prunus Cerasus)

Tart Cherry is dark blue Cherry, which contains large amount of Anthocyanins, especially Cyanidin-3-Glucosylrutinoside. Tart Cherry has positive impact on muscle soreness and pain, and it also improves sleep, by increasing Metanonin levels.

Tar Cherry has body weight and fat mass decreasing properties.

When rats on high fat diet were given in their daily diet 1% dried Tart Cherries, for 90 days, body weight decreased in the test group by 6.0% (517 g $\rightarrow$ 486 g; $p < 0.05$), compared to the control group. Body fat mass decreased in the test group by 9% (63% $\rightarrow$ 54%; $p < 0.05$), compared to the control group. Also in the test group triglycerides decreased by 15.1% ($p < 0.05$), total cholesterol decreased by 10.6% ($p < 0.05$), Glucose decreased by 15.8% ($p < 0.05$) and Insulin decreased by 20.2% ($p < 0.05$), compared to the control group (Seymour et.al. 2009).

Taurine

Taurine is a Suphur containing natural amino acid, which exists both in living cells and food. Taurine is known to decrease blood pressure and cholesterol. Taurine is a very cheap amino acid, which can be bought in Supermarkets.

Taurine has body weight and body fat mass decreasing properties.

When mice were given high fat diet and 5% Taurine in their daily food, for 18 weeks, body weight decreased by 26% ($p < 0.001$) and body fat-% decreased by 16% ($p < 0.001$) in test group, compared to the control group (Tsuboyama-Kasaoka et.al. 2006).

The body weight and body fat mass decreasing properties of Taurine has been verified in large number of experiments with mice and rats (Pina-Zentella et.al. 2012; Mikami et.al. 2012; Nakaya et.al. 2000; Du et.al. 2010; Mesallamy et.al. 2010; Nardelli et.al. 2011).

When volunteers were given 1.66 grams Taurine, 1 hour before 90 minutes bicycle exercise, Taurine increased fat oxidation by 16% ($p < 0.05$), compared to the control group (Rutherford et.al. 2010).

When 15 obese volunteers were given 3 grams Taurine daily, for 7 weeks, both body weight ($p < 0.05$) and triglycerides ($p < 0.05$) decreased significantly, compared to the 15 person control group (Zhang et.al. 2004). This was a double blind experiment.

Terminalia, fruit

(Terminalia Pallida, Terminalia Chebula, Terminalia Belerica)

Terminalia is a genus of large tropical trees. There are about 200 different Terminalia species. Especially in India the following famous Terminalia tree fruits are used in very many different illnesses: Bahera (Terminalia Bellerica), Haritaki (Terminalia Chebula) and Terminalia Pallida. All these fruits are known to decrease cholesterol, triglycerides and blood pressure.

Terminalia fruit has body weight decreasing properties.

When obese rats were given high fat diet and 100 mg/kg BW Terminalia Pallida fruit ethanol extract daily, for 30 days, body weight was 22% ($p < 0.0001$) lower in test group, compared to control group. Also total cholesterol, LDL-cholesterol and triglycerides were significantly ($p < 0.01$) lower, but HDL-cholesterol was significantly ($p < 0.01$) higher in test group, compared to control group (Sampathkumar et.al. 2011).

The body weight, total cholesterol and triglycerides decreasig properties has been verified also with Bahera fruit (Terminalia Bellerica) in experiments with mice (Makihara et.al. 2012) and with Haritaki (Terminalia Chebula) fruit in experiments with rats (Israni et.al. 2010).

Thistle

(Cirsium Oligophyllum, Cirsium Sp.)

There exists several tens of different Thistle species in the World. The leaves and roots of all these species are edible. Especially the leaves of the following Thistle species are eaten as vegetable: Cirsium Oligophyllum, Cirsium Pyrenaicum, Cirsium Vulgare and Cirsium Oleraceum. Thistle contains large amounts of flavonoids, especially Cirsimarin, which is known to decrease body weight and body fat mass.

Thistle leaves have body weight and fat mass decreasing properties.

When rats were given daily either water or 10% strong water-ethanol extract of Thistle, for 32 days, body weight decreased by 6.6% ($p < 0.05$) in test group, compared to control group. Subcutaneous fat mass decreased by 26.2% ($p < 0.05$) in test group, compared to control group. Also topical application of 2% strong extract for 7 days decreased subcutaneous fat mass by 23.3% ($p < 0.05$) (Mori et.al. 2009).

Three-leaved Ladybell, root

(Adenophora Triphylla)

Three-leaved Ladybell root is edible, and it is used in Korea against obesity. The root contains saponins. The root is also used in several lung diseases as a medicine.

Three-leaved Ladybell root has body weight decreasing properties.

When obese mice were given high fat diet and 75 mg/kg BW Three-leaved Ladybell root ethyl acetate extract daily, for 4 weeks, body weight in test group was 6.9% ($p < 0.05$) lower, compared to control group. Also triglycerides, total cholesterol and LDL-cholesterol were significantly lower in test group, compared to control group (Choi et.al. 2010).

Three-leaved Ladybell root extracts inhibits 3T3-L1 adipocyte differentiation and fat accumulation (Ahn et.al. 2012).

Thunberg's Geranium

(Geranium Thunbergii)

Thunberg's Geranium grows in China, Korea and Japan. It has been traditionally used as a medicinal plant in diarrhea.

Thunberg's Geranium has body weight and fat mass decreasing properties.

When obese rats were given high fat diet and 400 mg/kg BW extract made from 70% ethanol fraction of Thunberg's Geranium, daily for 6.5 weeks, body weight was 13% (p < 0.01) lower in test group, compared to control group. Total fat mass was 37% (p < 0.01) lower in test group, compared to control group. Also total cholesterol, LDL-cholesterol, triglycerides and Leptin were significantly (p < 0.01 in all parameters) lower, but Adiponectin was significantly (p < 0.05) higher in test group, compared to control group (Sung et.al. 2011).

Tienchi Ginseng

(Panax Notoginseng)

Tienchi Ginseng is cultivated in southern China, in Yunnan province. It is a very old medicinal plant, which increases blood circulation, lowers high blood pressure, and lowers high cholesterol levels. The active compounds are saponins and many different Ginsenoids.

Tienchi Ginseng has body weight and fat mass decreasing properties.

When diabetic mice were given Tienchi Ginseng saponins at a daily dose of 200 mg/kg BW, for 12 days, body weight in test group was 6.45%% (p < 0.001) lower, compared to control group. Body fat mass was 13.6% (p < 0.05) lower in test group, compared to control group. Also triglycerides were 14.7% (p < 0.05) and Leptin was 38.0% (p < 0.05) lower in test group, compared to control group (Yang et.al. 2010).

The body weight decreasing property of Tienchi Ginseng has been verified also in other experiments with mice (Yang et.al. 2009; Chen et.al. 2008).

Tiger nut

(Cyperus Esculentus)

Tiger nut is an ancient food crop. It has been cultivated in Asia and Africa over 5000 years. Its cultivation is extremely easy. Tiger nut contains large amounts of dietary fiber, protein and monounsaturated fatty acids.

Tiger nut has body weight and body fat mass decreasing properties.

When rats were given daily 500 mg/kg BW Tiger nut water extract, for 30 days, body weight in test group was 14.3% lower, compared to control group. Also blood sugar decreased in test group by 15.7% (p < 0.05), compared to contro group (Chukwuma et.al. 2010).

Also in another experiment with rats Tiger nut decreased significantly both body weight and body fat mass in test group, compared to control group (Moon et.al. 2012).

Tomato and Lycopene

(Lycopersicun Esculentum)

Tomato is known to everybody as a healthy vegetable. Lycopene is the most important carotenoid in Tomato. It is a strong antioxidant. Other good Lycopene sources are Guava, Watermelon and Red Grapefruit.

Tomato and Lycopene have body weight and fat mass decreasing properties.

When 16 type 2 diabetes patients were given 10 mg Lycopene daily, for 8 weeks, body weight decreased by 2.2 kg, fat-% decreased by 1.7% and waist circumferene decreased by 3.8 cm in Lycopene group, compared to the 16 volunteers control group (Neyestani et.al. 2007). This was a double blind experiment.

When rats were given high fat diet and either 8% Tomato paste, 24% raw Tomato or 0.1% Lycopene daily, for 8 weeks, body weight decreased in these test groups by 31.4% ($p < 0.05$), 31.7% ($p < 0.05$) and 30.7% ($p < 0.05$), compared to control group. Also total cholesterol, LDL-cholesterol, VLDL-cholesterol and triglycerides decreased significantly, but HDL-cholesterol increased significantly ($p < 0.05$ in all parameters), compared to control group (El-Nashar et.al. 2012).

The body weight, fat mass, LDL-cholesterol, VLDL-cholesterol, total cholesterol and triglycerides decreasing properties of Tomato and Lycopene has been verified in many experiments with hamsters, mice and rats (Friedman et.al. 2000; Phachonpai et.al. 2012; Kim et.al. 2012).

Tridax, leaves

(Tridax Procumbens)

Tridax is a small size flowering plant, which is regarded as a weed. It grows in America, Africa, Australia and Asia. Its English name is Coat Buttons and its Hindi language name is Ghamra. It has a large amount of medicinal uses. It is antihypertensive, antibacterial, hepatoprotective and antidiabetic. It contains large amounts of flavonoids, such as Quercetin, Luteolin and Isoquercetin (Mundada et.al. 2010).

Tridax leaves have body weight decreasing properties.

When rats were given high cholesterol diet and 20 mg/kg BW Tridax leaves water extract daily, for 7 days, body weight gain in test group was 36.0% ($p < 0.05$) lower, compared to controlgroup. Also triglycerides were 57.1% ($p < 0.05$), total cholesterol was 22.1% ($p < 0.05$), LDL-cholesterol was 26.3% ($p < 0.05$) and VLDL-cholesterol was 57.4% ($p < 0.05$) lower, but HDL-cholesterol was 12.6% ($p < 0.05$) higher in test group, compared to control group (Ikewuchi et.al. 2009).

Trifoliate orange, raw fruit

(Poncirus Trifoliata)

Trifoliate orange is a cold hardy citrus fruit. Its raw fruits are used medicinally in Asia, against viral infections and allergy.

Trifoliate orange raw fruit has body weight decreasing properties.

When rats were given normal diet and 200 mg/kg BW trifoliate orange raw fruit water extract daily, for 10 weeks, body weight in test group was 5.5% ($p < 0.05$) lower, compared to control group (Shim et.al. 2009).

Also in another experiment with rats fed high fat diet, trifoliate orange raw fruit decreased body weight gain by 40.6% ($p < 0.05$) in test group, compared to control group (Ban et.al. 2006).

Triphala

Triphala is a very famous mixture of 3 dried fruits, which has been used in India against different diseases over 3500 years. Triphala contains equal amounts of Amla fruit (Emblica Officinalis), Haritaki fruit (Terminalia Chebula) and Beleric fruit (Terminalia Bellerica). These are all known to decrease cholesterol and blood pressure.

Triphala has body weight decreasing properties.

When 31 obese volunteers were given 10 grams Triphala daily, for 12 weeks, body weight was 4.37 kg (96.89 kg → 92.52 kg; $p < 0.001$) lower in test group, but it increased by 0.45 kg (96.56 kg → 97.01 kg; $p > 0.05$) in the 31 person control group. Waist circumference was 3.5 cm ($p < 0.001$) lower in test group, but it increased by 0.5 cm ($p > 0.05$) in control group. Hip circumference was 2.9 cm ($p < 0.001$) lower in test group, but it increased by 0.4 cm ($p > 0.05$) in control group (Kamali et.al. 2012). This was a double blind experiment.

Also in experiments with rats Triphala decreases body weight (Srikumar et.al. 2005) and it also decreases triglycerides, total cholesterol, LDL-cholesterol and VLDL-cholesterol (Saravanan et.al. 2007).

Tsao-ko cardamon

(Amomum Tsao-ko)

and False cardamon, seeds

(Amomum Villosum)

Both Tsao-ko cardamom and False cardamom are ginger like plants, which belong to the Zingiberaceae family. The seeds are strongly aromatic and extremely popular spices in East-Asia, especially in China and Vietnam. They are used in many foods, especially in different soups. Medicinally they are used in stomach problems, diarrhea, throat infections and malaria. The Chinese name of Tsao-ko cardamom is CAO GUO and the Chinese name of False cardamom is SHA REN.

Tsao-ko cardamom and False cardamom seeds have body weight and body fat mass decreasing properties.

When mice were given ordinary diet and either 1% Tsao-ko cardamom seeds or 1% False cardamom seeds daily, for 90 days, body weight increased in control group by 9.75%, but it increased only by 2.09% in False cardamom group, and body weight decreased by 1.47% in Tsao-ko cardamom group. The weight changes in both cardamom groups were significantly ($p < 0.05$) lower, compared to control group. This 1% daily amount corresponds to about 5 grams of spice daily, in human nutrition (Yu et.al. 2007).

The body weight, body fat mass, triglycerides and total cholesterol decreasing properties of Tsao-ko cardamom has been verified in 2 other animal experiments (Yu et.al. 2008; Yu et.al. 2010).

Turnip

(Brassica Rapa)

Turnip is generally cultivated all around the World as a food plant.

Turnip has body weight and fat mass decreasing properties.

When obese mice on a high fat diet were given Turnip ethanol extract 50 mg/kg BW daily, for 8 weeks, body weight gain in the test group was 33.7% ($p < 0.05$) and body fat mass was 34.3% ($p < 0.05$) lower, than in the control group. Triglycerides were 17.3% ($p < 0.05$) lower in the test group, compared to the control group (An et.al. 2010).

The body weight, body fat and triglycerides decreasing properties of Turnip has been verified in many other experiment with rats and mice (Jung et.al. 2008; Rhee et.al. 2005; Choi et.al. 2006).

Ursolic acid

Ursolic acid is a natural triterpenoid, which exist in many plants and fruits. Especially apple skin contains large amounts of Ursolic acid.

Ursolic acid has body weight and fat mass decreasing properties.

When mice were given high fat diet and 0.14% Ursolic acid daily, for 6 weeks, body weight was 9% ($p < 0.05$) and fat mass was 27% ($p < 0.05$) lower in test group, compared to control group. Also blood glucose and heart rate were significantly ($p < 0.05$) lower, but running endurance and muscle strength were significantly ($p < 0.05$) higher in test group, compared to control group (Kunkel et.al. 2012).

The body weight, body fat mass, blood glucose and cholesterol decreasing properties of Ursolic acid has been verified in great many animal experiments (Jayaprakasam et.al. 2006; Sundaresan et.al. 2012; Rao et.al. 2011; Li et.al. 2010; Kim et.al. 2009; Kunkel et.al. 2011).

Vegetable Sesame, leaves

(Sesamum Radiatum)

Vegetable Sesame or Benniseed originates from Africa, where is is cultivated as an important vegetable for its edible leaves, seeds and oil. Vegetable Sesame is a close relative to our familiar Sesame, Sesamum Indicum, from which normally the seeds and oils are used.

Vegetable Sesame leaves have body weight decreasing properties.

When rats were given normal diet and 14 mg/kg BW Vegetable Sesame leaves water extract daily, for 4 weeks, body weight in test group was 10.0% ($p < 0.05$) lower, compared to control group. Also total cholesterol was 39% ($p < 0.05$), LDL-cholesterol was 82% ($p < 0.05$) and VLDL-cholesterol was 13% ($p < 0.05$) lower in test group, compared to control group (Shittu et.al. 2007).

Vegetarian diet

It is known, that vegetarians have clearly lower blood pressure, cholesterol levels and BMI values, than non-vegetarians or meat eaters.

When changing from non-vegetarian diet into vegetarian diet, large positive changes in blood pressure, cholesterol levels and BMI values can be noticed already within 2 weeks.

Vegetarian diet has body weight decreasing properties.

When 22343 male and 38649 females were studied in USA, it was noticed, that vegetarians have clearly the lowest BMI values, of all the studied different food eating groups. The BMI values were 23.6 kg/m2 for vegetarians, 25.7 for ovo vegetarians, 26.3 kg/m2 for pesco-vegetarians, 27.3 kg/m2 for semi-vegetarians and 28.8 kg/m2 for nonvegetarians (Tonstad et.al. 2009).

The same kind of results was noticed also in another meta-analysis, where it was found, that vegetarians have 2.0 lower BMI value, than other food eating groups. This means a 7.6 kg lower weight of male vegetarians and 3.3 kg lower weight for female vegetarians, compared to non-vegetarians (Sabate et.al. 2010).

In another research with 21105 male and females, the vegetarians had 5.9 kg lower weight for males and 4.7 kg lower weight for females, compared to non-vegetarians (Key et.al. 1996).

When 64 obese female were on vegetarian diet for 12 weeks, they lost 5.8 kg of body weight, being significantly ($p = 0.012$) more than the 3.8 kg in the control group (Barnard et.al. 2005). The daily calorific value was unlimited in both groups.

When 15 men with high cholesterol levels but normal blood pressure, were on a diet for 2 weeks, where they ate vegetarian food with high fiber content (40 g/1000 kcal), little salt (5 g/day), little cholesterol (25 mg/day), milk daily and 85 grams of fish once in a week, the following results were seen:
  - Body weight decreased by 2.6 kg (89.2 kg → 86.6 kg; $p < 0.05$)
  - Total cholesterol decreased by 21% ($p < 0.05$)
  - Triglycerides decreased by 44% ($p < 0.05$)
  - Systolic blood pressure decreased by 11.2 mmHg ($p < 0.05$)
  - Diastolic blood pressure decreased by 9.0 mmHg ($p < 0.05$)
(Barnard et.al. 1987).

Veldt Grape

(Cissus Quadrangularis)

Veldt Grape is a vine, which originates from Africa and Asia. Especially in India, it has been used for hundreds of years as a vegetable and medicinal plant. It has been used to heal broken bones, against asthma and as an anti-inflammatory agent. The plant is edible, and is used in India as a vegetable salad, all around the year.

Veldt Grape has body weight decreasing properties.

When 62 obese volunteers were given standardized Veldt Grape extract 1000 mg daily, for 8 weeks, body weight decreased by 6.9% ($p < 0.05$) in the group with BMI higher than 30, and 4.8% in the group, with BMI lower than 30, compared to the placebo group. Fat-% decreased by 6.0% and 4.7% in these groups, compared to the placebo group. (Oben et.al. 2006). This was a double blind experiment.

When 24 volunteers were given Veldt grape extract 300 mg daily, for 10 weeks, body weight decreased by 8.7 kg (8.82%; $p < 0.01$) and fat-% decreased by 4.73% ($p < 0.05$), compared to the placebo group (Oben et.al. 2008). This was a double blind experiment.

Velvet bean

(Mucuna Pruriens)

Velvet bean is a famous medicinal plant from India, where it is called Kevach in Hindi language. It is widely used as a sex stimulant. It is known to increase Testosterone and libido. The seeds contains very large amounts of the amino acid L-Dopa.

Velvet bean whole plant has body weight decreasing properties.

When obese rats were fed Methanol extract of whole Velvet bean plant, at a dose 200 mg/kg BW daily, for 9 weeks, body weight was 29.7% ($p < 0.05$) lower in test group, compared to control group. Also triglycerides, total cholesterol, LDL-cholesterol and VLDL-cholesterol were significantly ($p < 0.05$ in all parameters) lower, but HDL-cholesterol was significantly ($p < 0.05$) higher in test group, compared to control group (Kumar et.al. 2010).

Also in another experiment with rats, Flavonone fraction from the whole Velvet bean plant at a dose of 10 mg/kg BW daily, for 14 days, decreased body weight by 18.3% ($p < 0.001$) in test group, compared to control group (Kumar et.al. 2012).

Vernonia, Bitter leaf

(Vernonia Amygdalina)

Bitter leaf is a small tree or brush, which originates from tropical Africa. Its leaves are bitter and used as vegetable. They have also many medicinal properties. Bitter leaf is known to decrease triglycerides and cholesterol.

Bitter leaf has body weight and fat mass decreasing properties.

When obese rats were fed high calorific value food, and also either 5% or 10% of Bitter leaf in their daily diet for 4 weeks, body weight gain was 12.7% ($p < 0.05$) and 38.5% ($p < 0.05$) lower in test groups, compared to the control group with high calorific value food. Total fat mass was 28.0% ($p < 0.05$) and 30.0% ($p < 0.05$) lower in the test groups, compared to the control group. Also triglycerides and total cholesterol were 15% ($p < 0.05$) lower in the test groups, compared to the control group (Atangwho et.al. 2012).

The body weight decreasing property of Bitter leaf has been verified also in other experimetns with rats and rabbits (Ijeh et.al. 2011; Ong et.al. 2011; Adaramoye et.al. 2008).

With rats Bitter leaf decreased significantly triglycerides, LDL-cholesterol and total cholesterol, but increased HDL-cholesterol (Ugwu et.al. 2011).

When 39 obese volunteers were 30 days on a controlled diet, and they were given 4 – 8 times daily Bitter leaf tea, the average body weight decreased by 16 kg in this group (Anastasia et.al. 2011). This experiment did not have a control group.

Very Low Calorie Diet
(VLCD)

VLCD diet is defined as diets which contain energy levels less than 800 kcal daily. VLCD diet is usually used for 2 – 16 weeks, to get a rapid weight loss. Weight loss is usually between 1.5 kg – 2.5 kg per week (Mustjoki et.al. 2001). Also systolic and diastolic blood pressure, total cholesterol, LDL-cholesterol and triglycerides decrease significantly on VLCD diet (Mustjoki et.al. 2001).

VLCD diet has body weight and body fat mass decreasing properties.

When 17 obese females (BMI > 28) were on 500 – 600 kcal daily VLCD diet for 8 weeks, body weight decreased by 11% ($p < 0.01$). Also body fat mass ($p < 0.01$) decreased significantly (Svendsen et.al. 2012).

When 14 obese (BMI = 35) volunteers were on daily VLCD diet for 16 weeks, body weight decreased by 22% ($p < 0.05$) (Snel et.al. 2012). Also visceral and subcutaneous abdominal fat volume decreased by 47% ($p < 0.05$).

When 29 obese type II diabetes patients and 31 obese volunters were on 450 kcal daily VLCD diet for 15 days, BMI decreased in diabetes group by 2.0 units (35.3 → 33.3) and in the obese volunteer group by 2.4 units (40.5 → 38.1) (Rotella et.al. 1994).

When 9 obese (BMI = 33.4) female volunteers were on 500 – 600 kcal daily VLCD diet for 53 days, body weight decreased by 11.5% ($p < 0.05$) compared to baseline values (Rabol et.al. 2009).

When 8 obese children were on 240 kcal daily VLCD diet for 3 weeks, body weight decreased by 9.3 kg (82.5 kg → 73.2 kg). Also, when 8 obese children were on 320 kcal daily VLCD diet for 3 weeks, body weight decreased by 8.4 kg (89.3 kg → 80.9 kg) (Zwiauer et.al. 1987).

Large decreases in body weight can be achieved on VLCD diet already within 2 weeks, depending on the initial body weight and daily energy content.

Vietnamese Balm
(Elsholtzia Ciliata)

Vietnamese Balm is a salad plant, which is used in Korea, Japan, China and Vietnam. The leaves are used as a salad and the seeds are used as spice. The plant is anti-viral and anti-bacterial.

Vietnamese Balm has body weight and fat mass decreasing properties.

When obese mice were given high fat diet and ethanol extract of Vietnamese Balm at a dose of 400 mg/kg BW daily, for 6.5 weeks, body weight decreased by 10.6% ($p < 0.05$) and body fat mass decreased by 43.6% ($p < 0.05$) in test group, compared to control group. Also triglycerides, total cholesterol and Leptin decreased significantly ($p < 0.05$ in all parameters) in test group, compared to control group (Sung et.al. 2011).

Vinegar

Apple vinegar and rice vinegar are generally used in food making. Vinegar contains acetic acid. Vinegar is known to decrease blood pressure and cholesterol.

When 58 obese volunteers were given 30 ml Vinegar, containing 1500 mg acetic acid daily, for 12 weeks, body weight decreased in test group by 1.9 kg, being significantly ($p < 0.01$) different, compared to the control group, where body weight increased by 0.4 kg. Also triglycerides decreased by 26.4% ($p < 0.001$) and systolic blood pressure decreased by 4.56 mmHg ($p < 0.01$) in test group, compared to the control group (Kondo et.al. 2009). This was a double blind experiment.

The body weight decreasing and fatty acid oxidation increasing properties of Vinegar and acetic acid has been verified in many experiments with rats and fat cells (Hattori et.al. 2010; Kondo et.al. 2009; Yamashita et.al. 2007; Yamashita et.al. 2009; Fushimi et.al. 2006; Shuan-kui et.al. 2012).

Vitamin C

(Ascorbic acid)

Vitamin C is an essential, water soluble vitamin. Its recommended daily intake (RDA) is between 60-100 mg. It is totally safe, even in daily doses between 10 – 50 grams. It has many positive effects (in daily amounts over 1 grams): it increases immunity, increases sexual capacity, inhibits aromatase enzyme etc.

Vitamin C has body weight and fat mass decreasing properties.

When 19 severely obese volunteers were given 3.0 grams vitamin C daily, for 6 weeks, the body weight decreased significantly in test group by 2.5 kg ($p < 0.05$), which was much larger than the 1.0 kg decrease in 19 volunteers control group (Naylor et.al. 1985). This was a double blind experiment.

When comparing 118 volunteers, it was noticed, that there was a negative correlation between plasma vitamin C concentration, and body mass index BMI, body fat-% and waist circumference ($r = -0.383$ to -0.497; $p < 0.025$ in all parameters). (Johnston et.al. 2007). The higher the plasma vitamin C concentration, the lower were BMI, body fat-% and waist circumference.

When rats were on high fat diet, vitamin C decreased significantly both body weight and body fat-% in test group, compared to control group (Campion et.al. 2008).

When using vitamin C as a supplement, it should be taken 3 grams or more on daily bases.

Vitamin D3

(Cholecalciferol)

Vitamin D is an essential vitamin, which exists in food and can also be made in human skin by the effect of Sun light. It has a very important role together with Calcium in many cell functions.

D3 vitamin has body fat mass decreasing properties.

When 42 volunteers were given vitamin D3 25 micrograms daily, for 12 weeks, body fat mass decreased significantly ($p < 0.0001$) by 2.7 kg in test group, compared to the 0.47 kg decrease in the 43 volunteers control group. Also fat free mass increased significantly ($p < 0.0001$) by 1.8 kg in test group, compared to the 0.4 kg increase in the control group (Salehpour et.al. 2012). This was a double blind experiment.

When examining the plasma vitamin D level in 276 volunteers, it was noticed, that there was a negative correlation ($r=-0.480$; $p < 0.0001$) between vitamin D level and body mass index BMI, and also a negative correlation ($r=-0.480$; $p < 0.0001$) between vitamin D level and waist circumference (Tamer et.al. 2012). The higher the plasma vitamin D level, the lower are body weight and waist circumference.

Water

Water is essential for all life. The daily water need depends on many things: Body weight, age, work, ambient temperature, ambient humidity, exercise etc. Water is also very important, when trying to keep the ideal body weight for each person. In fact water is the cheapest and simplest method to decrease obesity. Body weight is dependent on water by many different ways. Water increases resting energy expenditure, decrease hunger feeling and decreases the energy density of food and increases satiety.

Water has body weight and body fat mass decreasing properties.

When 20 obese volunteers (BMI = 32.1) were given hypocaloric diet and 500 ml water before each meal daily, for 12 weeks, body weight decreases 2 kg ($p < 0.001$) more in test group, compared to 21 person (BMI = 31.8) placebo group without water, which was given the same hypocaloric diet. Body fat mass decreased in test group by 5.4 kg, but only 3.3 kg in the placebo group (Dennis et.al. 2010).

The same kind of results has been achieved also in another test with human volunteers (Stookey et.al. 2008).

Popkin (Popkin et.al. 2005) studied the daily water intake of 4755 adult persons. 87% of these adults drank daily water, 1.53 liter per average, and their daily energy intake was by average 9% (194 kcal) lower, than the energy intake of the other persons, who did not drink daily water.

When obese children were given cold (4 degres Celsius) water 10 ml/kg BW, the resting energy expenditure (REE) increased by 25%, 1 hour after drinking the cold water. This means the same as 1.2 kg weight reduction per year (Dubnov-Raz et.al. 2011).

The same REE increasing property of cold water has been verified also in other human experiments (Boschmann et.al. 2007).

When drinking 500 ml water before meal, the energy intake in meal was decreased by 12.9% (574 kcal → 500 kcal; $p = 0.004$) in human volunteers (Davy et.al. 2008).

Exactly the same kind of results has been achieved in other experiments with human volunteers (Lappalainen et.al. 1993; Rolls et.al. 1999; Walleghen et.al. 2007).

Watermelon

(Citrullus Lanatus)

Watermelon is known to everybody as a delicious fruit. Watermelon contains large amounts of the healthy compounds Lycopene and Citrulline amino acid. Watermelon and Citrulline are known to decrease blood pressure both in human and animal experiments. Watermelon contains only 23 kcal/100 g energy, so it is one of the least energy rich fruits.

Watermelon has body weight, body fat mass, LDL-cholesterol and total cholesterol decreasing properties.

When mice were given high fat diet and 2% Watermelon in their daily food, for 12 weeks, body weight was 12.2% ($p < 0.05$) and body fat mass was 24.0% ($p < 0.05$) lower in test group, compared to the control group. Also total cholesterol ($p < 0.05$) and LDL-cholesterol ($p < 0.05$) were significantly lower in the test group (Poduri et.al. 2012).

When obese rats were given daily either water or 63% strong Watermelon juice, for 4 weeks, weight gain was 24.0% ($p < 0.05$) lower in Watermelon juice group, compared to the water group. Body fat mass was 14.2% ($p < 0.05$) lower in Watermelon juice group, compared to the water group (Wu et.al. 2007).

The LDL-cholesterol decreasing but HDL-cholesterol increasing property of Watermelon has been verified in experiment with rats (Georgiana et.al. 2011).

Wax gourd

(Benincasa Hispida, Synoyme: Benincasa Cerifera)

Wax gourd is an edible vegetable, cultivated in many places around the World. It is known to lower cholesterol and it has diuretic properties.

Wax gourd has body weight and fat mass decreasing properties.

When rats were given high fat diet and 15% Wax gourd in their daily diet, for 4 weeks, body weight was 6.6% ($p < 0.05$) and fat mass was 11.3% ($p < 0.05$) lower in test group, compared to control group. Also triglycerides decreased by 49.3% ($p < 0.05$) in test group, compared to control group (Kang et.al. 2003).

The body weight, fat mass, triglycerides, total cholesterol and appetite suppressing effect of Wax gourd has been verified in many animal experiments (Wang et.al. 2000; Kumar et.al. 2004; Yagnik et.al. 2009; Niwano et.al. 2009).

Weeping Forsythia and Phillyrin

(Forsythia Suspensa)

The Chinese name of Weeping Forsythia is Liangiao. The dried fruits of Weeping Forsythia have been used over 2000 years in China against bacterial and viral diseases and as an anti-inflammatory medicine. The fruits and especially the leaves contain large amounts of lignans, such as Phillyrin and Forsythiaside. The leaves contain up to 4.3% Phillyrin.

Weeping Forsythia leaves and Phillyrin have body weight and fat mass decreasing properties.

In experiments with liver cells, Phillyrin decreases fat accumulation to hepatocytes and suppresses FAS activity (Do et.al. 2012).

When rats were given high fat diet and either 2.5% or 5.0% Weeping Forsythia leaves daily, body weight, fat mass and triglycerides were significantly ($p < 0.05$) lower, but Adiponectin was significantly ($p < 0.05$) higher in test group, compared to control group (Nishibe et.al. 2012).

In experiments with mice, Phillyrin decreases significantly body fat mass, triglycerides and total cholesterol (Zhao et.al. 2005).

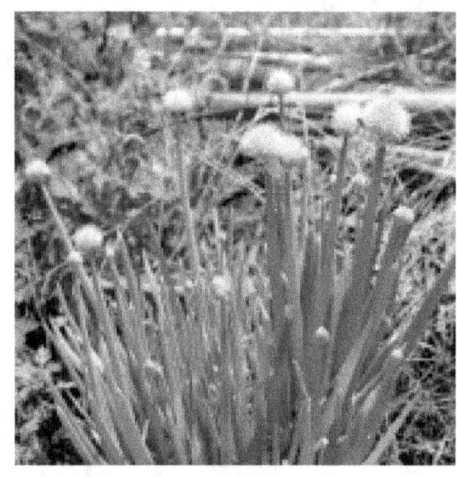

Welsh onion

(Allium Fistulosum)

Welsh onion is a very important vegetable, especially in China, Korea and Japan. Welsh onion contains large amounts of Flavonoids, especially Quercetin. Welsh onion is known to decrease blood pressure, triglycerides and total cholesterol.

Welsh onion has body weight decreasing properties.

When mice on a high fat diet were given Welsh onion ethanol extract 400 mg/kg in their daily diet, for 6.5 weeks, body weight was 10% ($p < 0.001$) lower in the test group, compared to the control group. Also triglycerides, total cholesterol and Leptin level decreased significantly ($p < 0.05$) in the test group, compared to the control group (Sung et.al. 2011).

When rats on a high fat diet were given 5% Welsh onion in their daily diet, for 4 weeks, body weight was 10% lower in the test group, compared to the control group. Also blood pressure was significantly ($p < 0.05$) lower in the test group, compared to the control group (Yamamoto et.al. 2005).

Welted Thistle

(Carduus Crispus)

Welted Thistle is a common plant in Europe and Asia. Its young leaves are edible. In Asia it is used in rheumatism, colds, stomach aches, atherosclerosis and cancer.

Welted Thistle aerial parts have body weight decreasing properties.

When rats were given high fat diet and 60 mg/kg BW Welted Thistle 70% ethanol extract daily, for 14 days, body weight decreased by 6.8% in test group, compared to control group. Also total cholesterol decreased by 12.5% and LDL-cholesterol decreased by 15.8% in test group, compared to control group (Davaakhuu et.al. 2010).

In experiments with fat cells, Welted Thistle significantly decreased fat accumulation in 3T3-L1 cells in a dose-dependent manner (Lee et.al. 2010).

Whey protein

Whey protein is manufactured as a by product of cheese processing. It contains large amounts of branched chain amino acids, BCAA, namely Leucine, Isoleucine and Valine. BCAA amino acids stimulate protein synthesis, and muscle cells can use them also as energy sources.

Whey protein has body weight decreasing properties.

When 31 volunteers were given 20 grams whey protein daily, for 12 weeks, both body weight ($p < 0.05$) and body fat-% ($p < 0.05$) decreased significantly, compared to the control group. The weight loss in whey protein group was 6.1% (Fredstedt et.al. 2008). This was a double blind experiment. Most of the volunteers lost fat by an average of 3.6 kg, during this 12 weeks test period, and total body mass loss was 5.2 kg. Muscle mass decreased by 1.35 kg less in test group, than in the control group, which shows the anabolic and protein synthesis stimulating effect of BCAA amino acids.

When 23 obese volunteers were given 56 grams whey protein daily, for 23 weeks, both body weight ($p < 0.006$) and body fat-% ($p < 0.005$) decreased significantly, compared to the control group. The average body mass reduction was 1.8 kg and the body fat mass decreased by 2.3 kg (Baer et.al. 2011). This was a double blind experiment.

When 13 bodybuilders were given daily whey protein, at a dose of 1.5 grams/kg body mass, for 10 weeks, body fat mass decreased by 1.5 kg, which was significantly ($p < 0.05$) more, than the 0.2 kg in the control group, which was given casein (Cribb et.al. 2006).

Also in experiments with rats and mice, whey protein decreases significantly both body weight and body fat mass, compared to the control groups (Huang et.al. 2008; Zhou et.al. 2011; Shi et.al. 2012; Siddiqui et.al. 2008; Belobrajdic et.al. 2004).

When 6 wrestlers were either in a low calorific diet or a low calorific diet and added BCAA amno acids, for 19 days, body weight decreased by 4.0 kg ($p < 0.05$), body fat-% decreased by 17.3% ($p < 0.05$) from original value, and waist fat content decreased by 34.4% ($p < 0.05$) from the original value. The changes were significantly larger, than in the low calorific control group (Mourier et.al. 1997).

When 68 obese volunteers were given whey protein 24.4 grams daily, for 8 weeks, body weight decreased by 2.8 kg ($p < 0.001$), BMI decreased by 1.0 kg/m2 ($p < 0.001$) and waist decreased by 7.1 cm ($p < 0.001$), compared to the control group (Sinnott et.al. 2009).

White kidney bean or Cannellini bean, water extract

(Phaseolus Vulgaris)

Cannellini beans are large, kidney looking beans, which are very popular food in Italy. They are also called White kidney beans, The Cannellini bean water extract inhibits very strongly the alfa-Amylase enzyme, which breaks down long chain complex carbohydrates. By this way the bean extract inhibits the absorption of sugars from complex carbohydrates in food, and they only increase the amount of stool.

White kidney bean water extract has body weight and body fat mass decreasing properties.

When 30 obese volunteers were given normal food and 445 mg standardized White kidney bean water extract daily, for 30 days, body weight in test group was 2.58 kg ($p < 0.001$) lower, compared to the 29 person control group. Also body fat mass was 2.24 kg ($p < 0.001$), waist circumference was 2.46 cm ($p < 0.001$) and hip circumference was 1.37 cm ($p < 0.001$) lower in test group, compared to control group. This was a double blind experiment (Celleno et.al. 2007).

The body weight and body fat mass decreasing properties of White kidney bean water extract has been verified in great many human double blind experiments (Udani et.al. 2007; Carai et.al. 2011; Kim et.al. 2004).

The alfa-Amylase inhibitors are taken before meals, and they are very effective, if the person eats a lot of carbohydrates with meal.

Whole grain barley

(Hordeum Vulgare)

Barley is a very important food. Whole grain barley contains very large amounts of beta-Glucans, which are known to decrease body weight, triglycerides and cholesterol.

Whole grain barley has body weight decreasing properties.

When obese rats were given either white rice or whole grain barley 50% of daily food, for 4 weeks, body weight gain in barley group was 18.48% ($p < 0.05$) lower, compared to the white rice group (Kim et.al. 2012).

The body weight decreasing properties of barley has been verified also in another experiment with rats (Sohn et.al. 2007).

In experiments with human volunteers, whole grain barley decreases significantly triglycerides ($p < 0.05$), total cholesterol ($p < 0.05$) and LDL-cholesterol ($p < 0.05$), compared to control group (Li et.al. 2003).

Whole grain oat

(Avena Sativa)

Oat is a very old and healthy food plant. Oat contains large amounts of beta-Glucans, which are known to decrease body weight, triglycerides and cholesterol.

When obese rats were given high fat diet together with 7.5% whole grain oat in daily food, for 8 weeks, body weight was 18.2% ($p < 0.05$) and body fat mass was 49.1% ($p < 0.01$) lower in oat group, compared to control group. Also triglycerides, total cholesterol and LDL-cholesterol were significantly lower, but HDL-cholesterol was significantly higher in oat group, compared to control group ($p < 0.05$ in all parameters) (Peng et.al. 2012).

Whole grain rice

(Oryza Sativa)

Rice is one of the most important cereal grains in the World. Especially the East-Asian countries use large amounts of rice in their daily food. Rice bran contains large amounts of healthy gamma-Oryzanol, Ferulic acid and gamma-Tocotrienol, which are known to decrease body weight and body fat.

Whole grain rice has body weight and fat mass decreasing properties.

When rats were given cholesterol rich food together with either 20% casein or 20% rice protein in their daily food, for 2 weeks, body weight was 5.1% ($p < 0.05$) and body fat mass was 15.4% ($p < 0.05$) lower in rice protein group, compared to casein protein group (Yang et.al. 2012).

When human volunteers were put on a 1070 kcal/day diet for 6 weeks, and 1 daily meal was replaced by either white rice or whole grain rice (giving 176 kcal/dose energy), body weight decreased 1.38 kg ($p < 0.05$) and body fat-% decreased by 1.20% ($p < 0.05$) more in whole grain rice group, compared to white rice group (Kim et.al. 2008).

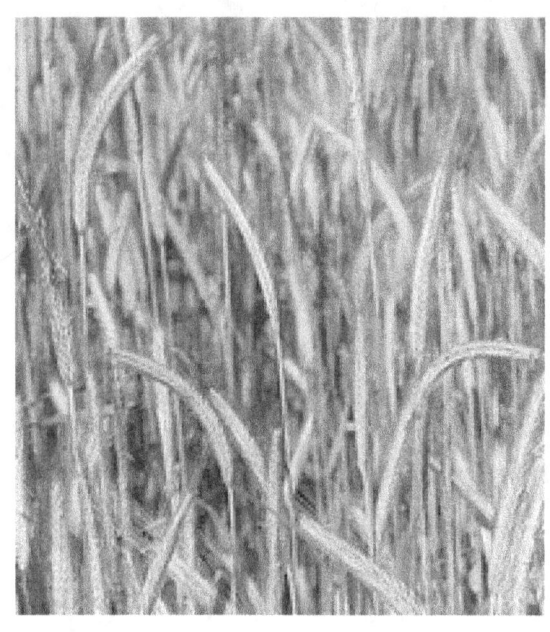

Whole grain rye

(Secale Cereale)

Rye is a very important food, which contains large amounts of healthy Lignans and fiber.

Whole grain rye has body weight and fat mass decreasing properties.

When mice were fed either whole grain rye or whole grain wheat 65% of their daily food, for 22 weeks, body weight was 8.3% ($p < 0.05$), fat mass was 31.5% ($p < 0.01$) and Leptin was 37% ($p < 0.05$) lower in whole grain rye group, compared to whole grain wheat group (Andersson et.al. 2010).

With human volunteers, rye bread breakfast decreases hunger before and after lunch, when compared to wheat bread breakfast (Isakkson et.al. 2009).

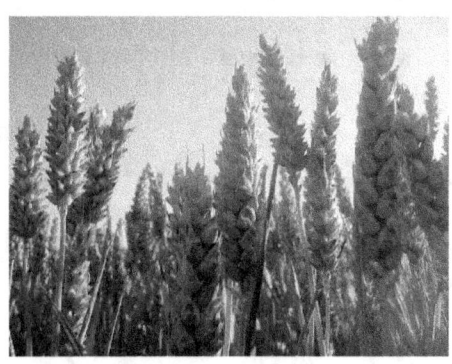

Whole grain wheat and wheat sprouts

(Triticum Aestivum)

Whole grain wheat contains all the nutrients in bran and germ, which have been removed from refined wheat.

Whole grain wheat and wheat sprouts have body weight and body fat mass decreasing properties.

When obese diabetic mice were given 100 mg/kg BW wheat sprout water extract daily, for 6 weeks, body weight in test group was 11.9% ($p < 0.05$) lower, compared to control group. Also blood sugar was 78.4% ($p < 0.05$), total cholesterol was 23.45% ($p < 0.05$) and triglycerides were 23.97% ($p < 0.05$) lower in test group, compared to control group (Lee et.al. 2011)

When 79 obese volunteers were given low calorie diet and either whole grain wheat or refined wheat daily, for 12 weeks, body weight was 0.9 kg, fat-% was 0.9% ($p = 0.04$) and LDL-cholesterol was 5% ($p = 0.02$) lower in whole grain wheat group, compared to refined wheat group (Kristensen et.al. 2012). The daily energy from wheat was 2 MJ.

When 14 healthy volunteers were given either whole grain wheat or refined wheat 48 grams daily, for 3 weeks, systolic blood pressure was 6 mmHg ($p = 0.015$) lower in whole grain wheat group, compared to refined wheat group (Bodinham et.al. 2011).

Wild Garlic

(Tulbaghia Violacea)

Wild Garlic is a fast growing plant from South-Africa. All parts of the plant are edible and used as a vegetable, and the rhizomes are also used as aphrodisiac in South-Africa.

Wild Garlic rhizomes have body weight decreasing properties.

When rats were fed very high cholesterol diet and 500 mg/kg BW Wild Garlic rhizome methanol extract daily, for 2 weeks, body weight in test group was 11.6% lower, compared to control group. Also triglycerides, total cholesterol, LDL-cholesterol and VLDL-cholesterol were all significantly ($p < 0.05$) lower, but HDL-cholesterol was significantly ($p < 0.05$) higher in test group, compared to control group (Olorunnisola et.al. 2012).

Wild rice

(Zizania Latifolia, Zizania Sp.)

Wild rice is much cultivated for food in China and Nort America. Wild rice grain has large amounts of protein, fiber and vitamins.

Wild rice has body weight and fat mass decreasing properties.

When rats were given 52.3% Wild rice daily, for 8 weeks, body weight in test group was 7.9% ($p < 0.05$) lower, compared to control group, which got ordinary white rice. Fat mass was significantly ($p < 0.05$) lower in test group, compared to control group. Also total cholesterol ($p < 0.05$) and triglycerides ($p < 0.05$) were significantly lower in test group, compared to control group (Zhang et.al. 2009).

Also in another experiment with rats Wild rice decreases significantly body weight, total cholesterol and triglycerides but increases HDL-cholesterol (Han et.al. 2012).

Yacon

(Smallanthus Sonchifolius)

Yacon originates from South-America, Peru, Equador, Argentina, Chile etc. It has been cultivated for thousands of yeas. It is a very popular root vegetable. The roots can weight up to 1 kg. The cultivation of Yacon is very easy, and it is now cultivated all around the World. Yacon roots contain up to 40 – 70% Fructo-oligosaccharides. Yacon has also large amounts of Polyphenols, up to 200 mg/100 g in roots. The most common of these are Chlorogenic acid, Ferulic acid and Quercetin. Yacon is known to decrease triglycerides and LDL-cholesterol.

Yacon has body weight reducing properties.

When 40 obese females were given daily Yacon Syrup made of the roots, containing 10 g/70 kg bodyweight Fructo-oligosaccharides, for 120 days, body weight decreased by 15.0 kg (91.2 kg → 76.2 kg; p < 0.05) in Yacon group, but it increased by 1.6 kg (90.7 kg → 92.3 kg) in the 15 obese female control group. Waist circumference decreased by 9.9 cm (105.1 cm → 95.2 cm; p < 0.05) in Yacon group, but it increased by 0.5 cm (101.4 cm → 101.9 cm) in the control group. Also LDL-cholesterol decreased by 28.8% (3.54 mmol/L → 2.52 mmol/L; p < 0.05) in the Yacon group, but it did not change in the control group (Genta et.al. 2009). This was a double blind experiment.

Yacon syrup is easily made from the root juice.

Yacon decreases body weight also in experiments with rats, compared to control group (Kim et.al. 2010). In this experiment Yacon decreased also both total cholesterol and LDL-cholesterol.

In experiments with diabetic rat, Yacon decreased both triglycerides (p < 0.05) and LDL-cholesterol (p < 0.05), compared to the control group (Habib et.al. 2011).

Yellow Loosestrife

(Lysimachia Vulgaris)

and Chinese Loosestrife

(Lysimachia Foenum-Graecum)

There exists several different Loostrife species in the World. In Europe there grows the familiar Yellow Loosestrife on wet places. It has long time been used as a herb in digestive problems, and its leaves are edible. The Chinese Loosestrife, Lysimachia Foenum-Graecum, grows in wet places in China, in Guanxi, Yunnan and Henan provinces. In Chinese it is called LING XIANG CAO. It is also used as a spice and as a medical herb in digestive problems etc.

Yellow Loosestrife and Chinese Loosestrife leaves have body weight and body fat mass decreasing properties.

In experiments with fat cells, Yellow Loosestrife strongly inhibits in vitro lipogenesis of adipose tissue (Choi et.al. 2010).

When mice were given high fat diet and 30 mg/kg BW Chinese Loosestrige ethanol extract daily, for 6 weeks, body weight was 18.4% (p < 0.01) and body fat mass was 23.8% (p < 0.01) lower in test group, compared to control group. Also triglycerides (p < 0.001) and Leptin (p < 0.01) were significantly lower, but Adinopectin (p < 0.05) was significantly higher in test group, compared to control group (Seo et.al. 2011).

The effective compound in Chinese Loosestrife is a triterpene saponin called Foenumoside B, which in experiments with mice on high fat diet, at a dose of 10 mg/kg BW daily for 42 days, decreased body weight by 16.7% (p < 0.001) and body fat mass by 33.8% (p < 0.01) in test group, compared to control group (Seo et.al. 2012).

YIN CHEN HAO

(Artemisia Capillaris)

YIN CHEN HAO or Capillary Wormwood in English, is a close relative to the common Wormwood, Artemisia Vulgaris. YIN CHEN HAO grows in China, Korea and Japan, and it is a very popular vegetable and medicinal plant, which is used in liver diseases, chronic hepatitis, abdominal pain, cough and as a diuretic.

When obese mice were given high fat diet together with either 0.05 g/kg BW or 0.10 g/kg BW YIN CHEN HAO water extract daily, for 12 weeks, body weight in test groups were 18.5% ($p < 0.05$) and 22.1% ($p < 0.05$) lower, than in the control group (Hong et.al. 2009).

The body weight and body fat mass decreasing properties of YIN CHEN HAO has been verified in 4 other experiments (Hong et.al. 2009; Kim et.al. 2007; Kim et.al. 2010; Lee et.al. 2008).

Yohimbine

(Pausinystalia Yohimbine)

Yohimbine is a an alkaloid, extracted from the African Pausinystalia Yohimbine tree bark. Yohimbine is a strong sex stimulant, and causes a strong erection. Yohimbine as a bark extract has been used as aphrodisiac in Africa hundreds of years before the discovery of Viagra.

Yohimbine has body fat mass decreasing properties.

When 10 sportsmen were given 20 mg Yohimbine daily, for 21 days, body fat-% decreased in Yohimbine group significantly by 2.2% (9.3% → 7.1%; $p < 0.05$), compared to the 10 sportsmen control group (Ostojic et.al. 2006).

Yomogi

(Artemisia Princeps)

Artemisia Princeps is called Yomogi in Japanese and Ssuk in Korea language. Yomogi is very popular vegetable in Japan, Korea and China. It has also medicinal properties. Its cultivation is very easy.

Yomogi has body weight and body fat mass decreasing properties.

When mice on a high fat diet were given 1% Yomogi in their daily diet, for 14 weeks, body weight ($p < 0.05$), body fat mass ($p < 0.05$) and blood sugar ($p < 0.05$) decreased significantly, compared to the control group (Yamamoto et.al. 2011). Yomogi also decreased hepatic FAS enzyme and it suppressed the high Leptin levels.

When Yomogi ethanol extract was given to type 2 diabetic, obese mice, body fat mass and the elevated plasma free fatty acids, triglycerides and total cholesterol decreased significantly, compared to the control group. Also FAS enzyme was decreased significantly (Jung et.al. 2009).

The anti-obesity effect of Yomogi has been verified also in a third experiment (Kim et.al. 2010).

Zinc

Zinc is an essential trace mineral in human nutrition. It has a very big role in human nutrition. It participates in over 200 enzyme reactions. Zinc is directly involved in biosynthesis of testosterone, Insulin and Thyroid hormones.

Zinc has body weight decreasing properties.

Serum Zinc concentration has a strong negative correlation with body weight in human obesity ($p < 0.01$): The more is the overweight, the less is the serum Zinc concentration, and vice versa. Also Zinc has a strong negative correlation with serum Leptin in obese volunteers (Konukoglu et.al. 2004; Ishikawa et.al. 2005; Chen et.al. 1991; Chen et.al. 1991; Chen et.al. 1988; Di Martino et.al. 1993).

In experiments with both top athletes and non-exercising volunteers, hard physical exercise decreased both serum Testosterone and Thyroid hormones. But when volunteers are given Zinc sulfate 3 mg/kg BW daily, for 4 weeks, the serum testosterone and Thyroid hormones do not decrease in hard physical exercise (Kilic 2007; Kilic et.al. 2006).

When type 2 diabetic volunteers were given 100 mg Zinc sulfate daily, for 12 weeks, triglycerides decreased by 14.0% ($p = 0.02$), total cholesterol decreased by 9.4% ($p = 0.01$) and VLDL-cholesterol decreased by 13.1% ($p = 0.03$), but HDL-cholesterol increased by 44.4% ($p = 0.002$) in test group, compared to control group. This was a double blind experiment with 30 volunteers (Partida-Hernandez et.al. 2006).

When type 2 diabetic volunteers were given 660 mg Zinc sulfate daily, for 6 weeks, body weight decreased by 5.57%, body mass index BMI decreased by 1.58 kg/m^2, triglycerides decreased by 39.3% ($P = 0.005$), total cholesterol decreased by 21.5% ($p = 0.02$), LDL-cholesterol decreased by 34.1% ($p = 0.01$) and systolic blood pressure decreased by 3.5% ($p = 0.02$) in test group, compared to control group. This was a double blind experiment with 40 volunteers (Afkhami et.al. 2009).

When 60 obese children were given 20 mg Zinc daily, for 8 weeks, body weight decreased in test group by an average of 1.98 kg ($p = 0.01$), but body weight increased in control group by an average of 2.49 kg. This was a double blind experiment (Hashemipour et.al. 2009).

References

Abdelbaky MS, Elmehiry HF, Ali NKM. Effect of some citrus peels on hypercholesterolemic rats. The 1st International and 4th Arab Annual Scientific Conference on: Academic Accreditation for Higher Specific Education Institutions and Programs in Egypt and Arab World "Reality and Expectation" - Faculty of Education Mansoura University – Egypt April, 8 – 9, 2009.

Abidov M, Ramazanov Z, Seifulla R, Grachev S. The effects of Xanthigen in the weight management of obese premenopausal women with non-alcoholic fatty liver disease and normal liver fat. Diabetes Obes Metab. 2010 Jan;12(1):72-81.

Abrams SA, Griffin IJ, Hawthorne KM, Ellis KJ. Effect of prebiotic supplementation and calcium intake on body mass index. J Pediatr. 2007 Sep;151(3):293-8.

Acheson KJ, Zahorska-Markiewicz B, Pittet, Anantharaman K, Jéquier E. Caffeine and coffee: their influence on metabolic rate and substrate utilization in normal weight and obese individuals. The American Journal of Clinical Nutrition 1980 May;33:989-997.

Achuthan CR, Padikkala J. Hypolipidemic effect of *Alpinia galanga* (Rasna) and *Kaempferia galanga* (Kachoori). Indian Journal of Clinical Biochemistry 1997;12(1):55-58.

Adaramoye OA, Akintayo O, Achem J, Fafunso MA. Lipid-lowering effects of methanolic extract of *Vernonia amygdalina* leaves in rats fed on high cholesterol diet. Vascular Health and Risk Management 2008;4(1):235-241.

Adeneye AA, Agbaje EO. Hypoglycemic and hypolipidemic effects of fresh leaf aqueous extract of *Cymbopogon citratus Stapf.* In rats. Journal of Ethnopharmacology 2007;112:440-444.

Adeneye AA, Benebo AS, Agbaje EO. Protective effect of the aqueous leaf and seed extract of *Phyllanthus amarus* on alcohol-induced hepatotoxicity in rats. West Afr. J. Pharmacol. Drug Res. 2007;23:42-50.

Adeneye AA. The leaf and seed aqueous extract of *Phyllanthus amarus* improves insulin resistance diabetes in experimental animal studies. Journal of Ethnopharmacology 2012;.

Afkhami M, Ardekani, Karimi M, Mohammadi SM, Nourani F. Effect of Zinc Sulfate Supplementation on Lipid and Glucose in Type 2 Diabetic Patients. Pakistan Journal of Nutrition 2008;7(4):550-553.

Agbafor KN, Akubugwo EI. Hypocholesterolaemic effect of ethanolic extract of fresh leaves of *Cymbopogon citratus* (lemongrass). African Journal of Biotechnology 2007 March;6(5):596-598.

Ahmed LA, Ramadan RS, Mohamed RA. Biochemical and Histopathological Studies on the Water Extracts of Marjoram and Chicory Herbs and Their Mixture in Obese Rats. Pakistan Journal of Nutrition 2009;8(10):1581-1587.

Ahmed SM, Manoj J. Anti-obesity activity of *Coccinia Indica* in female rats fed with cafeteria and atherogenic diets. Der Pharmacia Lettre 2012;4(5):1480-1485.

Ahn EK, Oh JS. Lupenone Isolated from Adenphora triphylla var. japonica Extract Inhibits Adipogenic Differentiation through the Downregulation of PPARγ in 3T3-L1 Cells. Phytother Res 2012 Jul 31.

Ahn M, Yang W, Kang S, Kang MC, Ko RK, Kim GO, Shin T. *Lindera erythrocarpa* Makino extract reduces obesity induced by high-fat diet in rats. Oriental Pharmacy and Experimental Medicine 2010;10(4):288-293.

Aji SB, Sandabe UK, Egbe-Nwiyi TN. Hypoglycemic, Anticholesterolemic and Body Weight-Lowering Effects of Aqueous Leaves Extract of *Olea hochstetteri* Bak. in Rats. Research Journal of Biological Sciences 2010;5(11):745-749.

Akaike M, Aihara KI, Yanagawa H, Iwase T, Yoshida S, Yakaishi Y, Tsuchiya K, Tamaki T, Matsumoto T, Sata M. A Randomized, Double-Blind, Pilot Study to evaluate the efficacy and safety of *Citrus sudachi* peel in metabolic syndrome. SA2012 XVI International Symposium on Atherosclerosis, Sydney, 2012, Poster #257.

Akase T, Shimada T, Terabayashi S, Ikeya Y, Sanada H, Aburada M. Antiobesity effects of Kaempferia parviflora in spontaneously obese type II diabetic mice. J Nat Med. 2011 Jan;65(1):73-80.

Akase T, Shimada T, Harasawa Y, Akase T, Ikeya Y, Nagai E, Iizuka S, Nakagami G, Iizaka S, Sanada H, Aburada M. Preventive Effects of *Salacia reticulata* on Obesity and Metabolic Disorders in TSOD Mice. Evidence-Based Complementary and Alternative Medicine 2011.

Akazome Y, Kametani N, Kanda T, Shimasaki H, Kobayashi S. Evaluation of Safety of Excessive Intake and Efficacy of Long-term Intake of Beverages Containing Apple Polyphenols. Journal of Oleo Science 2010;59(6):321-338.

Akpamu U, Nwaopara AO, Izunya AM, Oaikhena GA, O Okhiai, Idonije BO, Osifo UC. A comparative study on weight changes in rats fed with diet containing Yaji, Yaji-additives and Yaji-spices. Biology and Medicine 2011;3(5):6-15.

Al-Doghachi EHA. Hypolipidemic Effect of Volatile Oil of Two Varieties of Fennel *(Foeniculum Vulgare Mill.)* in Laboratory Rats. European Journal of Scientific Research 2012;82(1):58-64.

Al-Dwairi A, Pabona JMP, Simen RCM, Simmen FA. Cytosolic Malic Enzyme 1 (ME1) Mediates High Fat Diet-Induced Adiposity, Endocrine Profile, and Gastrointestinal Tract Proliferation-Associated Biomarkers in Male Mice. PLOS ONE 2012 Oct;7(10):1-13.

Al Hamedan WA. Protective Effect of *Lepidium sativum L.* Seeds Powder and Extract on Hypercholesterolemic Rats. Journal of American Science 2010;6(11):873-880.

Al-Harithy RN. Dehydroepiandrosterone sulfate levels in women. Relationships with body mass index, insulin and glucose levels. Saudi Med J. 2003 Aug;24(8):837-41.

Al-Qarawi AA, Al-Damegh MA, ElMougy SA. Effect of freeze dried extract of Olea europaea on the pituitary-thyroid axis in rats. Phytother Res 2002 May;16(3):286-7.

Al-Sayed HMA, Ashoush, IS, Salwa MA. Hypolipidemic Effect of Persimmon in Rats Fed High Fat Diet and its Use in Juice and Nectar Preparation. Alex. J. Fd. Sci. & Technol. 2009;6(2):11-18.

Al-Tellawy FM, El-Bahy AM, Mostafa UES, Ebrahiem YM, Hasan RH. Studies of effect of useing saffron, cyperus, honebee and their compination on rats suffering hyperlipdemia (II). The 6th Arab and 3rd International Annual Scientific Conference on: Development of Higher Specific Education Programs in Egypt and the Arab World in the Light of Knowledge Era Requirements. Faculty of Specific Education Mansoura University – Egypt Apr 13 – 14 2011.

Alagumanivasagam G, Muthu AK, Manavalan R. Hypolipidemic Effect of Methanolic Extract of whole plant of *Teramnus Iabialis* (Linn) on High Fat Diet Fed Rats. Journal of Pharmacy Research 2011;4(12):4663-4666.

Alam N, Amin R, Khan A, Ara I, Shim MJ, Lee MW, Lee UY, Lee TS. Comparative Effects of Oyster Mushrooms on Lipid Profle, Liver and Kidney Function in Hypercholesterolemic Rats. Mycobiology 2009;37(1):37-42.

Alam N, Yoon KN, Lee TS. Antihyperlipidemic activities of *Pleurotus ferulae* on biochemical and histological function in hypercholesterolemic rats. J Res Med Sci. 2011 June;1(6):776-786.

Alam N, Yoon KN, Lee TS, Lee UY. Hypolipidemic Activities of Dietary *Pleurotus ostreatus* in Hypercholesterolemic Rats. Mycobiology 2011;39(1):45-51.

Alam N, Yoon KN, Lee JS, Lee MW, Lee TS. *Pleurotus nebrodensis* Ameliorates Atherogenic Lipd and Histological Function in Hypercholesterolemic Rats. International Journal of Pharmacology 2011;7(4):455-462.

Alarcon-Aguilar FJ, Zamilpa A, Perez-Garcia MD, Almaza-Pere JC, Romero-Nuñez E, Campos-Sepulveda EA, Vazquez-Carrillo LI, Roman-Ramos R. Effect of *Hibiscus sabdariffa* on obesity in MSG mice. Journal of Ethnopharmacology 2007;114:66-71.

Alberdi G, Rodriguez VM, Miranda J, Macarulla MT, Arias N, Andrés-Lacueva C, Portillo MP. Changes in white adipose tissue metabolism induced by resveratrol in rats. Nutr Metab (Lond) 2011 May 10;8(1):29.

Algam TA, Atti KAA, Dousa BM, Elawad SM, Elseed AMF. Effect of Dietary Raw Chick Pea *(Cicer arietinum* L.) Seedson Broiler Performance and Blood Constituents. International Journal of Poultry Science 2012;11(4):294-297.

Alizadeh M, Daneghian S, Ghaffari A, Ostadrahimi A, Safaeiyan A, Estakhri R, Gargan BP. The effect of hypocaloric diet enriched in legumes with or without L-arginine and selenium on anthropometric measures in central obese women. J Res Med Sci. 2010 Nov-Dec;15(6):331-343.

Alizadeh M, Safaeiyan A, Ostadrahimi A, Estakhri R, Daneghian S, Ghaffari A, Gargari BP. Effect of L-arginine and selenium added to a hypocaloric diet enriched with legumes on cardiovascular disease risk factors in women with central obesity: a randomized, double-blind, placebo-controlled trial. Ann Nutr Metab 2012;60(2):157-68.

Allen DO, Ahmed B, Naseer K. Relationships between cyclic AMP levels and lipolysis in fat cells after isoproterenol and forskolin stimulation. J Pharmacol Exp Ther. 1986 Aug;238(2):659-64.

Allison DB, Gadbury G, Schwartz LG, Murugesan R, Kraker JL, Heshka S, Fontaine KR, Heymsfield SB. A novel soy-based meal replacement formula for weight loss among obese individuals: a randomized controlled clinical trial. European Journal of Clinical Nutrition 2003;57:514-522.

Amagase H, Nance DM. Lycium barbarum increases caloric expenditure and decreases waist circumference in healthy overweight men and women: pilot study. J Am Coll Nutr. 2011 Oct;30(5):304-9.

Amin KA, Nagy MA. Effect of Carnitine and herbal mixture extract on obesity induced by high fat dieet in rats. Diabetology & Metabolic Syndrome 2009;1:17s.

Amin R, Islam MZ, Sen M, Eva SN, Jesmin S, Nahar S. Anti-Obesity Effect Of Mushroom (Ganoderma Lucidum) On Experimentally Induced Obese Rats. Anwer Khan Modern Medical College Journal 2012;3(2):11-14.

An HJ, Chung HS, Jeong HJ, Lee SA, Kim HM, Baek SH. Reductive effect of body weight in rats fed a high-fat diet by Sense-line. Oriental Pharmacy and Experimental Medicine 2003;3(1):29-33.

An JY, Lee MS, Joo H, Kim CT, Kim Y. Reduction of Body Weight by Capsaicin is Associated with Inhibition of Glycerol-3-Phosphate Dehydrogenase Activity and Stimulation of Uncoupling Protein 2 mRNA Expression in Diet-induced Obese Rats. J Food Sci Nutr 2011;16:210-216.

An S, Han JI, Kim MJ, Park JS, Han JM, Baek NI, Chung HG, Choi MS, Lee KT, Jeong TS. Ethanolic Extracts of *Brassica campestris* spp. *Rapa* Roots Prevent High-Fat Diet-Induced Obesity via β_3-Adrenergic Regulatio of White Adipocyte Lipolytic Activity. J Med Food 2010;13(2):406-414.

Amini Z, Boyd B, Doucet J, Ribnicky DM, Stephens JM. St. John's Wort inhibits adipocyte differentiation and induces insulin resistance in adipocytes. Biochemical and Biophysical Research Communications 2009;388:146-149.

Anaka ON, Ozolua RI, Okpo SO. Effect of the aqueous seed extract of *Persea americana* mill (Lauraceae) on the blood pressure of sprague-dawley rats. African Journal of Pharmacy and Pharmacology 2009 Oct;3(10):485-490.

Anastasia UNU, Fred AC, Stanislaus NK, Anthonia OU. Excess Body Fat Elimination (Anti-Obesity) Effects of *Vernonia Amygdalina* Leaf Extract. American Journal of Pharmacology and Toxicology 2011;6(2):55-58.

Anbu J, Anjana A, Purushothaman K, Sumithra M, Suganya S, Bathula NK, Modak S. Evaluation of antihyperlipidemic activity of ethanolic extract of *Saussurae Lappa* in rats. International Journal of Pharma and Bio Sciences 2011 Dec;2(4):550-556.

Andersen T, Fogh J. Weight loss and delayed gastric emptying following a South American herbal preparation in overweight patients. J Hum Nutr Diet 2001 Jun;14(3):243-50.

Andersson U, Rosén L, Östman E, Ström K, Wierup N, Björck I, Holm C. Metabolic effects of whole grain wheat and whole grain rye in the C57BL/6J mouse. Nutrition 2010;26:230-239.

Andersson U, Henriksson E, Ström K, Alenfall J, Göransson O, Holm C. Rose hip exerts antidiabetic effects via a mechanism involving downregulation of the hepatic lipogenic program. Am J Physiol Endocrinol Metab 2011;300:111-121.

Ando C, Kobayashi T, Tsukamoto S, Hirata T, Yamaguchi Y, Ueda T. Anti-obesity Effects of *Eucommia ulmoides* Leaves. International Symposium on *Eucommia ulmoides* 2007;1(1):63-66.

Anno T, Oono H, Tomi H. Effects of Long-term Ingestion of Jelly Drink Containing *Garcinia cambogia* Extract and Partially Hydrolized Guar Gum on Obesity. J. Oleo Sci. 2004;53(4):197-205.

Antal M, Regöly-Mérei A, Biró L, Arató G, Schmidt J, Nagy K, Greiner E, Lásztity N, Szabó C, Péter S, Martos E. Effects of oligofructose containing diet in obese persons. Orv Hetil 2008 Oct 19;149(42):1989-95.

Antonio J, Colker CM, Torina GC, Shi Q, Brink W, Kalman D. Effects of a Standardized Guggulsterone Phosphate Supplement on Body Composition in Overweight Adults: A Pilot Study. Current Therapeutic Research 1999 Apr;60(4):220-227.

Aoi W, Naito Y, Takanami Y, Ishii T, Kawai Y, Akagiri S, Kato Y, Osawa T, Yoshikawa T. Astaxanthin improves muscle lipid metabolism in exercise via inhibitory effect of oxidative CPT I modification. Biochemical and Biophysical Research Communications 2008;366:892-897.

Aoki F, Honda S, Kishida H, Kitano M, Arai N, Tanaka H, Yokota S, Nakagawa K, Asakura T, Nakai Y, Mae T. Suppression by Licorice Flavonoids of Abdominal Fat Accumulation and Body Weight Gain in High-Fat Diet-Induced Obese C57BL/6J Mice. Biosci. Biotechnol. Biochem. 2007;71:60463-1-9.

Aoyama T, Fukui K, Nakamori T, Hashimoto Y, Yamamoto T, Takamatsu K, Sugano M. Effect of Soy and Milk Whey Protein Isolates and Their Hydrolysates on Weight Reduction in Genetically Obese Mice. Biosci. Biotechnol. Biochem. 2000;64(12):

2594-2600.

Aoyama T, Fukui K, Takamatsu K, Hashimoto Y, Yamamoto T. Soy protein isolate and its hydrolysate reduce body fat of dietary obese rats and genetically obese mice (yellow KK). Nutrition 2000 May;16(5):349-54.

Ara N, Rashid M, Amran MS. Comparison of hypotensive and hypolipidemic effects of *Catharanthus Roseus* leaves extract with atenolol on adrenaline induced hypertensive rats. Pak. J. Pharm. Sci. 2009;22(3):267-271.

Arakawa M, Masaki T, Nishimura J, Seike M, Yosimatsu H. The effects of branched-chain amino acd granules on the accumulation of tissue triglycerides and uncoupling proteins in diet-induced obese mice. Endocrine Journal 2011;58(3):161-170.

Arcari DP, Bartchewsky W, dos Santos TW, Oliveira KA, Funck A, Pedrazzoli J, de Souza MF, Saad MJ, Bastos DH, Gambero A, Carvalho Pde O, Ribeiro ML. Antiobesity effects of yerba mate extract *(Ilex paraguariensis)* in high-fat diet-induced obese mice. Obesity (Silver Spring) 2009 Dec;17(12):2127-33.

Arenas J, Huertas R, Campos Y, Diaz AE, Villalón JM, Vilas E. Effects of L-carnitine on the pyruvate dehydrogenase complex and carnitine palmitoyl transferase activities in muscle of endurance athletes. FEBS Lett. 1994 Mar 14;341(1):91-3.

Arima H, Oiso Y. Positive effect of baclofen on body weight reduction in obese subjects: a pilot study. Intern Med 2010;49(19):2043-7.

Armanini D, De Palo CB, Mattarello MJ, Spinella P, Zaccaria M, Ermolao A, Palermo M, Fiore C, Sartorato P, Francini-Pesenti F, Karbowiak I. Effect of licorice on the reduction of body fat mass in healthy subjects. J Endocrinol Invest 2003 Jul;26(7):646-50.

Arora P, Ansari SH, Nazish I. Study of antiobesity activity of grapes seeds extract. Journal of Pharmacy Research 2011;4(6): 1916-1920.

Arora P, Ansari SH, Nazish I. Study of antiobesity effects of ethanolic and water extracts of grapes seeds. J Complement Integr Med 2011 Jan;8(1)

Arora T, Loo RL, Anastasovska J, Gibson GR, Tuohy KM, Sharma RK, Swann JR, Deaville ER, Sleeth ML, Thomas EL, Holmes E, Bell JD, Frost G. Differential effects of two fermentable carbohydrates on central appetite regulation and body composition. PloS One 2012;7(8):1-10.

Arpornsuwan T, Changsri K, Roytrakul S, Punjanon T. The effects of the extracts from *Carthamus tinctorius* L. on gene expression related to cholesterol metabolism in rats. Songklanakarin J. Sci. Technol. 2010 Mar - Apr;32(2):129-136.

Asai A, Miyazawa T. Dietary curcuminoids prevent high-fat diet-induced lipid accumulation in rat liver and epididymal adipose tissue. J Nutr. 2001 Nov;131(11):2932-5.

Asdaq SM, Inamdar MN. Potential of Crocus sativus (saffron) and its constituent, crocin, as hypolipidemic and antioxidant in rats. Appl Biochem Biotechnol. 2010 Sep;162(2):358-72.

Asgary S, Najafi S, Najafi M, Kelishadi R, Rafieian-Kopaei M. Antiatherogenic potential of *Cornus mas* L. on inflammatory risk factors, lipid profile and apolipoproteins in dyslipidemic children. Research in Pharmaceutica Sciences 2012;7(5).

Ashakumary L, Rouyer I, Takahashi Y, Ide T, Fukuda N, Aoyama T, Hashimoto T, Mizugaki M, Sugano M. Sesamin, a sesame lignan, is a potent inducer of hepatic fatty acid oxidation in the rat. Metabolism 1999 Oct;48(10):1303-13.

Asnaashari S, Delazar A, Habibi B, Vasfi R, Nahar L, Hamedeyazdan S, Sarker SD. Essential oil from Citrus aurantifolia prevents ketotifen-induced weight-gain in mice. Phytother Res 2010 Dec;24(12):1893-7.

Asp NG, Bauer HG, Nilsson-Ehle P, Nyman M, Öste R. Wheat bran increases high-density-lipoprotein cholesterol in the rat. Br. J. Nutr. 1981;46:385-393.

Atangwho IJ, Edet EE, Uti DE, Obi AU, Asmawi MZ, Ahmad M. Biochemical and histological impact of *Vernonia amygdalina* supplemented diet in obese rats. Saudi Journal of Biological Sciences 2012;19:385-392.

Athesh K, Karthiga D, Brindha P. Anti-obesity effect of aqueous fruit extract of *Carica Papaya* L. in rats fed on high fat cafeteria diet. International Journal of Pharmacy and Pharmaceutical Sciences 2012;4(5):327-330.

Aubertin-Leheudre M, Lord C, Khalil A, Dionne IJ. Effect of 6 months of exercise and isoflavone supplementation on clinical cardiovascular risk factors in obese postmenopausal women: a randomized, double-blind study. Menopause: The Journal of The North American Menopause Society 2007;14(4):1-6.

Auvichayapat P, Prapochanung M, Tunkamnerdthai O, Sripanidkulchai BO, Auvichayapat N, Thinkhamrop B, Kunhasura S, Wongpratoom S, Sinawat S, Hongprapas P. Effectiveness of green tea on weight reduction in obese Thais: a randomized, controlled trial. Physiology & Behavior 2008;93:486-491.

Azizan NA, Ahmad R, Mohamed K, Ahmad MZ, Asmawi Z. The *in vivo* antihypertensive effects of standardized methanol extracts of *Orthosiphon stamineus* on spontaneous hypertensive rats: A preliminary study. African Journal of Pharmacy and Pharmacology 2012 Feb 15;6(6):376-379.

Azman F, Amom Z, Azlan A, Esa NM, Ali RM, Shah ZM, Kadir KK. Antiobesity effect of Tamarindus indica L. pulp aqueous extract in high-fat diet-induced obese rats. J Nat Med. 2012 Apr;66(2):333-42.

Babio N, Balanza R, Basulto J, Bullo M, Salas-Salvado J. Dietary fibre: influence on body weight, glycemic control and plasma cholesterol profile. Nutr Hosp 2010;25(3):327-340.

Badal RM, Badal D, Badal P, Khare A, Shrivastava J, Kumar V. Pharmacological Action of *Mentha piperita* on Lipid Profile in Fructose-Fed Rats. Iranian Journal of Pharmaceutical Research 2011;10(4):843-848.

Badmaev V, Majeed M, Conte AA, Parker JE. Diterpene Forskolin *(Coleus forskohlii, Benth.)*: A possible new compound for reduction of body weight by increasing lean body mass. Nutracos. 2002;1:6-7.

Baer DJ, Stoke KS, Paul DR, Harris GK, Rumpler WV, Clevidence BA. Whey protein but not soy protein supplementation alters body weight and composition in free-living overweight and obese adults. J Nutr 2011 Aug;141(8):1489-94.

Bahrami M, Ataie-Jafari A, Hosseini S, Foruzanfar MH, Rahmani M, Pajouhi M. Effects of natural honey consumption in diabetic patients: an 8-week randomized clinical trial. Int J Food Sci Nutr 2009 Nov;60(7):618-26.

Baiges I, Palmfeldt J, Blade C, Gregersen N, Arola L. Lipogenesis is Decreased by Grape Seed Proanthocyanidins According to Liver Proteomics of Rats Fed a High Fat Diet. Mol Cell Proteomics 2010 July;9(7):1499-1513.

Baile CA, Yang JY, Rayalam S, Hartzell DL, Lai CY, Andersen C, Della-Fera MA. Effect of resveratrol on fat mobilization. Ann N Y Acad Sci. 2011 Jan;1215:40-7.

Bak EJ, Park HG, Kim JM, Kim JM, Yoo YJ, Cha JH. Inhibitory effect of evodiamine alone and in combination with rosiglitazone on in vitro adipocyte differentiation and in vivo obesity related to diabetes. Int J Obes (Lond) 2010 Feb;34(2):250-60.

Bakare AA, Bassey RB, Okoko IE, Sanyaolu AO, Ashamu AE, Ademola AO. Effect of Lime Juice (Citrus Aurantifolia) on Histomorphological Alterations of the Ovaries and Uterus of Cyclic Sprague-Dawley Rats. Europea Journal of Scientific Research 2012;67(4):607-616.

Balakrishna K, Mangathayaru K, Kuruvilla S, Reddy CUM. Modulatory Effect of *Erythrina variegata* on Experimental Hyperlipidemia in Male Wistar Rats. Pharmacognosy Research 2009;1(4):202-207.

Balakrishna K, Mangathayaru K, Kuruvilla S. Effect of *Erythrina variegata* on experimental atherosclerosis in guinea pigs. Journal of Pharmacology & Pharmacotherapeutics 2011;2(4):285-287.

Balamurugan G, Muralidharan P. Antiobesity effect of *Bauhinia variegata* bark extract on female rats fed on hypercaloric diet. Bangladesh J Pharmacol 2010;5:8-12.

Balamurugan G, Shantha A. Effect of *Erythrina variegata* seed extract on hyperlipidemia elicited by high-fat diet in wistar rats. J Pharm Bioallied Sci. 2010 Oct - Dec;2(4):350-355.

Balasasirekha R, Lakshmi UK. Effect of cinnamon and garlic on hyperlipidemics. International Journal of Nutrition and Metabolism 2011 Aug;3(7):77-89.

Balasubramanian MN, Muralidharan P, Balamurugan G. Anti Hyperlipidemic Activity of *Pedalium murex* (Linn.) Fruits on High Fat Diet Fed Rats. International Journal of Pharmacology 2008;4(4):310-313.

Balcázar-Muñoz BR, Martinez-Abundis E, González-Ortiz M. Effect of oral inulin administration on lipid profile and insulin sensitivity in subjects with obesity and dyslipidemia. Rev Med Chil. 2003 Jun;131(6):597-604.

Bambhole VD, Jiddewar GG. Evaluation of Cyperus rotundus in the management of obesity and high blood pressure in human subjects. Nagarjun 1984;27(5):110-113.

Bambhole VD. Effect of some medicinal plant preparations of adipose tissue metabolism. Ancient Science of Life Oct 1988;VIII (2):117-124.

Bambhole VD, Kamalakar PL. Reduction of diet-induced obesity in rats with a herbal formulation. Ancient Science of Life Jul-Oct 1993;XIII (1 & 2):89-96.

Ban SS, Yoon HD, Shin OC, Shin YJ, Park CS, Park JH, Seo BI. The Effects of Artemisiae Capillaris, Ponciri Fructus and Cartaegi Fructus in Obese Rats Induced by High Fat Diet. Kor. J. Herbology 2006;21(3):55-67.

Bano F, Akthar N, Naz H. Effect of the aqueous extract of *Momordica charantia* on body weight of rats. Journal of Basic and Applied Sciences 2011;7(1):1-5.

Bao-Shan L Xiang-jun L, Xiao-qin L, Xian-min L, Zhi-gang Y. Effect of Feeding Broad Bean on the Growth, Flesh Quality and Protease Activity of *Allogynogenetic crucian carp*. Chinese Journal of Animal Nutrition 2007;19(5).

Baranowski M, Enns J, Blewett H, Yakandawala U, Zahradka P, Taylor CG. Dietary flaxseed oil reduces adipocyte size, adipose monocyte chemoattractant protein-1 levels and T-cell infiltration in obese, insulin-resistant rats. Cytokine 2012;59:382-391.

Barbalho SM, Spada APM, Oliveira EP, Paiva-Filho ME, Martuchi KA, Leite NC, Deus RM, Sasaki V, Braganti LS, Oshiiwa M. *Mentha piperita* Effects on Wistar Rats Plasma Lipids. Brazilian Archives of Biology and Technology 2009;52(5):1137-1143.

Barbalho SM, Machado FMVF, Oshiiwa M, Abreu M, Guiger EI, Tomazela P, Goulart RA. Investigation of the effects of peppermint *(Mentha piperita)* on the biochemical and anthropometric profile of university students. Ciênc. Tecnol. Aliment. Campinas 2011;31(3):584-588.

Barbalho SM, Souza MSS, Silva JCP, Mendes CG, Oliveira MGA, Costa T, Farinazzi-Machado FMV. Yellow passion fruit rind *(Passiflora edulis)*: an industrial waste or an adjuvant in the maintenance of glycemia and prevention of dyslipidemia?. Diabetes Research and Clinical Metabolism 2012;1(5).

Bargalló MV, Grau AA, Fernández-Larrea JD, Anguiano GP, Segarra MCB, Rovira MJS, Ferré LA, Olive MB. Moderate red-wine consumption partially prevents body weight gain in rats fed a hyperlipidic diet. Journal of Nutritional Biochemistry 2006;17: 139-142.

Barnard ND, Scialli AR, Turner-McGrievy G, Lanou AJ, Glass J. The effects of a low-fat, plant-based dietary intervention on body weight, metabolism, and insulin sensitivity. The American Journal of Medicine 2005;118:991-997.

Barnard RJ, Chaudhari JAHA, Miller JE, Kirschenbaum MA. Effects of a low-fat, low-cholesterol diet on serum lipids, platelet aggregration and thromboxane formation. Prostaglandins Leukotrienes and Medicine 1987;26:241-252.

Barrett ML, Udani JK. A proprietary alpha-amylase inhibitor from white bean (Phaseolus vulgaris): a review of clinical studies on weight loss and glycemic control. Nutr J 2011 Mar 17;10(24):1-10.

Barth SW, Koch TC, Watzl B, Dietrich H, Will F, Bub A. Moderate effects of apple juice consumption on obesity-related markers in obese men: impact of diet-gene interaction on body fat content. Eur J Nutr. 2011 Oct 25.

Basu A, Du M, Leyva MJ, Sanchez K, Betts NM, Wu M, Aston CE, Lyons TJ. Blueberries decrease cardiovascular risk factors in obese men and women with metabolic syndrome. J Nutr 2010 Sep;140(9):1582-7.

Battochio APR, Sartori MS, Coelho CAR. Water-soluble extract of *Coleus barbatus* modulates weight gain, energy utilization and lipid metabolism in secondary biliary cirrhosis: an experimental study in young rats. Acta Cirúrgica Brasileira 2005;20(3):229-236.

Baum HB, Biller BM, Finkelstein JS, Cannistraro KB, Oppenhein DS, Schoenfeld DA, Michel TH, Wittink H, Klibanski A. Effects of physiologic growth hormone therapy on bone density and body composition in patients with adult-onset growth hormone deficiency. A randomized, placebo-controlled trial. Ann Intern Med. 1996 Dec 1;125(11):883-90.

Baxheinrich A, Stratmann B, Lee-Barkey YH, Tschoepe D, Wahrburg U. Effects of a rapeseed oil-enriched hypoenergetic diet with a high content of α-linolenic acid on body weight and cardiovascular risk profile in patients with the metabolic syndrome. Br J Nutr 2012 Aug;108(4):682-91.

Beattie JH, Nicol F, Gordon MJ, Reid MD, Cantlay L, Horgan GW, Kwun IS, Ahn JY, Ha TY. Ginger phytochemicals mitigate the obesogenic effects of a high-fat diet in mice: a proteomic and biomarker network analysis. Mol Nutr Food Res 2011 Sep;55(2): 203-13.

Belal NM. Hepatoprotective Effect of Feeding Celery Leaves Mixed with Chicory Leaves and Barley Grains to Hypercholesterolemic Rats. Asian Journal of Clinical Nutrition 2011:1-11.

Belobrajdic DP, McIntosh GH, Owens JA. A High-Whey-Protein Diet Reduces Body Weight Gain and Alters Insulin Sensitivity

Relative to Red Meat in Wistar Rats. The Journal of Nutriton 2004;134(6):1454-1458.

Beltrán-Debón R, Rull A, Rodríguez-Sanabria F, Iswaldi I, Herranz-López M, Aragonès G, Camps J, Alonso-Villaverde C, Menéndez JA, Micol V, Segura-Carretero A, Joven J. Continuous administration of polyphenols from aqueous rooibos *(Aspalathus linearis)* extract ameliorates dietary-induced metabolic disturbances in hyperlipidemic mice. Phytomedicine 2011;18:414-424.

Benedini S, Perseghin G, Terruzzi I, Scifo P, Invernizzi PL, Del Maschio A, Lazzarin A, Luzi L. Effect of L-acetylcarnitine on body composition in HIV-related lipodystrophy. Horm Metab Res. 2009 Nov;41(11):840-5.

Beppu F, Niwano Y, Kyan R, Yasura K, Tamaki M, Nishino M, Midorikawa Y, Hamada H. Hypolipidemic Effects of Ethanol Extract of *Citrus depressa* and *Annona atemoya*, Typical Plant Foodstuffs in Okinawa, Japan on KKAy Mice Fed with Moderately High Fat Diet. Food Sci. Technol. Res. 2009;15(5):553-556.

Bernard A, Rigault C, Mazue F, Le Borgne F, Demarquoy J. L-carnitive supplementation and physical exercise restore age-associated decline in some mitochondrial functions in the rat. J Gerontol A Biol Sci Med Sci. 2008 Oct;63(10):1027-33.

Bharti D, Jagtap P, Undale V, Bhosale A. Aerial parts of Aqueous extract of Cynodon dactylon shows hypotensive effect in high fructose treated Wistar rats. International Journal of Research in Pharmaceutical and Biomedical Sciences 2012;3(2):585-591.

Bhatt AD, Dalal DG, Shah SJ, Joshi BA, Gajjar MN, Vaidya RA, Vaidya AB, Antarkar DS. Conceptual and methodologic challenges of assessing the short-term efficacy of Guggulu in obesity: data emergent from a naturalistic clinical trial. J Postgrad Med 1995;41(1):5-7.

Bhuvaneswari S, Arunkumar E, Viswanathan P, Anuradha CV. Astaxanthin restricts weight gain, promotes insulin sensitivity and curtails fatty liver disease in mice fed a obesity-promoting diet. Process Biochemistry 2010;45:1406-1414.

Bidkar JS, Ghanwat DD, Bhujbal MD, Dama GY. Anti-hyperlipidemic activity of Cucumis melo fruit peel extracts in high cholesterol diet induced hyperlipidemia in rats. J Complement Integr Med 2010 Sep 24;9(1).

Bigoniya P, Nishad R, Singh CS. Preventive effect of sesame seed cake on hyperglycemia and obesity against high fructose-diet induced Type 2 diabetes in rats. Food Chemistry 2012;133:1355-1361.

Birari R, Javia V, Bhutani KK. Antiobesity and lipid lowering effects of *Murraya koenigii* (L.) Spreng leaves extracts and mahanimbine on high fat diet induced obese rats. Fitoterapia 2010;81:1129-1133.

Birari RB, Gupta S, Mohan CG, Bhutani KK. Antiobesity and lipid lowering effects of *Glycyrrhiza* chalcones: Experimental and computational studies. Phytomedicine 2011;18:795-801.

Bird SP, Tarpenning KM, Marino FE. Effects of liquid carbohydrate/essenial amino acid ingestion on acute hormonal response during a single bout of resistance exercise in untrained men. Nutrition 2006;22:367-375.

Birketvedt GS, Aaseth J, Florholmen JR, Ryttig K. Long-term effect of fibre supplement and reduced energy intake on body weight and bloodlipids in overweight subjects. Acta Medica (Hradec Kralove) 2000;43(4):129-32.

Bisson JF, Daubié S, Hidalgo S, Guillemet D, Linarés E. Diuretic and antioxidant effects of Cacti-Nea, a dehydrated water extract from prickly pear fruit, in rats. Phytother Res.2010 Apr;24(4):587-94.

Blankson H, Stakkestad JA, Fagertun H, Thom E, Wadstein J, Gudmundsen O. Conjugated linoleic acid reduces bodyfat mass in overweight and obese humans. J Nutr 2000 Dec;130(12):2943-8.

Bocarsly ME, Powell ES, Avena NM, Hoebel BG. High-fructose corn syrup causes characteristics of obesity in rats: Increased body weight, body fat and triglyceride levels. Pharmacology, Biochemistry and Behavior 2010.

Bock de M, Derraik JGB, Brennan CM, Biggs JB, Smith GC, Cameron-Smith D, Wall CR, Cutfield WS. Psyllium Supplementation in Adolescents Imroves Fat Distribution & Lipid Profile: A Randomized, Participant-Blinded, Placebo-Controlled, Crossover Trial. PloS ONE 2012 Jul;7(7):1-6.

Bodinham CL, Hitchen KL, Youngman PJ, Frost GS, Robertson MD. Short-term effects of whole-grain wheat on appetite and food intake in healthy adults: a pilot study. Br J Nutr 2011 Aug;106(3):327-30.

Bojková B, Orendás P, Friedmanová L, Kassayová M, Datelinka I, Ahlersová E, Ahlers I. Prolonged melatonin administration in 6-month-old Sprague-Dwaley rats: metabolic alterations. Acta Physiol Hung. 2008 Mar;95(1):65-76.

Boschmann M, Steiniger J, Franke G, Birkenfeld AL, Luft FC, Jordan J. Water Drinking Induces Thermogenesis through Osmosensitive Mechanisms. The Journal of Clinical Endocrinology & Metabolism 2007;92(8):3334-3337.

Boutcher SH. High-Intensity Intermittent Exercise and Fat Loss. Journal of Obesity 2011:1-10.

Boxer RS, Kleppinger A, Brindisi J, Feinn R, Burleson JA, Kenny AM. Effects of dehydroepiandrosterone (DHEA) on cardiovascular risk factors in older women with frailty characteristics. Age and Ageing 2010;39:451-458.

Brai BIC, Odetola AA, Agmo PU. Effects of *Persea americana* leaf extracts on body weight and liver lipids in rats fed hyperlipidaemic diet. African Journal of Biotechnology 2007 Apr;6(8):1007-1011.

Brandhagen M, Forslund HB, Lissner L, Winkvist A, Lindroos AK, Carlsson LM, Sjöström L, Larsson I. Alcohol and macronutrient intake patterns are related to general and central adiposity. Eur J Clin Nutr. 2012 Mar;66(3):305-13.

Brant LHC, Cardozo FMF, Velarde LG, Boaventura GT. Impact of flaxseed intake upon metabolic syndrome indicators in female Wistar rats. Acta Cirúrgica Brasileira 2012;27(8):537-543.

Brewer CP, Dawson B, Wallman KE, Guelfi KJ. Effect of Repeated Sodium Phosphate Loading on Cycling Time Trial Performance and VO2peak. Int J Sport Nutr Exerc Metab 2012 Oct 30.

Buemann B, Astrup A. How does the body deal with energy from alcohol. Nutrition 2001 Jul - Aug;17(7-8):638-41.

Buonopane GJ, Kilara A, Smith JS, McCarthy RD. Effect of skim milk supplementation on blood cholesterol concentration, blood pressure, and triglycerides in a free-living human population. J Am Coll Nutr. 1992 Feb;11(1):56-67.

Buriro MA, Dttta A, Tayyab M. Effects of Nigella Sativa and Sunflower oil diet on weight of albino rats. Professional Med J. 2011;18(3):530-534.

Bustanji Y, Al-Masri IM, Mohammad M, Hudaib M, Tawaha K, Tarazi H, Alkhatib HS. Pancreatic lipase inhibition activity of trilactone terpenes of Ginkgo biloba. J Enzyme Inhib Med Chem 2011 Aug;26(4):453-9.

Buus NH, Hansson NC, Rodriguez-Rodriguez R, Stankevicius E, Andersen MR, Simonsen U. Antiatherogenic effects of oleanolic acid in apolipoprotein E knockout mice. European Journal of Pharmacology 2011;670:519-526.

Byars A, Keith S, Simpson W, Mooneyhan A, Greenwood M. The influence of a pre-exercise spors drink (PRX) on factors related to maximal aerobic performance. J Int Soc Sports Nutr 2010 Mar 11;7(12):1-6.

Cabioğlu MT. ElectroacupunctureTherapyfor Weight Loss Reduces Serum Total Cholesterol, Triglycerides, and LDL Cholesterol Levels in Obese Women. The American Journalof Chinese Medicine 2005;33(4):525-533.

Cade R, Conte M, Zauner C, Mars D, Peterson J, Lunne D, Hommen N, Packer D. Effects of phosphate loading on 2,3-diphosphoglycerate and maximal oxygen uptake. Med Sci Sports Exerc 1984 Jun;16(3):263-8.

Caimari A, Del Bas JM, Crescenti A, Arola L. Low doses of grape seed procyanidins reduce adiposity and improve the plasma lipid profile in hamsters. Int J Obes (Lond) 2012 May 15.

Calzadilla P, Sapochnik D, Cosentino S, Diz V, Dicelio L, Calvo JC, Guerra LN. N-Acetylcysteine Reduces Markers of Differentiation in 3T3-L1 Adipocytes. Int. J. Mol. Sci. 2011;12:6936-6951.

Campión J, Milagro FI, Fernández D, Martinez JA. Vitamin C supplementation influences body fat mass and steroidogenesis-related genes when fed high-fat diet. Int J Vitamin Nutr Res 2008 Mar;78(2):87-95.

Cani PD, Neyrinck AM, Maton N, Delzenne NM. Oligofructose Promotes Satiety in Rats Fed a High-Fat Diet: Involvement of Glucagon-Like Peptide-1. Obes Res. 2005;13:1000-1007.

Cani PD, Joly E, Horsmans Y, Delzenne NM. Oligofructose promotes satiety in healthy human: a pilot study. European Journal of Clinical Nutrition 2006;60:567-572.

Cangiano C, Ceci F, Cascino A, Ben MD, Laviano A Muscaritoli M, Antonucci F, Rossi-Fanelli F. Eating behavior and adherence to dietary prescriptions in obese adult subjects treated with 5-hydroxytryptophan. Am J Clin Nutr 1992;56:863-7.

Cao Q, Qu W, Deng Y, Zhang Z, Niu W, Pan Y. Effect of flavonoids from the seed and fruit residue of Hippophae rhamnoides L. on glycometabolism in mice. Zhong Yao Cal 2003 Oct;26(10):735-7.

Cao ZH, Gu DH, Lin QY, Xu ZQ, Huang QC, Rao H, Liu EW, Jia JJ, Ge CR. Effect of pu-erh tea on body fat and lipid profiles in rats with diet-induced obesity. Phytother Res 2011 Feb;25(2):234-8.

Carai MAM, Fantini N, Loi B, Colombo G, Gessa GL, Riva A, Bombardelli E, Morazzoni P. Multiple cycles of repeated treatments with a *Phaseolus vulgaris* dry extract reduce food intake and body weight in obese rats. British Journal of Nutrition 2011;106: 762-768.

Carbonelli MG, Di Renzo L, Bigioni M, Di Daniele N, De Lorenzo A, Fusco MA. Alpha-lipoic acid supplementation: a tool for obesity therapy?. Curr Pharm Des 2010;16(7):840-6.

Cardozo LFMF, Soares LL, Chagas MA, Boaventura GT. Maternal consumption of flaxseed during lactation affects weight and hemoglobin level of offspring in rats. J Pediatr (Rio J) 2010;86(2):126-130.

Carvajal-Zarrabal O, Waliszewski SM, Barradas-Dermitz DM, Orta-Flores Z, Hayward-Jones PM. Nolasco-Hipólito C, Angulo-Guerrero O, Sánchez-Ricaño R, Infanzón RM, Trujillo PR. The consumption of Hibiscus sabdariffa dried calyx ethanolic extract reduced lipid profile in rats. Plant Foods Hum Nutr. 2005 Dec;60(4):153-9.

Carvajal-Zarrabal O, Hayward-Jones PM, Orta-Flores Z, Nolasco-Hipólito C, Barradas-Dermitz DM, Aguilar-Uscange MG, Pedroza-Hernández MF. Effect of *Hibiscus sabdariffa* L. Dried Calyx Ethanol Extract on Fat Absorption-Excretion, and Body Weight Implication in Rats. Journal of Biomedicine and Biotechnology 2009.

Celleno L, Tolaini MV, D'Amore A, Perricone NV, Preuss HG. A Dietary Supplement Containing Standardized *Phaseolus vulgaris* Extract Influences Body Composition of Overweight Men and Women. Int. J. Med. Sci. 2007:4(1):45-52.

Center SA, Warner KL, Randolph JF, Sunvold GD, Vickers JR. Influence of dietary supplementation with (L)-carnitine on metabolic rate, fatty acid oxidation, body condition, and weight loss in overweight rats. Am J Vet Res 2012 Jul;73(7):1002-15.

Cha BR, Chae JS, Lee JH, Jang YS, Lee JH, Son JW. The Effect of a Potential Antiobesity-Supplement on Weight Loss and Visceral Fat Accumulation in Overweight Women. Korean J Nutr. 2003 Jun;36(5):483-90.

Cha JY, Jeong JJ, Park CS, Ahn HY, Moon H, Cho YS. Antiobesity activity of fermented Angelicae gigantis by high fat diet-induced obese rats. J Enzyme Inhib Med Chem. 2011 Sep 30.

Cha YS, Choi SK, Suh H, Lee SN, Cho D, Li K. Effects of carnitine coingested caffeine on carnitine metabolism and endurance capacity in athletes. J Nutr Sci Vitaminol (Tokyo) 2001 Dec;47(6):378-84.

Cha YS, Rhee SJ, Heo YR. Acanthopanax senticosus extract prepared from cultured cells decreases adiposity and obesity indices in C57BL/6J. J Med Food 2004;7(4):422-9.

Chan LL, Chen Q, Go AG, Lam EK, Li ET. Reduced adiposity in bitter melon (Momordica charantia)-fed rats is associated with increased lipid oxidative enzyme activities and uncouling protein expression. J Nutr. 2005 Nov;135(11):2517-23.

Chandrasekaran CV, Vijayalakshmi MA, Prakash K, Bansal VS, Meenakshi J. Review Article: Herbal Approach for Obesity Management. American Journal of Plant Sciences 2012;3:1003-1014.

Chang CJ, Tzeng TF, Liou SS, Chang YS, Liu IM. Kaempferol regulates the lipid-profile in high-fat diet-fed rats through an increase in hepatic PPARα levels. Planta Med 2011 Nov;77(17):1876-82.

Chang CJ, Tzeng TF, Liou SS, Chang YS, Liu IM. Myricetin Increases Hepatic Peroxisome Proliferator-Activated Receptor α Protein Expression and Decreases Plasma Lipids and Adiposity in Rats. Evidence-Based Complementary and Alternative Medicine 2012.

Chang CJ, Tzeng TF, Liou SS, Chang YS, Liu IM. Regulation of lipid disorders by ethanol extracts from *Zingiber zerumbet* in high-fat diet-induced rats. Food Chemistry 2012;132:460-467.

Chang HP, Wang ML, Chan MH, Chiu YS, Chen YH. Antiobesity activities of indole-3-carbinol in high-fat-diet-induced obese mice. Nutrition 2011;27:463-470.

Chang HP, Wang ML, Hsu CY, Liu ME, Chan MH, Chen YH. Suppression of inflammation-associated factors by indole-3-carbinol in mice fed high-fat diets and in isolated, co-cultured macrophages and adipocytes. International Journal of Obesity 2011;35: 1530-1538.

Chang UJ, Kim DG, Kim JM, Suh HJ, Oh SH. Weight Reduction Effet of Extract of Fermented Red Pepper on Female College Students. J. Korean Soc. Food Sci. Nutr. 2003;32(3):479-484.

Chang XX, Yan HM, Xu Q, Xia MF, Bian H, Zhu TF, Gao X. The effects of berberine on hyperhomocysteinemia and hyperlipidemia in rats fed with a long-term high-fat diet. Lipids Health Dis 2012 Jul 4;11(1):86.

Chantre P, Lairon D. Recent findings of green tea extract AR25 (Exolise) and its activity for the treatment of obesity. Phytomedicine 2002;9:3-8.

232

Chao CY, Yin MC, Huang CJ. Wild bitter gourd extract up-regulates mRNA expression of PPARα, PPARγ and their target genes in C57BL/6J mice. Journal of Ethnopharmacology 2011;135:156-161.

Charradi K, Sebai H, Elkahoui S, Hassine FB, Limam F, Aouani E. Grape Seed Extract Alleviates High-Fat Diet-Induced Obesity and Heart Dysfunction by Preventing Cardiac Siderosis. Cardiovasc Toxicol 2011;11:28-37.

Chatterjee A, Fernandez C, Khandalavala B, Golakoti T, Krishnaraju AV, Sengupta K, Lau FC, Bagchi D. Efficacy of a natural weight management herbal formulation in obese human subjects. American College of Nutrition. 51st Annual Meeting – New York, NY, USA Oct 7-9 2010;29(5):518.

Chen M, Shi XY, Xu B, Gu YH, Dong Q, Xu LF, Li KP, Zhang JB, Mu YY. Clinical observation on acupotomy for treatment of simple obesity. Zhongguo Zhen Jiu 2011 Jun;31(6):539-42.

Chen MD, Lin PY, Lin WH, Cheng V. Zinc in hair and serum of obese individuals in Taiwan. Am J Clin Nutr 1988 Nov;48(5): 1307-9.

Chen MD, Lin WH, Lin PY, Wang JJ, Tsou CT. Investigation on the relationships among blood zinc, copper, insulin and thyroid hormones in non-insulin dependent diabetes mellitus and obesity. Zhonghua Yi Xue Za Zhi (Taipei) 1991 Dec;48(6):431-8.

Chen MD, Lin PY, Lin WH. Investigation of the relationships between zinc and obesity. Gaoxiong Yi Xue Ke Xue Za Zhi 1991 Dec;7(12):628-34.

Chen Q, Chan LL, Li ET. Bitter melon (Momordica charantia) reduces adiposity, lowers serum insulin and normalizes glucose tolerance in rats fed a high fat diet. J Nutr 2003 Apr;133(4):1088-93.

Chen Q, Wang E, Ma L, Zhai P. Dietary resveratrol increases the expression of hepatic 7α-hydroxylase and ameliorates hypercholesterolemia in high-fat fedC57BL/6J mice. Lipids Health Dis. 2012 May 20;11(56):1-8.

Chen SC, Lin YH, Huang HP, Hsu WL, Houng JY, Huang CK. Effect of conjugated linoleic acid supplementation on weight loss and body fat composition in a Chinese population. Nutrition 2012;28:559-565.

Chen TJH, Blum K, Kaats G, Braverman ER, Eisenberg A, Sherman M, Davis K, Comings DE, Wood R, Pullin D, Arcuri V, Varshavski M, Mengucci JF, Blum SH, Downs BW, Meshkin B, Waite RL, Williams L, Schoolfield J, Prihoda TJ, White L. Chromium Picolinate (CrP) a putative anti-obesity nutrient induces changes in body composition as a function of the *Taq1* dopamine D2 receptor polymorphisms in a randomized double-blind placebo controlled study. Gene Ther Mol Biol 2007;11: 161-170.

Chen WP, Ho BY, Lee CL, Lee CH, Pan TM. Red mold rice prevents the development of obesity, dyslipidemia and hyperinsulinemia induced by high-fat diet. International Journal of Obesity 2008;32:1694-1704.

Chen ZH, Li J, Liu J, Zhao Y, Zhang P, Zhang MX, Zhang L. Saponins isolated from the root of Panax notoginseng showed significant anti-diabetic effects in KK-Ay mice. Am J Chin Med 2008;36(5):939-51.

Cheng W, Phillips B, Abumrad N. Effect of HMB on Fuel Utilization, Membrane Stability and Creatine Kinase Content of Cultured Muscle Cells. Faseb J. 1998;12:950.

Chepulis LM. The effect of honey compared to sucrose, mixed sugars, and a sugar-free diet on weight gain in young rats. J Food Sci 2007 Apr;72(3):224-9.

Chepulis L, Starkey N. The long-term effects of feeding honey compared with sucrose and a sugar-free diet on weight gain, lipid profiles, and DEXA measurements in rats. J Food Sci. 2008 Jan;73(1):1-7.

Cheskin LJ, Davis LM, Lipsky LM, Mitola AH, Lycan T, Mitchell V, Mickly B, Adkins E. Lack of energy compensation over 4 days when white button mushrooms are substituted for beef. Appetite 2008;51:50-57.

Chevassus H, Molinier N, Costa F, Galtier F, Renard E, Petit P. A fenugreek seed extract reduces spontaneous fat consumption in healthy volunteers. European Journal of Clinical Pharmacology 2009;65(12):1175-1178.

Chiang CT, Weng MS, Lin-Shiau SY, Kuo KL, Tsai YJ, Lin JK. Pu-erh tea supplementation suppresses fatty acid synthase expression in the rat liver through downregulating Akt and JNK signalings as demonstrated in human hepatoma HepG2 cells. Oncol Res. 2005;16(3):119-28.

Chidrawar VR, Patel KN, Sheth NR, Shiromwar SS, Trivedi P. Antiobesity effect of *Stellaria media* against drug induced obesity in Swiss albino mice. Ayu 2011 Oct-Dec;32(4):576-584.

Chidrawar VR, Patel KN, Chitme HR, Shiromwar SS, Shiromwar SS. Pre-clinical evolutionary study of *Clerodendrum phlomidis* as an anti-obesity agent against high fat diet induced C57BL/6J mice. Asian Pacific Journal of Tropical Biomedicine 2012:1-13.

Chien LW, Lin MH, Chung HY, Liu CF. Transcutaneous Electrical Stimulation of Acupoints Changes Body Composition and Heart Rate Variability in Postmenopausal Women with Obesity. Evidence-Based Complementary and Alternative Medicine 2011:1-7.

Chiolero A, Faeh D, Paccaud F, Cornuz J. Consequences of smoking for body weight, body fat distribution, and insulin resistance. Am J Clin Nutr. 2008 Apr;87(4):801-9.

Cho AS, Jeon SM, Kim MJ, Yeo J, Seo KI, Choi MS, Lee MK. Chlorogenic acid exhibits anti-obesity property and improves lipid metabolism in high-fat diet-induced-obese mice. Food and Chemical Toxicology 2010;48:937-943.

Cho JK, Lee SH, Lee JY, Kang HS. Randomized controlled trial of training intensity in adiposity. Int J Sports Med 2011 Jun;32(6):468-75.

Cho KD, Kim EJ, Kim MY, Kim JS, Han CK, Lee BH. Antiobesity and antidiabetic effects of Jerusalem artichoke and purple sweet potato in the diet-induced obese rats. FASEB J. 2010 Apr.

Cho S, Choi Y, Park S, Park T. Carvacrol prevents diet-induced obesity by modulating gene expressions involved in adipogenesis and inflammation in mice fed with high-fat diet. Journal of Nutritional Biochemistry 2012.

Cho SH, Choi SW, Lee HR, Lee JY, Lee WJ, Choi Y. Safety and Effects on Lipid Parameters of *Rubus coreanus* and *Atractylodes japonica* in Ovariectomized Rats. J. Food Sci. Nutr. 2004;9:361-366.

Cho SH, Lee JS, Thabane L, Lee J. Acupuncture for obesity: a systematic review and meta-analysis. International Journal of Obesity 2009;33:183-196.

Cho SI. Effects of the Rehmanniae Radix Preparat on Ovariectomized Rats. Kor. J. Herbology 2005;20(4):61-67.

Cho SJ, Jung UJ, Choi MS. Differential effects of low-dose resveratrol on adiposity and hepatic steatosis in diet-induced obese mice. Br J Nutr. 2012 Mar 14;1-10.

Cho SY, Jeong HW, Sohn JH, Seo DB, Kim WG, Lee SJ. An Ethanol Extract of *Artemisia iwayomogi* Activates PPARδ Leading to

Activation of Fatty Acid Oxidation in Skeletal Muscle. PloS ONE 2012 Mar;7(3):1-8.

Cho YJ, Hou WN. Effects of Dietary Bong-ip (Morus alba L.), Gam-chi (Glycyrrhizae glabra), Sol-ip (Pinus densiflora) and Dang-gi (Angelica gigas) on Serum Composition in Rats. Koren J. Food Culture 2005;20(1):123-129.

Cho YO, Kong EY. The Effect of *Allium* Vegetable Intake on the Utilization and Recuperation of Plasma Fuel in Acute-Exercising Rats. Nutritional Sciences 2003 Aug;6(3):155-159.

Choi CS, Chung HK, Choi MK, Kang MH. Effects of grape pomace on the antioxidant defense system in diet-induced hypercholesterolemic rabbits. Nutrition Research and Practice 2010;4(2):114-120.

Choi H, Myung KH. Comparative Study of Red Wine and Korean Black Raspberry Wine in Adipocyte Differentiation and Cardiovascular Disease Related Gene Expression. Food Sci. Biotechnol. 2005;14(4):514-517.

Choi H, Eo H, Park K, Jin M, Park EJ, Kim SH, Park JE, Kim S. A water-soluble extract from *Cucurbita moschata* shows anti-obesity effects by controlling lipid metabolism in a high fat diet-induced obesity mouse model. Biochemical and Biophysical Research Communications 2007;359:419-425.

Choi HD, Kim YS, Choi IW, Park YK, Park YD. Hypotensive Effect of Germinated Brown Rice on Spontaneously Hypertensive Rats. Korean J. Food Sci. Technol. 2006;38(3):448-451.

Choi HJ, Han MJ, Baek NI, Kim DH, Jung HG, Kim NJ. Hepatoprotective Effects of *Brassica rapa* (Turnip) on d-Galactosamine Induced Liver Injured Rats. Kor. J. Pharmacogn. 2006;37(4):258-265.

Choi HJ, Chung MJ, Ham SS. Antiobese and hypocholesterolaemic effects of an *Adenophora triphylla* extract in HepG2 cells and high fat diet-induced obese mice. Food Chemistry 2010;119:437-444.

Choi I, Park Y, Choi H, Lee EH. Anti-adipogenic activity of rutin in 3T3-L1 cells and mice fed with high-fat diet. Biofactors 2006;26(4):273-81.

Choi I, Seog H, Park Y, Kim Y, Choi H. Suppressive effects of germinated buckwheat on development of fatty liver in mice fed with high-fat diet. Phytomedicine 2007;14:563-567.

Choi J, Lee KT, Kim WB, Park KK, Chung WY, Lee JH, Lim SC, Jung HJ, Park HJ. Effect of *Allium victorialis* var. *Platyphyllum* Leaves on Triton WR-1339-Induced and Poloxamer-407-Induced Hyperlipidemic Rats and on Diet-Induced Obesity Rats. Kor. J. Pharmacogn. 2005;36(2):109-115.

Choi JS, Kim H, Jung MH, Hong S, Song J. Consumption of barley-glucan ameliorates fatty liver and insulin resistance in mice fed a high-fat diet. Mol Nutr Food Res. 2010 Jul;54(7):1004-13.

Choi JY, JeonJE, Jang SY, Jeong YJ, Jeon SM, Park HJ, Choi MS. Differential effects of powdered whole soy milk and its hydrolysate and antiobesity and antihyperlipidemic response to high-fat treatment in C57BL/6N mice. J Agric Food Chem 2011 Mar 23;59(6):2584-91.

Choi KH, Shon JH, Choi IS, Choi YJ, Bae CSJ, Kim MH. The Effect of Mulberry Fruits Extracts on Blood Flow Improvement in Ovariectomized Rats. Journal of Life Science 2007;17(4):575-580.

Choi MS, Jung UJ, Kim HJ, Do GM, Jeon SM, Kim MJ, Lee MK. Du-zhong (Eucommia ulmoides Oliver) leaf extract mediates hypolipidemic action in hamsters fed a high-fat diet. Am J Chin Med. 2008;36(1):81-93.

Choi PS, Kwon JY, Han MR, Kim MH, Kim SH, Chang MJ. Effect of Raw versus Flavor, Browning and Caking reduced Onion (*Allium cepa* L.) on Blood Pressure of Spontaneously Hypertensive Rats. Korean J. Food Culture 2008;23(1):55-61.

Choi SH, Kim HJ, Kwon MJ, Baek YH, Song YO. The Effect of *Kimchi* Pill Supplementation on Plasma Lipid Concentration in healthy people. J. Korean. Soc. Food Sci. Nutr- 2001;30(5):913-920.

Choi SY, Ko HC, Ko SY, Hwang JH, Park JG, Kang SH, Han SH, Yun SH, Kim SJ. Correlation between Flavonoid Content and the NO Production Inhibitory Activity of Peel Extracts from Various Citrus Fruits. Biol. Pharm. Bull. 2007;30(4):772-778.

Choi Y, Kim Y, Park S, Lee KW, Park T. Indole-3-carbinol prevents diet-induced obesity through modulation of multiple genes related to adipogenesis, thermogenesis or inflammation in the visceral adipose tissue of mice. Journal of Nutrition Biochemistry 2012.

Choi YJ, Park SY, Kim JY, Won KC, Kim BR, Son JK, Lee SH, Kim YW. Combined Treatment of betulinic Acid, a PTP1B Inhibitor, with Orthosiphon stamineus Extract Decreases Body Weight in High-Fat-Fed Mice. J Med Food 2012 Dec 20.

Choi YS, Choi KD, Kim SD, Owens P, Chung CS. Extracts of Korean Medicinal Plant Extracts Alter Lipogenesis of Pig Adipose Tissue and Differentiation of Pig Preadipocytes *In vitro*. Journal of Animal Science and Technology 2010;52(5):383-388.

Chon JW, Sung JH, Hwang EJ, Park YK. Chlorella methanol extract reduces lipid accumulation in and increases the number of apoptotic 3T3-L1 cells. Ann N Y Acad Sci. 2009 Aug;1171:183-9.

Chon SU, Heo BG, Park YS, Kim DK, Gorinstein S. Total phenolics level, antioxidant activities and cytotoxicity of young sprouts of some traditional Korean salad plants. Plant Foods Hum Nutr. 2009 Mar;64(1):25-31.

Chou YC, Wang SY, Chen GC, Lin YS, Chao PM. The Functional Assessment of *Alpinia pricei* on Metabolic Syndrome Induced by Sucrose-containing Drinking Water in Mice. Phytotherapy Research 2009;23:558-563.

Chrubasik C, Maier T, Dawid C, Torda T, Schieber A, Hofmann T, Chrubasik S. An observational study and quantification of the actives in a supplement with Sambucus nigra and Asparagus officinalis used for weight reduction. Phytother Res. 2008 Jul;22(7):913-8.

Chu SL, Fu H, Yang JX, Liu GX, Dou P, Zhang L, Tu PF, Wang XM. A randomized double-blind placebo-controlled study of Pu'er tea extract on the regulation on meabolic syndrome. Chin J Integr Med 2011 Jul;17(7):492-8.

Chukwuma ER, Obioma N, Christopher OI. The Phytochemical Composition and Some Biochemical Effects of Nigerian Tigernut (*Cyperus esculentus L.*) Tuber. Pakistan Journal of Nutrition 2010;9(7):709-715.

Chung MY, Rho MC, Lee SW, Park HR, Kim K, Lee IA, Kim DH, Jeune KH, Lee HS, Kim YK. Inhibition of diacylglycerol acyltransferase by betulinic acid from Ainus hirsuta. Planta Med. 2006 Feb;72(3):267-9.

Cicero AF, Derosa G, Manca M, Bove M, Borghi C, Gaddi AV. Different effect of psyllium and guar dietary supplementation on blood pressure control in hypertensive overweight patients: a six-month, randomized clinical trial. Clin Exp Hypertens 2007 Aug;29(6):383-94.

Cignarella A, Nastasi M, Cavalli E, Puglisi L. Novel lipid-lowering properties of *Vaccinium myrtillus* L. leaves, a traditional antidiabetic treatment, in several models of rat dyslipidaemia: a comparison with ciprofibrata. Thrombosis Research

1996;84(5):311-322.

Ciortea R, Costin N, Braicu I, Haragâs D, Hudacsko A, Bondor C, Mihu D, Mihu CM. Effect of melatonin on intra-abdominal fat in correlation with endometrial proliferation in ovariectomized rats. Anticancer Res. 2011 Aug;31(8):2637-43.

Clemmensen C, Madsen AN, Smajilovic S, Holst B, Bräuner-Osborne H. L-Arginine improves multiple physiological parameters in mice exposed to diet-induced metabolic disturbances. Amino Acids 2012 Sep;43(3):1265-75.

Clifton PM, Bastiaans K, Keogh JB. High protein diets decrease total and abdominal fat and improve CVD risk profile in overweight and obese men and women with elevated triacylglycerol. Nutr Metab Cardiovasc Dis. 2009 Oct;19(8):548-54.

Colditz GA, Giovannucci E, Rimm EB, Stampfer MJ, Rosner B, Speizer FE, Gordis E, Willett WC. Alcohol intake in relation to diet and obesity in women and men. Am J Clin Nutr. 1991 Jul;54(1):49-55.

Colker CM, Kalman DS, Torina GC, Perlis T, Street C. Effects of *Citrus aurantium* Extract, Caffeine, and St. John's Wort on Body Fat Loss, Lipid Levels, and Mood States in Overweight Healthy Adults. Current Therapeutic Research 1999 Mar;60(3):145-153.

Cong WN, Tao RY, Tian JY, Zhao J, Liu Q, Ye F. Egb761, an extract of *Ginkgo biloba* leaves, reduces insulin resistance in a high-fat-fed mouse model. Acta Pharmaceutica Sinica B 2011;1(1):14-20.

Cortez MY, Torgan CE, Jr Brozinick JT, Miller RH, Ivy JL. Effects of pyruvate and dihydroxyacetone consumption on the growth and metabolic state of obese Zucker rats. Am J. Clin. Nutr. 1991;53:847-53.

Costa ACR, Rosado EL, Soares-Mota M. Influence of the dietary intake of medium chain triglycerides on body composition, energy expenditure and satiety; a systematic review. Nutr Hosp 2012;27(1):103-108.

Costa JA, Alfenas RCG. The consumption of low glycemic meals reduces abdominal obesity in subjects with excess body weight. Nutr Hosp. 2012;27(4):1178-1183.

Couet C, Delarue J, Ritz P, Antoine JM, Lamisse F. Effect of dietary fish oil on body fat mass and basal fat oxidation in healthy adults. International Journal of Obesity 1997;21:637-643.

Couturier K, Batandier C, Awada M, Hininger-Favier I, Canini F, Anderson RA, Leverve X, Roussel AM. Cinnamon improves insulin sensitivity and alters the body composition in an animal model of the metabolic syndrome. Archives of Biochemistry and Biophysics 2010;501:158-161.

Cox CL, Stanhope KL, Schwarz JM, Graham JL, Hatcher B, Griffen SC, Bremer AA, Berglund L, McGahan JP, Havel PJ, Keim NL. Consumption of fructose-sweetened beverages for 10 weeks reduces net fat oxidation and energy expenditure in overweight/obese men and women. Eur J Clin Nutr. 2012 Feb;66(2):201-8.

Crawford V, Scheckenbach R, Preuss HG. Effects of niacin-bound chromium supplementation on body composition in overweight African-American women. Diabetes, Obesity and Metabolism 1999;1:331-337.

Crespo N, Esteve-Garcia E. Dietary Linseed Oil Produces Lower Abdominal Fat Deposition but Higher De Novo Fatty Acid Synthesis in Broiler Chickens. Poultry Science 2002;81:1555-1562.

Cribb PJ, Hayes A. Effect of supplement timing and resistance exercise on skeletal muscle hypertrophy. Med Sci Sports Exerc 2006 Nov;38(11):1918-25.

Cribb PJ, Williams AD, Carey MF, Hayes A. The effect of whey isolate and resistance training on strength, body composition, and plasma glutamine. Int J Sport Nutr Exerc Metab. 2006 Oct;16(5):494-509.

Croze ML, Vella RE, Pillon NJ, Soula HA, Hadji L, Guichardant M, Soulage CO. Chronic treatment with *myo*-inositol reduces white adipose tissue accretion and improves insulin sensitivity in female mice. Journal of Nutrition Biochemistry 2012.

Cui BK, Liu S, Lin XJ, Wang J, Li SH, Wang QB, Li SP. Effects of *Lycium Barbarum* Aqueous and Ethanol Extracts on High-Fat-Diet Induced Oxidative Stress in Rat Liver Tissue. Molecules 2011;16:9116-9128.

Da-Silva WS, Harney JW, Kim BW, Li J, Bianco SDC, Crescenzi A, Christoffolete MA, Huang SA, Bianco AC. The Small Polyphenolic Molecule Kaempferol Increases Cellular Energy Expenditure and Thyroid Hormone Activation. Diabetes 2007 March;56:767-775.

Dai DL, Shen W, Yu HF, Guan XQ, Yi YF. Effect of Cordyceps Sinensison Uncoupling Protein 2 in Experimental Rats with Nonalcoholic Fatty Liver. Journal of Health Science 2006;52(4):390-396.

Daily JW, Hongu N, Mynatt RL, Sachan DS. Choline supplementation increases tissue concentrations of carnitine and lowers body fat in guinea pigs. J. Nutr. Biochem. 1998;9:464-470.

Daleprane JB, Batista A, Pachero JT, da Silva AFE, Costa CA, Resende ÂC, Boaventura GT. Dietary flaxseed supplementation improves endothelial fuction in the mesenteric arterial bed. Food Research International 2010;43:2052-2056.

Dallas C, Gerbi A, Tenca G, Juchaux F, Bernard FX. Lipolytic effect of a polyphenolic citrus dry extract of red orange, grapefruit, orange (SINETROL) in human body fat adipocytes. Mechanism of action by inhibition of cAMP-phosphodiesterase (PDE). Phytomedicine 2008;15:783-792.

Daniel T,Tan BKH. The Mechanism underlying the hypocholesterolaemic activity of aqueous celery extract, its butanol and aqueous fractions in genetically hypercholesterolaemic rico rats. Life Sciences 2000;66(8):755-767.

Dashti HM, Bo-Abbas YY, Asfar SK, Mathew TC, Hussein T, Behbahani A, Khoursheed MA, Al-Sayer HM, Al-Zaid NS. Ketogenic Diet Modifies the Risk Factors of Heart Disease in Obese Patients. Nutrition 2003;19:901-902.

Dashti HM, Mathew TC, Hussein T, Asfar SK, Behbahani A, Khoursheed MA, Al-Sayer HM, Bo-Abbas YY, Al-Zaid NS. Long-term effects of a ketogenic diet in obese patients. Exp Clin Cardiol. 2004;9(3):200-5.

Dashti HM, Al-Zaid NS, Mathew TC, Al-Mousawi M, Talib H, Asfar SK, Behbahani AI. Long term effects of ketogenic diet in obese subjects with high cholesterol level. Mol Cell Biochem. 2006 Jun;286(1-2):1-9.

Dashti HM, Mathew TC, Khadada M, Al-Mousawi M, Talib H, Asfar SK, Behbahani AI, Al-Zaid NS. Beneficial effects of ketogenic diet in obese diabetic subjects. Mol Cell Biochem. 2007 Aug;302(1-2):249-56.

Datau EA, Wardhana, Surachmanto EE, Pandelaki K, Langi JA, Fias. Efficacy of Nigella Sativa on Serum Free Testosterone and Metabolic Disturbances in Central Obese Male. Acta Med Indones – Indones J Inern Med 2010;42(3):130-134.

Davaakhuu G, Sukhdolgor J, Gereltu B. Lipid Lowering Effect of Ethanolic Extract of *Carduus crispus* L. on Hypercholesterolemic Rats. Mongolian Journal of Biological Sciences 2010;8(2):49-51.

Dave S, Kaur NJ, Nanduri R, Dkhar HK, Kumar A, Gupta P. Inhibition of Adipogenesis and Induction of Apoptosis and Lipolysis by Stem Bromelain in 3T3-L1 Adipocytes. PloS ONE 2012 Jan;7(1):1-12.

Davis J, Iqbal MJ, Steinle J, Oitker J, Higginbotham DA, Peterson RG, Banz WJ. Soy protein influences the development of the metabolic syndrome in male obese ZDFxSHHF rats. Horm Metab Res. 2005 May;37(5):316-25.

Davy BM, Dennis EA, Dengo AL, Wilson KL, Davy KP. Water consumption reduces energy intake at a breakfast meal in obese older adults. J Am Diet Assoc 2008 Jul;108(7):1236-9.

De Melo CL, Queiroz MG, Arruda Filho AC, Rodrigues AM, de Sousa DF, Almeida JG, Pessoa OD, Silveira ER, Menezes DB, Melo TS, Santos FA, Rao VS. Betulinic acid, a natural pentacyclic triterpenoid, prevents abdominal fat accumulation in mice fed a high-fat diet. J Agric Food Chem 2009 Oct 14;57(19):8776-81.

De Oliveira MC, Sichieri R, Moura AS. Weight Loss Associated With a Daily Intake of Three Apples or Three Pears Among Overweight Women. Nutrition 2003;19:253-256.

De Wit N, Derrien M, Bosch-Vermeulen H, Oosterink E, Keshtkar S, Duval C, de Vogel-van den Bosch J, Kleerebezem M, Müller M, van der Meer R. Saturated fat stimulates obesity and hepatic steatosis and affects gut microbiota composition by an enhanced overflow of dietary fat to the distal intestine. Am J Physiol Gastrointest Liver Physiol. 2012 Sep 1;303(5):589-99.

Decorde K, Teissèdre PL, Sutra T, Ventura E,Cristol JP, Rouanet JM. Chardonnay grape seed procyanidin extract supplementation prevents high-fat diet-induced obesity in hamsters by improving adipokine imbalance and oxidative stress markers. Mol. Nutr. Food Res. 2009 May;53(5):659-66.

Decorde K, Agne A, Lacan D, Ramos J, Fouret G, Ventura E, Feillet-Coudray C, Cristol JP, Rouanet JM. Preventive Effect of a Melon Extract Rich in Superoxide Scavenging Activity on Abdominal and Liver Fat and Adipokine Imbalance in High-Fat-Fed Hamsters. J. Agric. Food Chem. 2009;57(14):6461-6467.

Décordé K, Ventura E, Lacan D, Ramos J, Cristol JP, Rouanet JM. An SOD rich melon extract Extramel® prevents aortic lipids and liver steatosis in diet-induced model of atherosclerosis. Nutrition, Metabolism & Cardiovascular Disease 2010;20:301-307.

Deibert P, König D, Schmidt-Trucksaess A, Zaenker KS, Frey I, Landmann U, Berg A. Weight loss without losing muscle massin pre-obese and obese subjects induced by a high-soy-protein diet. Int J Obes Relat Metab Disord. 2004 Oct;28(10):1349-52.

Deng G, Yu YR. Radix Astragali improves impaired endothelial dependent vasodilation in obese rat. Sichuan Da Xue Xue Bao Yi Xue Ban 2009 Jul;40(4):608-11.

Dennis EA, Dengo AL, Comber DL, Flack KD, Savla J, Davy KP, Davy BM. Water consumption increases weight loss during a hypocaloric diet intervention in middle-aged and older adults. Obesity (Silver Spring) 2010 Feb;18(2):300-7.

Deshaies Y, Begin F, Savoie L, Vachon C. Attenuation of the Meal-Induced Increase in Plasma Lipids and Adipose Tissue Lipoprotein Lipase by Guar Gum in Rats. J Nutr. 1990;120:64-70.

Dharnarjan SK, Arumugam KM. Comparative evaluation of flavone from Mucuna pruriens and coumarin from Ionidium suffruticosum for hypolipidemic activity in rats fed with high Fat diet. Lipids in Health and Disease 2012;11:126.

Di Martino G, Matera MG, De Martino B, Vacca C, Di Martino S, Rossi F. Relationship between zinc and obesity. J Med. 1993;24(2-3):177-83.

Dinesh D, Vaneeta J, Sunil S, Kumar HR. Evaluation of antiobesity activity of *Tinospora* Cordifolia stems in rats. Dhingra Dinesh 2011;2(1):306-311.

Ding X, Fan S, Lu Y, Zhang Y, Gu M, Zhang L, Liu G, Guo L, Jiang D, Lu X, Li Y, Zhou Z, Huang C. Citrus ichangensis peel extract exhibits anti-metabolic disorder effects by the inhibition of PPAR? and LXR signaling in high-fat diet-induced C57BL/6 mouse. Evidence-Based Complementary and Alternative Medicine 2012 29 Nov.

Ding YJ, Tang KJ, Li FI, Hu QI. Effects of Gypenosides from *Gynostemma pentaphyllum* supplementation on exercise-induced fatigue in mice. African Journal of Agricultural Research 2010 Apr 18;5(8):707-711.

Diniz YS, Rocha KKHR, Souza GA, Galhardi CM, Ebaid GMX, Rodrigues HG, Filho JLVB, Cicogna AC, Novelli ELB. Effects of N-acetylcysteine on sucrose-rich diet-induced hyerglycaemia, dyslipidemia and oxidative stress in rats. European Journal of Pharmacology 2006;543:151-157.

Do MT, Kim HG, Choi JH, Khanal T, Park BH, Tran TP, Hwang YP, Na MK, Jeong HG. Phillyrin attenuates high glucose-induced lipid accumulation in human HepG2 hepaocytes through the activation of LKB1/AMP-activated protein kinase-dependent signalling. Food Chemistry 2012;136:415-425.

Dodin S, Cunnane SC, Mâsse B, Lemay A, Jacques H, Asselin G, Tremblay-Mercier J, Marc I, Lamarche B, Légaré F, Forest JC. Flaxseed on cardiovascular disease markers in healthy menopausal women: a randomized, double-blind, placebo-controlled trial. Nutrition 2008;24:23-30.

Donato J, Pedrosa RG, Cruzat VF, Pires ISO, Chem B, Tirapegui J. Effects of leucine supplementation on the body composition and protein status of rats submitted to food restriction. Nutrition 2006;22:520-527.

Dove ER, Hodgson JM,Puddey IB, Beilin LJ, Lee YP, Mori TA. Skim milk compared with a fruit drink acutely reduces appetite and energy intake in overweight men and women. Am J Clin Nutr 2009 Jul;90(1):70-5.

Dow CA, Going SB, Chow HHS, Patil BS, Thomson CA. The effects of daily consumption of grapefruit on body weight, lipids, and blood pressure in healthy, overweight adults. Metabolism Clinical and Experimental 2012.

Dragull K, Breksa III AP, Cain B. Synephrine Content of Juice from Satsuma Mandarins *(Citrus unshiu* Marcovitch). J. Agric. Food Chem 2008;56:8874-8878.

Du H, You JS, Zhao X, Park JY, Kim SH, Chang KJ. Antiobesity and hypolipidemic effects of lotus leaf hot water extract with taurine supplementation in rats fed a high fat diet. Journal of Biomedical Science 2010;17(42):1-5.

Du H, Zhao X, You JS, Park JY, Kim SH, Chang KJ. Antioxidant and hepatic protective effects of lotus root hot water extract with taurine supplementation in rats fed a high fat diet. Journal of Biomedical Science 2010;17(1):539.

Du J, Li JM. BAS/BSCR23 Apocynin treatment reduces high-fat diet-induced obesity and hypertension but has no significant effect on hyperglycaemia. Heart 2010;96(17).

Du R, Xue J, Wang HB, Zhang Y, Xie ML. Osthol ameliorates fat milk-induced fatty liver in mice by regulation of hepatic sterol regulatory element-binding protein-1c/2-mediated target gene expression. European Journal of Pharmacology 2011;666:183-188.

Du XM, Sun NY, Tamura T, Mohri A, Sugiura M, Yoshizawa T, Irino N, Hayashi J, Shoyama Y. Higher Yielding Isolation of Kinsenoside in *Anoectochilus* and Its Anti-hyperliposis Effect. Biol. Pharm. Bull. 2001;24(1):65-69.

Du XM, Sun NY, Hayashi J, Chen Y, Sugiura M, Shoyama Y. Hepatoprotective and antihyperliposis activities of *in vitro* cultured

236

Anoectochilus formosanus. Phytother. Res. 2003;17:30-33.

Du XM, Sun NY, Furusho N, Hayashi J, Shoyama Y. Effect of in vitro cultured Anoectochilus formosanus on lipid metabolism in clinical uses. Am J Chin Med. 2007;35(5):735-41.

Du XM, Irino N, Furusho N, Hayashi J, Shoyama Y. Pharmacologically active compounds in the Anoectochilus and Goodyear species. J Nat Med. 2008 Apr;62(2):132-48.

Dubnov-Raz G, Constantini NW, Yariv H, Nice S, Shapira N. Influence of water drinking on resting energy expenditure in overweight children. Int J Obes (Lond). 2011 Oct;35(10):1295-300.

Dulloo AG, Duret C, Rohrer D, Girardier L, Mensi N, Fathi M, Chantre P, Vandermander J. Efficacy of a green tea extrac rich in catechin polyphenols and caffeine in increasing 24-h energy expenditure and fat oxidation in humans. Am J Clin Nutr 1999 Dec;70(6):1040-5.

Earnest CP. Exercise interval training: An improved stimulus for improving the physiology of pre-diabetes. Medical Hypotheses 2008;71:752-761.

Ebaid GMX, Seiva FRF, Rocha KKHR, Souza GA, Novelli ELB. Effects of olive oil and its minor phenolic constituents on obesity-induced cardiac metabolic changes. Nutrition Journal 2010;9:46.

Eddouks M, Lemhadri A, Michel JB. Hypolipidemic activity of aqueous extract of *Capparis spinosa* L. in normal and diabetic rats. Journal of Ethnopharmacology 2005;98:345-350.

Eddouks M, Maghrani M, Zeggwagh NA, Michel JB. Study of the hypoglycaemic activity of *Lepidium sativum* L. aqueous extract in normal and diabetic rats. Journal of Ethnopharmacology 2005;97:391-395.

Edijala JK, Asagba SO, Eriyamremu GE, Atomatofa U. Comparative Effect of Garden Egg Fruit, Oat and Apple on Serum Lipid Profile in Rats Fed a High Cholesterol Diet. Pakistan Journal of Nutrition 2005;4(4):245-249.

Ejaz A, Wu D, Kwan P, Meydani M. Curcumin inhibits adipogenesis in 3T3-L1 adipocytes and angiogenesis and obesity in C57/BL mice. J Nutr 2009 May;139(5):919-25.

El-Gengaihi SE, Salem A, Bashandi SA, Ibrahim NA Abd el-Hamid SR. Hypolipidemic effect of some vegetable oils in rats. Food, Agriculture & Environment 2004;2(2):88-93.

El-Kherbawy GM, Ibrahem ES, Zaki SA. Effects of Parsley and Coriander leaves on hypercholesterolemic rats. The 6th Arab and 3rd International Annual Scientific Conference on: Development of Higher Specific Education Programs in Egypt and the Arab Word in the Light of Knowledge Era Requirements. Faculty of Specific Education Mansoura University – Egypt, April, 13-14,2011.

El-Kewawy HEM, Al-Firdous FA, Nagib RM. Beneficial Effects of some beverage consumption and Orlist drug on Diet Induced Obesity in Experimental Rate. Life Science Journal 2011;8(2):667-675.

El-Nashar NN, Abduljawad SH. Impact effect of lycopene and tomato-based products network on cardio-protective biomarkers *in vivo*. Functional Foods in Health and Disease 2012;2(5):151-165.

El-Razek FHA, Hassan AA. Nutritional Value and Hypoglycemic Effect of Prickly Cactus Pear *(Opuntia Ficus-Indica)* Fruit Juice in Alloxan-Induced Diabetic Rats. Australian Journal of Basic and Applied Sciences 2011;5(10):356-377.

El-Sayed MIK. Effects of *Portulaca oleracea* L. seeds in treatment of type-2 diabetes mellitus patients as adjunctive and alternative therapy. Journal of Ethnopharmacology 2011;137:643-651.

El-Shebini SM, Hanna LM, Topouzada ST, Hegazi SM, Metwalli OM. The Role of Pectin as a Slimming Agent. J Clin. Biochem. Nutr. 1988;4:255-262.

El-Shobaki FA, El-Bahay AM, Esmail RSA, Abd El Megeid AA, Esmail NS. Effect of Figs Fruit *(Ficus carica* L.) and its Leaves on Hyperglycemia in Alloxan Diabetic Rats. World Journal of Dairy & Food Sciences 2010;5(1):47-57.

Ello-Martin JA, Roe LS, Ledikwe JH, Beach AM, Rolls BJ. Dietary energy density in the treatment of obesity: a year-long trial comparing 2 weight-loss diets. Am J Clin Nutr. 2007 Jun;85(6):1465-77.

Eller LK, Reimer RA. A high calcium, skim milk powder diet results in a lower fat mass in male, energy-restricted, obese rats more than a low calcium, casein, or soy protein diet. J Nutr. 2010 Jul;140(7):1234-41.

Elliott SS, Keim NL, Stern JS, Teff K, Havel PJ. Fructose, weight gain, and the insulin resistance syndrome. Am J Clin Nutr. 2002 Nov;76(5):911-22.

Elkayam A, Mirelma D, Peleg E, Wilchek M, Miron T, Rabinkov A, Oron-Herman M, Rosenthal T. The effects of allicin on weight in fructose-induced hyperinsulinemic, hyperlipidemic, hypertensive rats. Am J Hypertens 2003 Dec;16(12):1053-6.

Elshorbagy AK, Valdivia-Garcia M, Mattocks DAL, Plummer JD, Orentreich DS, Orentreich N, Refsum H, Perrone CE. Effect of taurine and N-acetylcysteine on methionine restriction-mediated adiposity resistance. Metabolism Clinical and Experimental 2012.

Ennouri M, Fetoui H, Bourret E, Zeghal N, Guermazi F, Attia H. Evaluation of some biological parameters of *Opuntia ficus indica.* 2. Influence of seed supplemented diet on rats. Bioresource Technology 2006;97:2136-2140.

Estakhr J, Javdan N, Najafi S. Anti-Hyperlipidemic Activity of Ethanolic Extract of Salvia Hypoleuca in Rats. Pharmacologyonline 2011;3:773-776.

Etoundi CB, Kuaté D, Ngondi JL, Oben J. Anti-amylase, anti-lipase and antioxidant effects of aqueous extracts of some Cameroonian spices. Journal of Natural Produts 2010;3:165-171.

Eun-Ju Y, Young-Sook C, Myung-Sook C, Myoung-Nam W, Myung-Joo K, Mi-Yae S, Mi-Kyung L. Effect of Young Barley Leaf on Lipid Contents and Hepatic Lipid-Regulating Enzyme Activities in Mice Fed High-Fat Diet. Korean J Nutr 2009;42(1):14-22.

Faghih SH, Abadi AR, Hedayati M, Kimiagar SM. Comparison of the effects of cows' milk, fortified soy milk, and calcium supplement on weight and fat loss in premenopausal overweight and obese women. Nutr Metab Cardiovasc Dis. 2011 Jul;21(7):499-503.

Fajcsak Z, Gabor A, Kovacs V, Martos E. The effects of 6-week low glycemic load diet based on low glycemic index foods in overweight/obese children – pilot study. J Am Coll Nutr. 2008 Feb;27(1):12-21.

Fan S, Zhang Y, Hu N, Sun Q, Ding X, Li G, Zheng B, Gu M, Huang F, Sun YQ, Zhou Z, Lu X, Huang C, Ji G. Extract of Kuding Tea Prevents High-Fat Diet-Induced Metabolic Disorders in C57BL/6 Mice via Liver X Receptor (LXR) β Antagonism. PloS One 2012 Dec;7(12):1-12.

Farinazzi-Machado FMV, Barbalho SM, Oshiiwa M, Goulart R, Pessan Junior O. Use of cereal bars with quinoa *(Chenopodium quinoa* W.) to reduce risk factors related to cardiovascular diseases. Ciênc. Tecnol. Aliment. Campinas. 2012;32(2):239-244.

Figueiredo AS, Modesto-Filho J. Efeito do uso da farinha desengordurada do *Sesamum indicum* L nos niveis glicêmicos em diabéticas tipo 2. Brazilian Journal of Pharmacology 2008;18(1):77-83.

Flegal KM, Troiano RP, Pamuk ER, Kuczmarski RJ, Campbell SM. The influence of smoking cessation on the prevalence of overweight in the United States. N Engl J Med. 1995 Nov 2;333(18):1165-70.

Folland JP, Stern R, Brickley G. Sodium phosphate loading improves laboratory cycling time-trial performance in trained cyclists. J Sci Med Sport 2008 Sep;11(5):464-8.

Foster EB, Fisher G, Sartin JL, Elsasser TH, Wu G, Cowan W, Pascoe DD. Acute regulation of IGF-I by alterations in post-exercise macronutrients. Amino Acids 2012 Apr;42(4):1405-16.

Foster-Schubert KE, Alfano CM, Duggan CR, Xiao L, Campbell KL, Kong A, Bain CE, Wang CY, Blackburn GL, McTiernan A. Effect of diet and exercise, alone or combined, on weight and body composition in overweight-to-obese postmenopausal women. Obesity (Silver Spring) 2012 Aug;20(8):1628-38.

Foucault AS, Mathé V, Lafont R, Even P, Dioh W, Veillet S, Tomé D, Huneau JF, Hermier D, Quignard-Boulangé A. Quinoa extract enriched in 20-hydroxyecdysone protects mice from diet-induced obesity and modulates adipokines expression. Obesity (Silver Spring) 2012 Feb;20(2):270-7.

Franco JG, Lisboa PC, Lima NS, Amaral TAS, Peixoto-Silva N, Resende AC, Oliveira E, Passos MCF, Moura EG. Resveratrol attenuates oxidative stress and prevents steatosis and hypertension in obese rats programmed by early weaning. Journal of Nutritional Biochemistry 2012.

Frati-Munari AC, Fernández-Harp JA, Becerril M, Chávez-Negrete A, Bañales-Ham M. Decrease in serum lipids, glycemia and body weight by Plantago psyllium in obese and diabetic patients. Arch Invest Med (Mex) 1983;14(3):259-68.

Freise C, Erben U, Neuman U, Kim K, Zeitz M, Somasundaram R, Ruehl M. An active extract of *Lindera obtusiloba* inhibits adipogenesis via sustained Wnt signaling and exerts anti-inflammatory effects in the 3T3-L1 preadipocytes. Journal of Nutritional Biochemistry 2010;21:1170-1177.

Frestedt JL, Zenk JL, Kuskowski MA, Ward LS, Bastian ED. A whey-protein supplement increases fat loss and spares lean muscle in obese subjects: a randomized human clinical study. Nutrition & Metabolism 2008;5:8.

Freudenberg A, Petzke KJ, Klaus S. Comparison of high-protein diets and leucine supplementation in the prevention of metabolic syndrome and related disorders in mice. Journal of Nutritional Biochemistry 2012.

Freudenberg A, Petzke KJ, Klaus S. Dietary L: -leucine and L: -alanine supplementation have similar acute effects in the prevention of high-fat diet-induced obesity. Amino Acids 2012 Jul 31.

Fried A, Manske SL, Eller LK, Lorincz C, Reimer RA, Zernicke RF. Skim milk powder enhances trabecular bone architecture compared with casein or whey in diet-induced obese rats. Nutrition 2012;28:331-335.

Friedman M, Fitch TE, Levin CE, Yokoyama WH. Feeding Tomatoes to Hamsters Reduces their Plasma Low-density Lipoprotein Cholesterol and Triglycerides. Journal of Food Science 2000;65(5):890-897.

Frühbeck G, Monreal I, Santidrián S. Hormonal implications of the hypocholesterolemic effect of intake of field beans (*Vicia faba* L.) by young men with hypercholesterolemia. Am J Clin Nutr 1997;66:1452-60.

Fu WJ, Haynes TE, Kohli R, Hu J, Shi W, Spencer TE, Carroll RJ, Meininger CJ, Wu G. Dietary L-arginine supplementation reduces fat mass in Zucker diabetic fatty rats. J Nutr. 2005 Apr;135(4):714-21.

Fuhrman B, Volkova N, Kaplan M, Presser D, Attias J, Hayek T, Aviram M. Antiatherosclerotic Effects of Licorice Extract Supplementation on Hypercholesterolemic Patients: Increased Resistance of LDL to Atherogenic Modifications, Reduced Plasma Lipid Levels, and Decreased Systolic Blood Pressure. Nutrition 2002;18:268-273.

Fujikawa T, Hirata T, Wada A, Kawamura N, Yamaguchi Y, Fujimura K, Ueda T, Yurugi Y, Soya H, Nishibe S. Chronic administration of Eucommia leaf stimulates metabolic function of rats across several organs. British Journal of Nutrition 2010;104:1868-1877.

Fujioka K, Greenway F, Sheard J, Ying Y. The effects of grapefruit on weight and insulin resistance: relationship to the metabolic syndrome. J Med Food 2006 Spring;9(1):49-54.

Fujita H, Yamagami T. Antihypercholesterolemic effect of Chinese black tea extract in human subjects with borderline hypercholesterolemia. Nutrition Research 2008;28:450-456.

Fujita H, Yamagami T. Efficacy and safety of Chinese black tea (Pu-Ehr) extract in healthy and hypercholesterolemic subjects. Ann Nutr Metab 2008;53(1):33-42.

Fukuchi Y, Hiramitsu M, Okada M, Hayashi S, Nabeno Y, Osawa T, Naito M. Lemon Polyphenols Suppress Diet-induced Obesity by Up-Regulation of mRNA Levels of the Enzymes Involved in β-Oxidation in Mouse White Adipose Tissue. J. Clin. Biochem. Nutr. 2008 Nov;43:201-209.

Fukuda I, Tsutsui M, Yoshida T, Toda T, Tsuda T, Ashida H. Oral toxicological studies of black soybean *(Glycine max)* hull extract: Acute studies in rats and mice, and chronic studies in mice. Food and Chemical Toxicology 2011;49:3272-3278.

Fukumitsu S, Aida K, Ueno N, Ozawa S, Takahashi Y, Kobori M. Flaxseed lignan attenuates high-fat diet-induced fat accumulation an induces adiponectin expression in mice. British Journal of Nutrition 2008;100:669-676.

Fushimi T, Suruga K, Oshima Y, Fukiharu M, Tsukamoto Y, Goda T. Dietary acetic acid reduces serum cholesterol and triacylglycerols in rats fed a cholesterol-rich diet. British Journal of Nutrition 2006;95:916-924.

Gaafar AM, Yossef HE, Ibrahim HH. Protective effects of mushroom and their ethyl extract on aging compared with L-carnitine. International Journal of Nutrition and Metabolism 2010 Aug;2(4):63-69.

Gaamoussi F, Israili ZH, Lyoussi B. Hypoglycemic and hypolipidemic effects of an aqueous extract of Chamaerops humilis leaves in obese, hyperglycemic and hyperlipidemic Meriones shawi rats. Pak J Pharm Sci 2010 Apr;23(2):212-9.

Gadir WSA, Ali AM, Bakhiet AO. Susceptibility of Bovans Chicks to Low Levels of Dietary Cassia Italica Fruits and *Ocimum basilicum* Leaves or their Mixture. Journal of Animal and Veterinary Advances 2006;5(6):468-471.

Galisteo M, Sánchez M, Vera R, González M, Anguera M, Duarte J, Zarzuelo A. A diet supplemented with husks of Plantago ovata reduces the development of endothelial dysfunction, hypertension, and obesity by affecting adiponectin and TNF-alpha in obese Zucker rats. J Nutr 2005 Oct;135(10):2399-404.

Galisteo M, Morón R, Rivera L, Romero R, Anguera A, Zarzuelo A. *Plantago ovata* husks-supplemented diet ameliorates metabolic

238

alterations in obese Zucker rats through activation of AMP-activated protein kinase. Comparative study with other dietary fibers. Clinical Nutrition 2010;29:261-267.

Gao D, Li Q, Liu Z, Feng J, Li J, Han Z, Duan Y. Antidiabetic potential of Rhodiola sachalinensis root extract in streptozotocin-induced diabetic rats. Methods Find Exp Clin Pharmacol 2009 Jul-Aug;31(6):375-81.

Gao D, Li Q, Gao Z, Wang L. Antidiabetic Effects of *Corni Fructus* Extract in Streptozotocin-Induced Diabetic Rats. Yonsei Med J 2012;53(4):691-700.

Gao XL, He L, Zhang XJ, Ding M. Effect of acupuncture on serum insulin level in the patient of simple obesity. Zhongguo Zhen Jiu 2007 Oct;27(10):738-40.

Gao XX, Meng XJ, Li JH. Study on function of active polysaccharide from Schisandra Chinensis (Turcz) Baill in reducing weight and fat. Sci. Technol. Food Industry 2008;11:248-250.

Garg C, Ansari SH, Khan SA, Garg M. Effect of *Foeniculum vulgare* Mill. Fruits in Obesity and Associated Cardiovascular Disorders Demonstrated in High Fat Diet Fed Albino Rats. Journal of Pharmaceutical and Biomedical Sciences (JPBMS) 2011;8(19):1-5.

Gauhar R, Hwang SL, Jeong SS, Kim JE, Song H, Park DC, Song KS, Kim TY, Oh WK, Huh TL. Heat-processed Gynostemma pentaphyllum extract improves obesity in ob/ob mice by activating AMP-activated protein kinase. Biotechnol Lett 2012 Sep;34(9):1607-16.

Gaullier JM, Halse J, Høye K, Kristiansen K, Fagertun H, Vik H, Gudmundsen O. Conjugated linoleic acid supplementation for 1 y reduces body fat mass in healthy overweight humans. Am J Clin Nutr 2004 Jun;79(6):1118-25.

Gaullier JM, Halse J, Høye K, Kristiansen K, Fagertun H, Vik H, Gudmundsen O. Supplementation with conjugated linoleic acid for 24 months is well tolerated by and reduces body fat mass in healthy, overweight humans. J Nutr 2005 Apr;135(4):778-84.

Gaullier JM, Halse J, Høivik HO, Høye K, Syvertsen C, Nurminiemi M, Hassfeld C, Einerhand A, O'Shea M, Gudmundsen O. Six months supplementation with conjugated linoleic acid induces regional-specific fat mass decreases in overweight and obese. British Journal of Nutrition 2007;97:550-560.

Geetha M, Reddy SK, Krupanidhi AM, Muralikrishna KS, Patil N, Prashanth P. Effect of Fenugreek on Total Body and Organ Weights: A Study on Mice. Pharmacologyonline 2011;3:747-752.

Genazzani AD, Stomati M, Strucchi C, Puccetti S, Luisi S, Genazzani AR. Oral dehydroepiandrosterone supplementation modulates spontaneous and growth hormone-releasing hormone-induced growth hormone and insulin-like growth factor-1 secretion in early and late postmenopausal women. Fertility and sterility 2001 Aug;76(2):241-248.

Genazzani AR, Inglese S, Lombardi I, Pieri M, Bernardi F, Genazzani AD, Rovati L, Luisi M. Long-term low-dose dehydroepiandrosterone replacement therapy in aging males with partial androgen deficiency. Aging Male 2004 Jun;7(2):133-43.

Genta S, Cabrera W, Habib N, Pons J, Carillo IM, Grau A, Sánchez S. Yacon syrup: Beneficial effects on obesity and insulin resistance in humans. Clinical Nutrition 2009;28:182-187.

Georgina EO, Kingsley O, Esosa US, Helen NK, Frank AO, Anthony OC. Comparative evaluation of antioxidant effects of watermelon and orange, and their effects on some serum lipid profile of Wister albino rats. International Journal of Nutrition and Metabolism 2011 Sep;3(8):97-102.

Geraedts MCP, Troost FJ, Munsters MJM, Stegen JHCH, de Ridder RJ, Conchillo JM, Kruimel JW, Masclee AAM, Saris WHM. Intraduodenal Administration of Intact Pea Protein Effectively Reduces Food Intake in Both Lean and Obese Male Subjects. PloS 2011 Sep;6(9):1-7.

Gerli S, Papaleo E, Ferrari A, Di Renzo GC. Randomized, double blind placebo-controlled trial: effects of Myo-inositol on ovarian function and metabolic factors in woen with PCOS. European Review for Medical and Pharmacological Sciences 2007;11:347-354.

Ghule BV, Ghante MH, Saoji AN, Yeole PG. Antihyperlipidemic effect of the methanolic extract from *Lagenaria siceraria* Stand. fruit in hyperlipidemic rats. Journal of Ethnopharmacology 2009;124:333-337.

Girotti C, Ginet M, Demarne FC, Lagarde M, Géloën A. Lipolytic activity of cirsimarin extracted from Microtea debilis. Planta Med 2005 Dec;71(12):1170-2.

Godard MP, Johnson BA, Richmond SR. Body composition and hormonal adaptations associated with forskolin consumption in overweight and obese men. Obes Res. 2005 Aug;13(8):1335-43.

Gómez-Santos C, Hernández-Morante JJ, Tébar FJ, Granero E, Garaulet M. Differential effect of oral dehydroepiandrosterone-sulphate on metabolic syndrome features in pre- and postmenopausal obese women. Clin Endocrinol (Oxf) 2012 Oct;77(4):548-54.

Gong J, Peng C, Chen T, Gao B, Zhou H. Effects of theabrownin from pu-erh tea on the metabolism of serum lipids in rats: mechanism of action. J Food Sci 2010 Aug 1;75(6):182-9.

Goto T, Teraminami A, Lee JY, Ohyama K, Funakoshi K, Kim YI, Hirai S, Uemura T, Yuf R, Takahashi N, Kawada T. Tiliroside, a glycosidic flavonoid, ameliorates obesity-induced metabolic disorders via activation of adiponectin signaling followed by enhancement of fatty acid oxidation in liver and skeletal muscle in obese-diabetic mice. Journal of Nutritional Biochemistry 2012;23:768-776.

Gout B, Bourges C, Paineau-Dubreuil S. Satiereal, a *Crocus sativus* L. extract, reduces snacking and increases satiety in a randomized placebo-controlled study of mildly overweight, healthy women. Nutrition Research 2010;30:305-313.

Goyal RK, Kadnur SV. Beneficial effects of *Zingiber officinale* on goldthioglucose induced obesity. Fitoterapia 2006;77:160-163.

Grant G, Dorward PM, BuchanWC, Armour JC, Pusztai A. Consumption of diets containing raw soya beans *(Glycine max)*, kidney beans *(Phaseolus vulgaris)*, cowpeas *(Vigna unguiculata)* or lupin seeds *(Lupinus angustifolius)* by rats for up to 700 days: effects on body composition and organ weights. British Journal of Nutrition 1995;73:17-29.

Grube B, Chong PW, Lau KZ, Orzechowski HD. A Natural Fiber Complex Reduces Body Weight in the Overweight and Obese: A Double-Blind, Randomized, Placebo-Controlled Study. Obesity (Silver Spring) 2012 Jun 25.

Gualano AB, Bozza T, Lopes De Campos P, Roschel H, Dos Santos Costa A, Luiz Marquezi M, Benatti F, Herbert Lancha Junior A. Branched-chain amino acids supplementation enhances exercise capacity and lipid oxidation during endurance exercise after muscle glycogen depletion. J Sports Med Phys Fitness 2011 Mar;51(1):82-8.

Gudej J, Tomczyk M. Determination of Flavonoids, Tannins and Ellagic Acid in Leaves from *Rubus* L. Species. Arch Pharm Res 2004;27(11):1114-1119.

Guo AJ, Choi RC, Cheung AW, Li J, Chen IX, Dong TT, Tsim KW, Lau BW. Stimulation of Apolipoprotein A-IV expression in Caco-2/TC7 enterocytes and reduction of triglyceride formation in 3T3-L1 adipocytes by potential anti-obesity Chinese herbal medicines. Chin Med. 2009 Mar 26;4(5).

Guo F, Huang C, Liao X, Wang Y, He Y, Feng R, Li Y, Sun C. Beneficial effects of mangiferin on hyperlipidemia in high-fat-fed hamsters. Mol Nutr Food Res 2011 Dec;55(12):1809-18.

Guo H, Li D, Ling W, Feng X, Xia M. Anthocyanin inhibits high glucose-induced hepatic mtGPAT1 activation and prevents fatty acid synthesis through PKCς. J Lipid Res 2011 May;52(5):908-22.

Guo HX, Liu DH, Ma Y, Liu JF, Wang Y, Du ZY, Wang X, Shen JK, Peng HI. Long-term baicalin administration ameliorates metabolic disorders and hepatic steatosis in rats given a high-fat diet. Acta Pharmacologica Sinica 2009;30:1505-1512.

Guo H, Liu G, Zhong R, Wang Y, Wang D, Xia M. Cyanidin-3-O-β-glucoside regulates fatty acid metabolism via an AMP-activated protein kinase-dependent signaling pathway in human HepG2 cells. Lipids in Health and Disease 2012;11:10.

Guo P, Kai Q, Gao J, Lian ZQ, Wu CM, Wu CA, Zhu HB. Cordycepin Prevents Hyperlipidemia in Hamsters Fed a High-Fat Diet via Activation of AMP-Activated Protein Kinase. J Pharmacol 2010;113:395-403.

Gupta P, Mehla J, Gupta YK. Antiobesity effect of Safoof Mohazzil, a polyherbal formulation, in cafeteria diet induced obesity in rats. Indian Journal of Experimental Biology 2012;50:776-784.

Gupta UC, Jain GC. Hypolipidemic Effect of *Ginkgo biloba* Extract in Hypercholesterolemic Rats. Asian J. Exp. Sci. 2006;20(1):69-76.

Gwak JH, Lee JH, Lee SJ, Park HW, Kim Y, Hyun YJ. The Effect of L-Carnitine and Isoflavone Supplementation on Weight Reduction and Visceral Fat Accumulation in Overweight Women. Korean J Nutr. 2007 Oct;40(7):630-638.

Ha CH, So WY. Effects of Combined Exercise Training on Body Composition and Metabolic Syndrome Factors. Iranian J Publ Health 2012 Aug;41(8):20-26.

Ha DT, Trung TN, Thu NB, On TV, Nam NH, Men CV, Phuong TT, Bae K. Adlay Seed Extract *(Coix lachryma-jobi* L.) Decreased Adipocyte Differentiation and Increased Glucose Uptake in 3T3-L1 Cells. Journal of Medicinal Food 2010 Dec;13(6):1331-1339.

Ha US, Koh JS, Woo JC, Kim SJ, Kim SJ, Jang H, Yong BI, Hwang SY, Kim SW. The Effect of Cyanidin-3-O-β-d-glucopyranoside on the Penile Erection and Corpus Cavernosum in a Rat Model of Diabetic Erectile Dysfunction. Korean J Androl. 2011 Aug;29(2):127-133.

Ha YL, Jeong SB. Effects of Conjugated Linoleic Acid on Body Fat Reduction and Physical Exercise Enhancement of Obese Male Middle School Students. Journal of Life Science 2010;20(12):1844-1850.

Habib NC, Honoré SM, Genta SB, Sánchez SS. Hypolipidemic effect of *Smallanthus sonchifolius* (yacon) roots on diabetic rats: Biochemical approach. Chemico-Biological Interactions 2011;194:31-39.

Hackney KJ, Bruenger AJ, Lemmer JT. Timing protein intake increases energy expenditure 24 h after resistance training. Med Sci Sports Exerc 2010 May;42(5):998-1003.

Hafidi ME, Pérez I, Zamora J, Soto V, Carvajal-Sandoval G, Baños G. Glycine intake decreases plasma free fatty acids, adipose cell size, and blood pressure in sucrose-fed rats. Am J Physiol Regul Integr Comp Physiol 2004;287:1387-1393.

Hagberg JM, Coyle EF. Physiologic Comparison of Competitive Racewalking and Running. Int. J. Sports Med. 1984;5:74-77.

Hahm TS, Park SJ, Lo M. Effects of germination on chemical composition and functional properties of sesame *(Sesamum indicum* L.) seeds. Bioresource Technology 2009;100:1643-1647.

Hamza N, Berke B, Cheze C, Le Carrec R, Umar A, Agli AN, Lassalle R, Jove J, Gin H, Moore N. Preventive and curative effect of *Trigonella foenum-graecum* L. seeds in C57BL/6J models of type 2 diabetes induced by high-fat diet. Journal of Ethnopharmacology 2012.

Han HK, Yoon SJ, Kim GH. Effects of Compositae Plats on Plasma Glucose and Lipid Level in Streptozotocin Induced Diabetic Rats. J Korean Soc Food Sci Nutr 2009;38(6):674-682.

Han JR, Deng B, Sun J, Chen CG, Corkey BE, Kirkland JL, Ma J, Guo W. Effects of dietary medium-chain triglyceride on weight loss and insulin sensitivity in a group of moderately overweight free-living type 2 diabetic Chinese subjects. Metabolism Clinical and Experimental 2007;56:985-991.

Han LK, Takaku T, Li J, Kimura Y, Okuda H. Anti-obesity action of oolong tea. Int J Obes Relat Metab Disord 1999 Jan;23(1): 98-105.

Han LK, Xu BJ, Kimura Y, Zheng Y, Okuda H. Platycodi radix affects lipid metabolism in mice with high fat diet-induced obesity. J Nutr 2000 Nov;130(11):2760-4.

Han LK, Zheng YN, Xu BJ, Okuda H, Kimura Y. Saponins from platycodi radix ameliorate high fat diet-induced obesity in mice. J Nutr 2002 Aug;132(8):2241-5.

Han LK, Sumiyoshi M, Zhang J, Liu MX, Zhang XF, Zheng YN, Okuda H, Kimura Y. Anti-obesity action of Salix matsudana leaves (Part 1). Anti-obesity action by polyphenols of Salix matsudana in high fat-diet trated rodent animals. Phytother Res. 2003 Dec;17(10):1188-94.

Han LK, Sumiyoshi M, Zheng YN, Okuda H, Kimura Y. Anti-obesity action of Salix matsudana leaves (Part 2). Isolation of anti-obesity effectors from polyphenol fractions of Salix matsudana. Phytother Res. 2003 Dec;17(10):1195-8.

Han LK, Gong XJ, Kawano S, Saito M, Kimura Y, Okuda H. Antiobesity Actions of *Zingiber officinale* Roscoe. Yakuoaku Zasshi 2005;125(2):213-217.

Han LK, Morimoto C, Yu RH, Okuda H. Effects of Coleus *forskohlii* on Fat Storage in Ovariectomized Rats. Yakugaku Zasshi 2005;125(5):449-453.

Han LK, Zheng YN, Yoshikawa M, Okuda H, Kimura Y. Anti-obesity effects of chikusetsusaponins isolated from *Panax japonicus* rhizomes. BMC Complementary and Alternative Medicine 2005;5(9):1-10.

Han S, Oh KS, Yoon Y, Park JS, Park YS, Han JH, Jeong AL, Lee S, Park M, Choi YA, Lim JS, Yang Y. Herbal extract THI improves metabolic abnormality in mice fed a high-fat diet. Nutrition Research and Practice 2011;5(3):198-204.

Han SF, Zhang H, Zhai CK. Protective potentials of wild rice *(Zizania latifolia* (Griseb) Turcz) against obesity and lipotoxicity induced by a high-fat/cholesterol diet in rats. Food and Chemical Toxicology 2012;50:2263-2269.

Han Y, Jung HW, Park YK. The roots of Atractylodes japonica Koidzumi promote adipogenic differentiation via activation of the insulin signaling pathway in 3T3-L1 cells. BMC Complementary and Alternative Medicine 2012;12:154.

Handa T, Yamaguchi K, Sono Y, Yazawa K. Effects of Fenugreek Seed Extract in Obese Mice Fed a High-Fat Diet. Biosci. Biotechnol. Biochem. 2005;69(6):1186-1188.

Handayani D, Chen J, Meyer BJ, Huang XF. Dietary Shiitake Mushroom *(Lentinus edodes)* Prevents Fat Deposition and Lowers Triglyceride in Rats Fed a High-Fat Diet. Journal of Obesity 2011:1-8.

Handayani D, Meyer BJ, Chen J, Tang P, Kwok PCL, Chan HK, Huang XF. The Comparison of the Effect of Oat and Shiitake Mushroom Powder to Prevent Body Weight Gain in Rats Fed High Fat Diet. Food and Nutrition Sciences 2012;3:1009-1019.

Hansen PA, Han DH, Nolte LA, Chen M, Holloszy JO. DHEA protects against visceral obesity and muscle insulin resistance in rats fed a high-fat diet. Am J Physiol 1997 Nov;273(5 Pt 2):1704-8.

Hao J, Shen W, Yu G, Jia H, Li X, Feng Z, Wang Y, Weber P, Wertz K, Sharman E, Liu J. Hydroxytyrosol promotes mitochondrial biogenesis and mitochondrial function in 3T3-L1 adipocytes. Journal of Nutritional Biochemistry 2010;21:634-644.

Harach T, Aprikian O, Monnard I, Moulin J, Membrez M, Béolor JC, Raab T, Macé K, Darimont C. Rosemary (Rosmarinus officinalis L.) leaf extract limits weight gain and liver steatosis in mice fed a high-fat diet. Planta Med. 2010 Apr;76(6):566-71.

Harada U, Chikama A, Saito S, Takase H, Nagao T, Hase T, Tokimitsu I. Effects of the Long-Term Ingestion of Tea Catechins on Energy Expenditure and Dietary Fat Oxidation in Healthy Subjects. Journal of Health Science 2005;51(2):248-252.

Haramizu S, Kawabata F, Ohnuki K, Inoue N, Watanabe T, Yazawa S, Fushiki T. Capsiate, a non-pungent capsaicin analog, reduces body fat without weight rebound like swimming exercise in mice. Biomedical Research 2011;32(4):279-284.

Harbilas D, Brault A, Vallerand D, Martineau LC, Saleem A, Arnason JT, Musallam L, Haddad PS. *Populus balsamifera* L. (Salicaceae) mitigates the development of obesity and improves insulin sensitivity in a diet-induced obese mouse model. Journal of Ethnopharmacology 2012;141:1012-1020.

Hariri N, Gougeon R, Thibault L. A highly saturated fat-rich diet is more obesogenic than diets with lower saturated fat content. Nutr Res 2010 Sep;30(9):632-43.

Harnafi H, Aziz M, Amrani S. Sweet basil *(Ocimum basilicum* L.) improves lipid metabolism in hypercholesterolemic rats. E-SPEN, the European e-Journal of Clinical Nutrition and Metabolism 2009;4:181-186.

Hasegawa N. Stimulation of Lipolysis by Pycnogenol. Phytotherapy research 1999;13:619-620.

Hashemipour M, Kelishadi R, Shapouri J, Sarrafzadegan N, Amini M, Tavakoli N, Movahedian-Attar A, Mirmoghtadaee P, Poursafa P. Effect of zinc supplementation on insulin resistance and components of the metabolic syndrome in prepubertal obese children. Hormones 2009;8(4):279-285.

Hassanali Z, Ametaj BN, Field CJ, Proctor SD, Vine DF. Dietary supplementation of n-3 PUFA reduces weight gain and improves postprandial lipaemia and the associated inflammatory response in the obese JCR:LA-cp rat. Diabetes Obes Metab 2010 Feb;12(2):139-47.

Hattori M, Kondo T, Kishi M, Yamagami K. A Single Oral Administration of Acetic Acid Increased Energy Expenditure in C57BL/6J Mice. Biosci. Biotechnol. Biochem. 2010;74(10):2158-2159.

Hayamizu K, Ishii Y, Kaneko I, Shen M, Sakaguchi H, Okuhara Y, Shigematsu N, Miyazaki S, Shimasaki H. Effects of Long-term Administration of *Garcinia cambogia* extract on Visceral Fat Accumulation in Humans: A Placebo-controlled Double Blind Trial. J. Oleo Sci. 2001;50(10):805-812.

Hayamizu K, Ishii Y, Kaneko I, Shen M, Okuhara Y, Shigematsu N, Tomi H, Furuse M, Yoshino G, Shimasaki H. Effects of *Garcinia cambogia* (Hydroxycitric Acid) on Visceral Fat Accumulation: A Double-Blind, Randomized, Placebo-Controlled Trial. Current Therapeutic Research 2003 Sep-Oct;64(8):551-567.

He CC, Hui RR, Tezuka Y, Kadota S, Li JX. Osteoprotective effect of extract from *Achyranthes bidentata* in ovariectomized rats. Journal of Ethnopharmacology 2010;127:229-234.

He L, Gao XL, Deng HX, Zhao YX. Effects of acupuncture on body mass index and waist-hip ratio in the patient of simple obesity. Zhongguo Zhen Jiu 2008 Feb;28(2):95-7.

He RR, Chen L, Lin BH, Matsui Y, Yao XS, Kurihara H. Beneficial effects of oolong tea consumption on diet-induced overweight and obese subjects. Chin J Integr Med 2009 Feb;15(1):34-41.

Helal EGE, Eid FA, El-Wahsh AMSEA. Effect of fennel *(Foeniculum vulgare)* on hyperlipidemic rats. The Egyptian Journal of Hospital Medicine 2011 Apr;43:212-225.

Hermsdorff HH, Zulet MA, Abete I, Martinez JA. A legume-based hypocaloric diet reduces proinflammatory status and improves metabolic features in overweight/obese subjects. Eur J Nutr. 2011 Feb;50(1):61-9.

Heydari M, Freund J, Boutcher SH. The Effect of High-Intensity Intermittent Exercise on Body Composition of Overweight Young Males. Journal of Obesity 2012:1-8.

Hidaka S, Okamoto Y, Arita M. A hot water extract of Chlorella pyrenoidosa reduces body weight and serum lipids in ovariectomized rats. Phytother Res. 2004 Feb;18(2):164-8.

Hill AM, Buckley JD, Murphy KJ, Howe PRC. Combining fish-oil supplements with regular aerobic exercise improves body composition and cardiovascular disease risk factors. Am J Clin Nutr 2007;85:1267-74.

Hirata T, Kobayashi T, Wada A, Ueda T, Fujikawa T, Miyashita H, Ikeda T, Tsukamoto S, Nohara T. Anti-obesity compounds in green leaves of *Eucommia ulmoides.* Bioorganic & Medicinal Chemistry Letters 2011;21:1786-1791.

Hisashi M, Kiyofumi N, Osamu M, Norihisa N, Masayuki Y. Inhibitory effects of a constituent from *Rosa canina* on accumulation of visceral adipose tissues. Journal of the Pharmaceutical Society of Japan 2006;126(3):92-93.

Hiwatashi K, Kosaka Y, Suzuki N, Hata K, Mukaiyama T, Sakamoto K, Shirakawa H, Komai M. Yamabushitake Mushroom *(Hericium erinaceus)* Improved Lipid Metabolism in Mice Fed a High-Fat Diet. Biosci. Biotechnol. Biochem. 2010;74(7): 1447-1451.

Ho JN, Son ME, Lim WC, Lim ST, Cho HY. Anti-Obesity Effects of Germinated Brown Rice Extract through Down-Regulation of Lipogenic Genes in High Fat Diet-Induced Obese Mice. Biosci. Biotechnol. Biochem. 2012;76(6):1068-1074.

Ho JN, Jang JY, Yoon HG, Kim Y, Kim S, Jun W, Lee J. Anti-obesity effects of a standardised ethanol extract from *Curcuma longa* L. fermented with *Aspergillus oryzae* in *ob/ob* mice and primary mouse adipocytes. Journal of the Science of Food and Agriculture 2012 Jul;92(9):1833-1840.

Ho SS, Dhaliwal SS, Hills AP, Pal S. The effect of 12 weeks of aerobic, resistance or combination exercise training on cardiovascular risk factors in the overweight and obese in a randomized trial. BMC Public Health 2012;12(704):1-10.

Hoffman JR, Ratamess NA, Ross R, Shanklin M, Kang J, Faigenbaum AD. Effect of a pre-exercise energy supplement on the acute hormonal response to resistance exercise. J Strength Cond Res. 2008 May;22(3):874-82.

Hoffman JR, Ratamess NA, Tranchina CP, Rashti SL, Kang J, Faigenbaum AD. Effect of a proprietary protein supplement on recovery indices following resistance exercise in strength/power athletes. Amino Acids 2010 Mar;38(3):771-8.

Homady MH, Hussain HH, Tarawneh KA, Shakhanbeh JM, Al-Raheil IA, Brain PF. Effects of Oral Applications of Some Medicinal Plant Extracts Used in Jordan on Social Aggression as Well as Testicular and Preputial Gland Structures in Male Mice. Pakistan Journal of Biologial Sciences 2000;3(3):398-402.

Hong HJ, Jin JY, Yang H, Kang WY, Kim DG, Lee S, Choi Y, Kim JH, Han CH, Lee YJ. Dangyuja *(Citrus grandis* Osbeck) Peel Improves Lipid Profiles and Alleviates Hypertension in Rats Fed a High-Fat Diet. Lab. Anim. Res. 2010;26(4):361-367.

Hong JH, Hwang EY, Kim HJ, Jeong YJ, Lee IS. Artemisia capillaris inhibits lipid accumulation in 3T3-L1 adipocytes and obesity in C57BL/6J mice fed a high fat diet. J Med Food 2009 Aug;12(4):736-45.

Hong JH, Cha YS, Rhee SJ. Effects of the Cellcultured *Acanthopanax senticosus* Extract on Antioxidative Defense System and Membrane Fluidity in the Liver of Type 2 Diabetes Mouse. J. Clin. Biochem. Nutr. 2009 Jul;45:101-109.

Hong JH, Lee IS. Effects of *Artemisia capillaris* ethyl acetate fraction on oxidative stress and antioxidant enzyme in high-fat diet induced obese mice. Chemico-Biological Interaction 2009;179:88-93.

Hong S, Park J, Sohn JS, Kim J, Kim MK. Effects of *Garcinia cambogia* Extract Feeding on Body Weight and Lipid Profiles in Rats Fed a High-carbohydrate or High-fat Diet. Food Sci. Biotechnol. 2009;18(3):649-654.

Hongu N, Sachan DS. Caffeine, carnitine and choline supplementation of rats decreases body fat and serum leptin concentration as does exercise. J Nutr. 2000 Feb;130(2):152-7.

Hottenrott K, Ludyga S, Schulze S. Effects of high intensity training and continuous endurance training on aerobic capacity and body composition in recreationally active runners. Journal of Sports Science and Medicine 2012;11:483-488.

Hou Y, Shao W, Xiao R, Xu K, Ma Z, Johnstone BH, Du Y. Pu-erh tea aqueous extracts lower atherosclerotic risk factors in rat hyperlipidemia model. Experimental Gerontology 2009;44:434-439.

Howarth NC, Saltzman E, Roberts SB. Dietary fiber and weight regulation. Nutr Rev. 2001 May;59(5):129-39.

Hsu CL, Yen GC. Effects of flavonoids and phenolic acids on the inhibition of adipogenesis in 3T3-L1 adipocytes. J Agric Food Chem 2007 Oct 17;55(21):8404-10.

Hsu CL, Wu CH, Huang SL, Yen GC. Phenolic compounds rutin and o-coumaric acid ameliorate obesity induced by high-fat diet in rats. J Agric Food Chem 2009 Jan 28;57(2):425-31.

Hsu SC, Huang CJ. Reduced fat mass in rats fed a high oleic acid-rich safflower oil diet is associated with changes in expression of hepatic PPARalpha and adipose SREBP-1c-regulated genes. J Nutr. 2006 Jul;136(7):1779-85.

Hu WL, Chang CH, Hung YC. Clinical observations on laser acupuncture in simple obesity therapy. Am J Chin Med 2010;38(5):861-7.

Hu X, Li Y, Li C, Fu Y, Cai F, Chen Q, Li D. Combination of fucoxanthin and conjugated linoleic acid attenuates body weight gain and improves lipid metabolism in high-fat diet-induced obese rats. Archives of Biochemistry and Bophysics 2012;519:59-65.

Hu Y, Davies GE. Berberine inhibits adipogenesis in high-fat diet-induced obesity mice. Fitoterapia 2010;81:358-366.

Hu Y, Fahmy H, Zjawiony JK, Davies GE. Inhibitory effect and transcriptional impact of berberine and evodiamine on human white preadiocyte differentation. Fitoterapia 2010;81:259-268.

Hu Y, Ehli EA, Kittelsrud J, Ronan PJ, Munger K, Downey T, Bohlen K, Callahan L, Munson V, Jahnke M, Marshall LL, Nelson K, Huizena P, Hansen R, Soundy TJ, Davies GE. Lipid-lowering effect of berberine in human subjects and rats. Phytomedicine 2012;19:861-867.

Huang BW, Chiang MT, Yao HT, Chiang W. The effect of adlay oil on plasma lipids, insulin and leptin in rat. Phytomedicine 2005;12:433-439.

Huang HC, Lin JK. Pu-erh tea, green tea, and black tea suppresses hyperlipidemia, hyperleptinemia and fatty acid synthase through activating AMPK in rats fed a high-fructose diet. Food Funct 2012 Feb;3(2):170-7.

Huang HL, Hong YW, Wong YH, Chen YN, Chyuan JH, Huang CJ, Chao PM. Bitter melon *(Momordica charantia L.)* inhibits adipocyte hypertrophy and down regulates lipogenic gene expressio in adipose tissue of diet-induced obese rats. British Journal of Nutrition 2008;99:230-239.

Huang LC, Pan WY. Comparison of effect and cost-benefit analysis between acupoint catgut-embedding and electroacupuncture on simple obesity. Zhongguo Zhen Jiu 2011 Oct;31(10):883-6.

Huang XF, Liu Y, Rahardjo GL, Mclennan PL, Tapsell LC, Buttemer WA. Effects of diets high in whey, soy, red meat and milk protein on body weight maintenance in diet-induced obesity in mice. Nutrition & Dietetics 2008;65(3):53-59.

Huang XF, Yu Y, Beck EJ, South T, Li Y, Batterham MJ, Tapsell LC, Chen J. Diet high in oat β-glucan activates the gut-hypothalamic (PYY$_3$□$_3$□-NPY) axis and increases satiety in diet-induced obesity in mice. Mol Nutr Food Res. 2011 Jul;55(7):1118-21.

Huang YW, Liu Y, Dushenkov S, Ho CT, Huang MT. Anti-obesity effects of epigallocatechin-3-gallate, orange peel extract, black tea extract, caffeine and their combinations in a mouse model. Journal of Functional Foods 2009;1:304-310.

Hung W, Liu TH, Chen CY, Chang CK. Effect of β-hydroxy-β-methylbutyrate supplementation during energy restriction in female Judo athletes. J Exerc Sci Fit 2010;8(1):50-53.

Hunter GR, Weinsier RL, Bamman MM, Larson DE. A role for high intensity exercise on energy balance and weight control. International Journal of Obesity 1998;22:489-493.

Husain GM, Chatterjee SS, Singh PN, Kumar V. Hypolipidemic and Antiobesity-Like Activity of Standardised Extract of *Hypericum perforatum* L. in Rats. International Scholarly Research Network 2011.

Hussein A. Purslane Extract Effects on Obesity-Induced Diabetic Rats Fed a High-Fat Diet. Mal J Nutr 2010;16(3):419-429.

Hussein AM, Hussein AEM. Biochemical effects of Resveratrol and Curcumin combination on obese diabetic rats. Molecular & Clinical Pharmacology 2013;4(1):1-10.

Hussein AMS, Amal SAE, Amany MH, Abeer AA, Gamal HR. Physiochemical, Sensory and Nutritional Properties of corn-fenugreek Flour Composite biscuits. Australian Journal of Basic and Applied Sciences 2011;5(4):84-95.

Hussein G, Nakagawa T, Goto H, Shimada Y, Matsumoto K, Sankawa U, Watanabe H. Astaxanthin ameliorates features of metabolic syndrome in SHR/NDmcr-*cp*. Life Sciences 2007;80:522-529.

Hussein GME, Matsuda H, Nakamura S, Hamao M, Akiyama T, Tamura K, Yoshikawa M. Mate Tea *(Ilex paraguariensis)* Promotes Satiety and Body Weight Lowering in Mice: Involvement of Glucagon-Like Peptide-1. Biol. Pharm. Bull. 2011;34(12):1849-1855.

Hussein GME, Matsuda H, Nakamura S, Hamao M, Akiyama T, Tamura K, Yoshikawa M. Protective and ameliorative effects of mate *(Ilex paraguariensis)* on metabolic syndrome in TSOD mice. Phytomedicine 2011;19:88-97.

Hussein MA. Anti-obesity, antiatherogenic, anti-diabetic and antioxidant activities of *J. montana* ethanolic formulation in obese diabetic rats fed high-fat diet. Free Radicals and Antioxidants 2011 Jan-Mar;1(1):49-60.

Hussein MA, El-Maksoud HA. Biochemical effects of Resveratrol and curcumin combination on obese diabetic rats. Molecular & Clinical Pharmacology 2013;4(1):1-10.

Hussein MR, Ahmed OG, Hassan AF, Ahmed MA. Intake of melatonin is associated with amelioration of physiological changes, both metabolic and morphological pathologies associated with obesity: and animal model. Int. J. Exp. Path. 2007;88:19-29.

Hwang JH, Kim JD. Inhibitory Effects of *Corni Fructus* Extract on Angiogenesis and Adipogenesis. Korean J Physiol Pharmacol 2011 Feb;15(1):43-51.

Hwang JS, Suk JM, Choi HM, Shin I, Hwang SJ, Park JY, Kim SO, Seo BI, Kim MR. Effects of CJB Water Extract on Obesity-Related Factors in Hypothalamus of Rats Fed High-Fat Diet. Kor. J. Herbology 2012;27(5):99-107.

Hwang JT, Kim SH, Hur HJ, Kim HJ, Park JH, Sung MJ, Yang HJ, Ryu SY, Kim YS, Cha MR, Kim MS, Kwon DY. Decursin, an active compound isolated from Angelica gigas, inhibits fat accumulation, reduces adipocytokine secretion and improves glucose tolerance in mice fed a high-fat diet. Phytother Res. 2012 May;26(5):633-8.

Hwang YP, Choi JH, Han EH, Kim HG, Wee JH, Jung KO, Jung KH, Kwon KI, Jeong TC, Chung YC, Jeong HG. Purple sweet potato anthocyanins attenuate hepatic lipid accumulation through activating adenosine monophosphate-activated protein kinase in human HepG2 cells and obese mice. Nutrition Research 2011;31:896-906.

Ibarra A, Cases J, Roller M, Chiralt-Boix A, Coussaert A, Ripoll C. Carnosic acid-rich rosemary (Rosmarinus officinalis L.) leaf extract limits weight gain and improves cholesterol levels and glycaemia in mice on a high-fat diet. Br J Nutr. 2011 Oct;106(8):1182-9.

Ibarra A, Bai N, He K, Bily A, Cases J, Roller M, Sang S. *Fraxinus excelsior* seed extract FraxilPure™ limits weight gains and hyperglycemia in high-fat diet-induced obese mice. Phytomedicine 2011;18:479-485.

Ichi I, Hori H, Takashima Y, Adachi N, Kataoka R, Okihara K, Hashimoto S, Kojo S. The beneficial effect of propolis on fat accumulation and lipid metabolism in rats fed a high-fat diet. J Food Sci. 2009 Jun;74(5):127-31.

Ide T, Murata M, Sugano M. Stimulation of the activities of hepatic fatty acid oxidation enzymes by dietary fat rich in alpha-linolenic acid in rats. J Lipid Res 1996 Mar;37(3):448-63.

Ide T, Kobayashi H, Ashakumary L, Rouyer IA, Takahashi Y, Aoyama T, Hashimoto T, Mizugaki M. Comparative effects of perilla and fish oils on the activity and gene expression of fatty acid oxidation enzymes in rat liver. Biochim Biophys Acta 2000 May 6;1485(1):23-35.

Ide T. Effect of dietary alpha-linolenic acid on the activity and gene expression of hepatic fatty acid oxidation enzymes. Biofactors 2000;13(1-4):9-14.

Ide T, Hong DD, Ranasinghe P, Takahashi Y, Kushiro M, Sugano M. Interaction of dietary fat types and sesamin on hepatic fatty acid oxidation in rats. Biochim Biophys Acta 2004 Jun 1;1682(1-3):80-91.

Ide T, Lim JS, Odbayar TO, Nakashima Y. Comparative Study of Sesame Lignans (Sesamin, Episesamin and Sesamolin) Affecting Gene Expression Profile and Fatty Acid Oxidation in Rat Liver. J Nutr Sci Vitaminol 2009;55:31-43.

Ide T, Ono Y, Kawashima H, Kiso Y. Interrelated effects of dihomo-γ-linolenic and arachidonic acids, and sesamin on hepatic fatty acid synthesis and oxidation in rats. Br J Nutr 2012 Feb 28:1-14.

Iio A, Ohguchi K, Inoue H, Maruyama H, Araki Y, Nozawa Y, Ito M. Ethanolic extracts of Brazilian red propolis promote adipocyte differentiation through PPARγ activation. Phytomedicine 2010;17:974-979.

Ijeh II, Akomas SC. Effect of oral administration of ethanolic extract of *Vernonia amygdalina* on the exocrine functions in weanling rabbits. Continental J. Biomedical Sciences 2011;5(2):3-6.

Ikeuchi M, Yamaguchi K, Nishimura T, Yazawa K. Effects of *Anoectochilus formosanus* on Endurance Capacity in Mice. J Nutr Sci Vitaminol 2005;51:40-44.

Ikeuchi M, Koyama T, Takahashi J, Yazawa K. Effects of Astaxanthin Supplementation on Exercise-Induced Fatigue in Mice. Biol. Pharm. Bull. 2006;29(10):2106-2110.

Ikeuchi M, Yamaguchi K, Koyama T, Sono Y, Yazawa K. Effects of Fenugreek Seeds *(Trigonella foenum greaecum)* Extract on Enudrance Capacity in Mice. J Nutr Sci Vitaminol 2006;52:287-292 .

Ikeuchi M, Koyama T, Takahashi J, Yazawa K. Effects of Astaxanthin in Obese Mice Fed a High-Fat Diet. Biosci. Biotechnol. Biochem. 2007;71(4):893-899.

Ikewuchi CJ, Ikewuchi CC. Alteration of Plasma Lipid Profile and Atherogenic Indices of Cholesterol Loaded Rats by *Tridax Procumbens* Linn: Implications for the Management of Obesity and Cardiovascular Diseases. Biokemistri 2009 Dec;21(2):95-99.

Im R, Mano H, Nakatani S, Shimizu J, Wada M. Aqueous Extract of Kotahla Himbutu *(Salacia reticulata)* Stems Promotes Oxygen Consumption and Supresses Body Fat Accumulation in Mice. Journal of Health Science 2008;54(6):645-653.

Imafidon KE, Lucky OO. Biochemical Evaluation of the Tradomedicinal Uses of the Seeds of *Persea americana* Mill., (Family: Lauraceae). World Journal of Medical Sciences 2009;4(2):143-146.

Imafidon KE. Liver Function Status of Hypertensive and Normotensive Rats Administered *Persea americana* Mill. (Avocado) Seeds. Academic Journal of Plant Sciences 2010;3(3):130-133.

Inoue N, Matsunaga Y, Satoh H, Takahashi M. Enhanced Energy Expenditure and Fat Oxidation in Humans with High BMI Scores by the Ingestion of Novel and Non-Pungent Capsaicin Analogues (Capsinoids). Biosci. Biotechnol. Biochem. 2007;71(2):380-389.

Irving BA, Davis CK, Brock DW, Weltman JY, Swift D, Barrett EJ, Gaesser GA, Weltman A. Effect of exercise training intensity on abdominal visceral fat and body composition. Med Sci Sports Exerc. 2008 Nov;40(11):1863-1872.

Irving BA, Weltman JY, Patrie JT, Davis CK, Brock DW, Swift D, Barrett EJ, Gaesser GA, Weltman A. Effects of Exercise Training Intensity on Nocturnal Growth Hormone Secretion in Obese Adults with the Metabolic Syndrome. J Clin Endocrinol Metab 2009 Jun;94(6):1979-1986.

Isaksson H, Fredriksson H, Andersson R, Olsson J, Åman P. Effect of rye bread breakfasts on subjective hunger and satiety: a randomized controlled trial. Nutrition Journal 2009;8:39.

Ishihara K, Oyaizu S, Onui K, Lim K, Fushiki T. Chronic (-)-hydroxycitrate administration spares carbohydrate utilization and promotes lipid oxidation during exercise in mice. J Nutr. 2000 Dec;130(12):2990-5.

Ishikawa Y, Kudo H, Kagawa Y, Sakamoto S. Increased Plasma Levels of Zinc in Obese Adult Females on a Weight-loss Program Based on a Hypocaloric Balanced Diet. In vivo 2005;19:1035-1038.

Israni DA, Patel KV, Gandhi TR. Anti-hyperlipidemic activity of aqueous extract of *Terminalia Chebula* & Gaumutra in high cholesterol diet fed rats. Pharma Science Monitor 2010;1(1):48-59.

Ivy JL, Cortez MY, Chandler RM, Byrne HK, Miller RH. Effects of pyruvate on the metabolism and insulin resistance of obese Zucker rats. Am J. Clin. Nutr. 1994;59:331-7.

Iwami M, Shimooka R, Shimazu T. Effects of L-carnitine on energy metabolism in rats. Physiology of human nutrition 2006 Apr;59(2):107-113

Iwamoto M, Imai K, Ohta H, Shirouchi B, Sato M. Supplementation of highly concentrated beta-cryptoxanthin in a satsuma mandarin beverage improves adipocytokine profiles in obese Japanese women. Lipids in Health and Disease 2012;11:52.

Iwashita K, Yamaki K, Tsushida T. Effect of Flavonoids on the Differentiation of 3T3-L1 Adipocytes. Food Sci. Technol. Res. 2001;7(2):154-160.

Iwashita K, Yamaki K, Tsushida T. Mioga (*Zingiber mioga* Rosc.) Extract Prevents 3T3-L1 Differentiation into Adipocytes and Obesity in Mice. Food Sci. Technol. Res. 2001;7(2):164-170.

Iwashita S, Mikus C, Baier S, Flakoll PJ. Glutamine Supplementation Increases Postprandial Energy Expenditure and Fat Oxidation in Humans. Journal of Parenteral and Enteral Nutrition 2006;30(2):76-80.

Iweala EEJ, Akubugwo EI, Okeke CU. Effects of ethanolic extract of *Allium sativum Linn. Liliaceae* (Garlic) on serum cholesterol and blood sugar levels of albino rabbits. Plant Product Research Journal 2005;9:14-18.

Iyare EE, Adegoke OA, Nwagha UI. Mechanism of the decreased food consumption and weight gain in rats following consumption of aqueous extract of the calyx of *Hibiscus sabdariffa* during pregnacy. Asian Pacific Journal of Tropical Medicine 2010:185-188.

Iyare EE, Adegoke OA. Gestational Outcome in Rats That Consumed Aqueous Extract of *Hibiscus sabdariffa* During Pregnancy. Pakistan Journal of Nutrition 2011;10(4):350-354.

Jaakola L, Määttä-Riihinen K, Kärenlampi S, Hohtola A. Activation of flavonoid biosynthesis by solar radiation in bilberry (*Vaccinium myrtillus* L.) leaves. Planta 2004 Mar;218(5):721-8.

Jadeja RN, Thounaojam MC, Ansarullah, Patel VB, Devkar RV, Ramachandran AV. Protective effect of Clerodendron glandulosum extract against experimentally induced metabolic syndrome in rats. Pharm Biol 2010 Dec;48(12):1312-9.

Jadeja RN, Thounaojam MC, Ramani UV, Devkar RV, Ramachandran AV. Anti-obesity potential of *Clerodendron glandulosum* Coleb leaf aqueous extract. Journal of Ethnopharmacology 2011;135:338-343.

Jamieson JA, Ryz NR,Taylor CG, Weiler HA. Dietary long-chain inulin reduces abdominal fat but has no effect on bone density in growing female rats. British Journal of Nutrition 2008;100:451-459.

Janebro DI, Quieroz MSR, Ramos AT, Sabaa-Srur AUO, Cunha MAL, Diniz MFFM. Efeito da farinha da casca do maracujá-amarelo *(Passiflora edulis* f. *flavicarpa* Deg.) nos niveis glicêmicos e lipidicos de pacientes diabéticos tipo 2. Revista Brasileira de Farmacognosia Brazilian Journal of Pharmacognosy 2008 Dez;18(1):724-732.

Jang EH, Moon JS, Ko JH, Ahn CW, Lee HH, Shin JK, Park CS, Kang JH. Novel black soy peptides with antiobesity effects: activation of leptin-like signaling and AMP-activated protein kinase. Int J Obes (Lond). 2008 Jul;32(7):1161-70.

Jang JJ, Choi HJ. Effects of *Artemisia Iwayomogi* Oligosaccharide on the Blood Lipids, Abdominal Adipose Tissues and Leptin Levels in the Obese Rats. Korean J Nutrition 2003;36(5):437-445.

Javadi M, Everts H, Hovenier R, Kocsis S, Lankhorst AE, Lemmens AG, Schonewille JT, Terpstra AHM, Beynen AC. The effect of six different C18 fatty acids on body fat energy metabolism in mice. British Journal of Nutrition 2004 Sep;92(3):391-399.

Javadi M, Geelen MJ, Lemmens AG, Lankhorst A, Schonewille JT, Terpstra AH, Beynen AC. The influence of dietary linoleic and alpha-linolenic acid on body composition and the activities of key enzymes of hepatic lipogenesis and fatty acid oxidation in mice. J Anim Physiol Anim Nutr (Berl) 2007 Feb;91(1-2):11-8.

Javdan N, Estakhr J. Evaluation of the effect of salvia hypoleuca on the expression of cytokines: IL-6, IL-10 and TNF-α in high fat diet-fed mice towards a cure for diabetes mellitus. Pharmacologyonline 2011;2:842-852.

Jayaprakasam B, Olson LK, Schutzki RE, Tai MH, Nair MG. Amelioration of obesity and glucose intolerance in high-fat-fed C57BL/6 mice by anthocyanins and ursolic acid in Cornelian cherry (Cornus mas). J Agric Food Chem 2006 Jan 11;54(1):243-8.

Jeon G, Choi Y, Lee SM, Kim Y, Jeong HS, Lee J. Anti-obesity activity of methanol extract from hot pepper *(Capsicum annuum* L.) seeds in 3T3-L1 adipocyte. Food Science and Biotechnology 2010;19(4):1123-1127.

Jeon JR, Kim JY. Effects of Pine Needle Extract on Differentiation of 3T3-L1 Preadipocytes and Obesity in High-Fat Diet Fed Rats. Biol. Pharm. Bull. 2006;29(10):2111-2115.

Jeon SM, Kim HJ, Woo MN, Lee MK, Shin YC, Park YB, Choi MS. Fucoxanthin-rich seaweed extract suppresses body weight gain and improves lipid metabolism in high-fat-fed C57BL/6J mice. Biotechnol J. 2010 Sep;5(9):961-9.

Jeong H, Yang BK, Jeong YT, Kim GN, Jeong YS, Kim SM, Mehta P, Song CH. Hypolipidemic Effects of Biopolymers Extracted from Culture Broth, Mycelia, and Fruiting Bodies of *Auricularia auricula-judae* in Dietary-induced Hyperlipidemic Rats. Mycobiology 2007;35(1):16-20.

Jeong S, Chae K, Jung YS, Rho YH, Lee J, Ha J, Yoon KH, Kim GC, Oh KS, Shin SS, Yoon M. The Korean traditional medicine Gyeongshingangjeehwan inhibits obesity through the regulation of leptin and PPARα action in OLETF rats. Journal of Ethnopharmacology 2008;119:245-251.

Jeong SM, Kang MJ, Choi HN, Kim JH, Kim JI. Quercetin ameliorates hyperglycemia and dyslipidemia and improves antioxidant status in type 2 diabetic db/db mice. Nutrition Research and Practice *(Nutr Res Pract)* 2012;6(3):201-207.

Jetté L, Harvey L, Eugeni K, Levens N. 4-Hydroxyisoleucine: a plant-derived treatment for metabolic syndrome. Curr Opin Investig Drugs 2009 Apr;10(4):353-8.

Jiabing W, Chengkui C, Ping C, Xingmei L, Miao X, Xiaoyan M, Xin L. Effects of Extract from Sibirae angustata (Rchd). Hand.-Mazz on Lipid Metabolism in Rats with Simple Obesity. Traditional Chinese Drug Research & Clinical Pharmacology 2012.

Jiao L, Chi ZH. Electroacupuncture for treatment of simple obesity complicated with fatty liver. Zhongguo Zhen Jiu 2008 Mar;28(3):183-6.

Jiang HF, Li XR, Tang C. Effect of purple sweet potato flavonoids on metabolism of glucose and lipids in diabetic rats. Zhejiang Da Xue Xue Bao Yi Xue Ban 2011 Jul;40(4):374-9.

Jiangwei M, Zengyong Q, Xia X. Aqueous extract of *Astragalus mongholicus* ameliorates high cholesterol diet induced oxidative injury in experimental rats models. Journal of Medicinal Plants Research 2011 March;5(5):855-858.

Jing L, Da-Xiang L, Hua-Dong W, Ren-Bin Q, Yong-Mei F, Yang-Ping W. Effect of glycine on body weight and lipid metabolism in mice. Chinese Journal of Pathophysiology 2005;21(6):1143-1146.

Jing L, Zhang NX, Mo W, Wan R, Ma CG, Li X, Gu YL, Yang XY, Tang QQ. *Rehmannia* inhibits adipocyte differentiation and adipogenesis. Biochemical and Biophysical Research Communications 2008;371:185-190.

Jitpukdeebodintra S, Jangwang A. Instant noodles with pectin for weight reduction. Journal of Food, Agriculture & Environment 2009;7(3 & 4):126-129.

Jobgen W, Meininger CJ, Jobgen SC, Li P, Lee MJ, Smith SB, Spencer TE, Fried SK, Wu G. Dietary L-arginine supplementation reduces white fat gain and enhances skeletal muscle and brown fat masses in diet-induced obese rats. J Nutr. 2009 Feb;139(2): 230-7.

Jouad H, Lemhadri A, Maghrani M, Zeggwagh NA, Eddouks M. Cholesterol-lowering activity of the aqueous extract of *Spergularia purpurea* in normal and recent-onset diabetic rats. Journal of Ethnopharmacology 2003;87:43-49.

Jouad H, Lemhadri A, Maghrani M. Effects of a high-protein ketogenic diet on hunger, appetite, and weight loss in obese men feeding ad libitum. Am J Clin Nutr 2008;87:44-55.

Johnkennedy N, Adamma E, Austin A, Chukwunyere NE. Influence of Xylopia Athiopica Fruits on Some Hematological and Biochemical Profile. Al Ameen J Med Sci 2011;4(2):191-196.

Johnstone AM, Horgan GW, Murison SD, Bremner DM, Lobley GE. Effects of a high-protein ketogenic diet on hunger, appetite, and weight loss in obese men feeding ad libitum. Am J Clin Nutr 2008;87:44-55.

Johnstone CS, Beezhold BL, Mostow B, Swan PD. Plasma vitamin C is inversely related to body mass index and waist circumference but not to plasma adiponectin in nonsmoking adults. J Nutr 2007 Jul;137(7):1757-62.

Jorge PA, Neyra LC, Osaki RM, de Almeida E, Bragagnolo N. Effect of eggplant on plasma lipid levels, lipid peroxidation nd reversion of endothelial dysfunction in experimental hypercholesterolemia. Arg Bras Cardiol 1998 Feb;70(2):87-91.

Ju JH, Yoon HS, Park HJ, Kim MY, Shin HK, Park KY, Yang JO, Sohn MS, Do MS. Anti-obesity and antioxidative effects of purple sweet potato extract in 3T3-L1 adipocytes in vitro. J Med Food 2011 Oct;14(10):1097-106.

Juan YC, Kuo YH, Chang CC, Zhang LJ, Lin YY, Hsu CY, Liu HK. Administration of a decoction of sucrose- and polysaccharide-rich radix astragali (huang qi) ameliorated insulin resistance and Fatty liver but affected Beta-cell function in type 2 diabetic rats. Evid Based Complement Alternat Med 2011;2011:349807.

Junbao Y, Long J, Jiangbi W, Yonghui D, Tianzhen Z, Songyi Q, Wei L. Inhibitive effect of Semen Cassiae on the weight gain in rats with nutritive obesity. Zhong Yao Chai 2004 Apr;27(4):281-4.

Jung CH, Cho I, Ahn J, Jeon TI, Ha TY. Quercetin Reduces High-Fat Diet-Induced Fat Accumulation in the Liver by Regulating Lipid Metabolism Genes. Phytother Res 2012 Mar 23.

Jung CH, Ahn J, Jeon TI, Kim TW, Ha TY. *Syzygium aromaticum* ethanol extract reduces high-fat diet-induced obesity in mice through downregulation of adipogenic and lipogenic gene expression. Experimental and therapeutic medicine 2012;4:409-414.

Jung HK, Jeong YS, Park CD, Park CH, Hong JH. Inhibitory Effect of Citrus Peel Extract on Lipid Accumulation of 3T3-L1 Adipocytes. J. Korean Soc. Appl. Biol. Chem. 2011;54(2):169-176.

Jung KA, Han D, Kwon EK, Lee CH, Kim YE. Antifatigue effect of Rubus coreanus Miquel extract in mice. J Med Food 2007 Dec;10(4):689-93.

Jung UJ, Baek NI, Chung HG, Bang MH, Jeong TS, Lee KT, Kang YJ, Lee MK, Kim HJ, Yeo J, Choi MS. Effects of the ethanol extract of the roots of *Brassica rapa* on glucose and lipid metabolism in C57BL/KsJ-*db/db* mice. Clinical Nutrition 2008;27: 158-167.

Jung UJ, Baek NI, Chung HG, Jeong TS, Lee KT, Lee MK, Choi MS. Antilipogenic and hypolipidemic effects of ethanol extracts from two variants of Artemisia princeps Pampanini in obese diabetic mice. J Med Food 2009 Dec;12(6):1238-44.

Jung YM, Lee SH, Lee DS, You MJ, Chung IK, Cheon WH, Kwon YS, Lee YJ, Ku SK. Fermented garlic protects diabetic, obese mice when fed a high-fat diet by antioxidant effects. Nutrition Research 2011;31:387-396.

Jönssön T, Ahrén B, Pacini G, Sundler F, Wierup N, Steen S, Sjöberg T, Ugander M, Frostegård J, Göransson L, Lindeberg S. A Paleolithic diet confers higher insulin sensitivity, lower C-reactive protein and lower blood pressure than a cereal-based diet in domestic pigs. Nutr Metab (Lond) 2006 Nov 2;3:39.

Jönssön T, Granfeldt Y, Ahrén B, Branell UC, Pålsson G, Hansson A, Söderström M. Beneficial effects of a Paleolithic diet on cardiovascular risk factors in type 2 diabetes: a randomized cross-over pilot study. Cardiovasc Diabetol 2009 Jul 16;8:35.

Jönsson T, Granfeldt Y, Erlanson-Albertsson C, Ahrén B, Lindeberg S. A paleolithic diet is more satiating per calorie than a mediterranean-like diet in individuals with ischemic heart disease. Nutrition & Metabolism 2010;7:85.

Kaats GR, Blum K, Fisher JA, Adelman JA. Effects of Chromium Picolinate supplementation on body compositio: a randomized, double-masked, placebo-controlled study. Current Therapeutic Research 1996 Oct;57(10):747-756.

Kaats GR, Blum K, Pullin D, Keith SC, Wood R. A randomized, double-masked, placebo-controlled study of the effects of Chromium Picolinate supplementation on body composition: a replication and extension of a previous study. Current Therapeutic Research 1998 Jun;59(6):379-388.

Kabir M, Skurnik G, Naour N, Pechtner V, Meugnier E, Rome S, Quignard-Boulangé A, Vidal H, Slama G, Clément K, Guerre-

Millo M, Rizkalla SW. Treatment for 2 mo with n-3 polyunsaturated fatty acids reduces adiposity and some atherogenic factors but not improve insulin sensitivity in women with type 2 diabetes: a randomized controlled study. Am J Clin Nutr 2007;86:1670-9.

Kabir Y, Kimura S, Tamura T. Dietary Effect of *Ganoderma lucidum* Mushroom on Blood Pressure and Lipid Levels in Spontaneously Hypertensive Rats (SHR). J. Nutr. Sci. Vitaminol. 1988;34:433-438.

Kabir Y, Ide T. Activity of hepatic fatty acid oxidation enzymes in rats fed alpha-linolenic acid. Biochim Biophys Acta 1996 Nov 22;1304(2):105-19.

Kaciuba-Uscilko H, Nazar K, Chwalbinska-Moneta J, Ziemba A, Kruk B, Szczepanik J, Titow-Stupnicka E, Bicz B. Effect of phosphate supplementation on metabolic and neuroendocrine responses to exercise and oral glucose load in obese women during weight reduction. J Physiol Pharmacol 1993 Dec;44(4):425-40.

Kalman D, Colker CM, Stark R, Minsch A, Wilets I, Antonio J. Effect of Pyruvate supplementation on body composition and mood. Current Therapeutic Research 1998 Nov;59(11):793-802.

Kalman D, Colker CM, Wilets I, Roufs JB, Antonio J. The Effects of Pyruvate Supplementation on Body Composition in Overweight Individuals. Nutrition 1999;15:337-340.

Kalman DS, Colker CM, Swain MA, Torina GC, Shi Q. A Randomized, Double-Blind, Placebo-Controlled Study of 3-Acetyl-7-Oxo-Dehydroepiandrosterone in Healthy Overweight Adults. Current Therapeutic Research 2000 Jul;61(7):435-442.

Kamalakkannan S, Rajendran R, Venkatesh RV, Clayton P, Akbarsha MA. Antiobesogenic and Antiatherosclerotic Properties f *Caralluma fimbriata* Extract. Journal of Nutrition and Metabolism 2010.

Kamali SH, Khalaj AR, Hasani-Ranjbar S, Esfehani MM, Kamalinejad M, Omidmalayeri S, Kamali SA. Efficacy of 'Itrifal Saghir', a combination of three medicinal plants in the treatment of obesity; A randomized controlled trial. DARU Journal of Pharmaceutical Sciences 2012;20:33.

Kamesh V, Sumathi T. Effect of *Bacopa monniera* linn. in attenuating hepatic oxidative stress in hypercholesterolemic induced rats. Asian Journal of Pharmaceutical and Clinical Research 2012;5(3):90-95.

Kamiya T, Matsuzuka Y, Kusaba N, Ikeguchi M, Takagaki K, Kondo K. Preliminary Research for the Anti-obesity Effect of Puerariae Flos Extract in Humans. Journal of Health Science 2011;57(6):521-531.

Kamiya T, Takano A, Matsuzuka Y, Kusaba N, Ikeguchi M, Takagaki K, Kondo K. Consumption of *Pueraria* Flower Extract Reduces Body Mass Index *via* Decrease in the Visceral Fat Area in Obese Humans. Biosci. Biotechnol. Biochem. 2012;76(8):1-5.

Kamiya T, Sameshima-Kamiya M, Nagamine R, Tsubata M, Ikeguchi M, Takagaki K, Shimada T, Aburada M. The Crude Extract from *Puerariae* Flower Exerts Antiobesity and Antifatty Liver Effects in High-Fat Diet-Induced Obese Mice. Evidence-Based Complementary and Alternative Medicine 2012:1-6.

Kamiya T, Nagamine R, Sameshima-Kamiya M, Tsubata M, Ikeguchi M, Takagaki K. The Isoflavone-Rich Fraction of the Crude Extract of the *Puerariae* Flower Increases Oxygen Consumption and BAT UCP1 Expression in High-Fat Diet-Fed Mice. Global Journal of Health Science 2012;4(5):147-155.

Kamphuis MMJW, Lejeune MPGM, Saris WHM, Westerterp-Plantenga MS. The effect of conjugated linoleic acid supplementation after weight loss on body weight regain, body composition, and resting metabolic rate in overweight subjects. International Journal of Obesity 2003;27:840-847.

Kan WC, Wang HY, Chien CC, Li SL, Chen YC, Chang LH, Cheng CH, Tsai WC, Hwang JC, Su SB, Huang LH, Chuu JJ. Effects of Extract from Solid-State Fermented *Cordyceps sinensis* on Type 2 Diabetes Mellitus. Evidence-Based Complementary and Alternative Medicine 2012.

Kang DG, Hur TY, Lee GM, Oh H, Kwon TO, Sohn EJ, Lee HS. Effects of Cudrania tricuspidata water extract on blood pressure and renal functions in NO-dependent hypertension. Life Sci. 2002 Apr 19;70(22):2599-609.

Kang JH, Goto T, Han IS, Kawada T, Kim YM, Yu R. Dietary capsaicin reduces obesity-induced insulin resistance and hepatic steatosis in obese mice fed a high-fat diet. Obesity (Silver Spring) 2010 Apr;18(4):780-7.

Kang KJ, Lim SJ, Jeong JG, Han HK, Choi SS, Kim MH, Kwon SY. Effects of Wax Guard on Weight, Triglyceride, Leptin and Fat Cell Size in Rats Fed on a High Fat Diet. Korean J Nutr. 2003 Jun;36(5):446-451.

Kang MH, Park WJ, Choi MK. Anti-Obesity and Hypolipidemic Effets of *Lycium chinense* Leaf Powder in Obese Rats. Journal of Medicinal Food 2010 Aug;13(4):801-807.

Kang SA, Jang KH, Hong K, Choi WA, Jung KH, Lee IY. Effects of Dietary β-Glucan on Adiposity and Serum Lipids Levels in Obese Rats Induced by High Fat Diet. J. Korean Soc. Food. Sci. Nutr 2002;31(6):1052-1057.

Kang SB, Gao XL, Wang SJ, Wang YJ. Acupuncture for treatment of simple obesity and its effect on serum leptin level of the patient. Zhongguo Zhen Jiu 2005 Apr;25(4):243-5.

Kang SI, Shin HS, Kim HM, Hong YS, Yoon SA, Kang SW, Kim JH, Ko HC, Kim SJ. Anti-Obesity Properties of a *Sasa quelpaertensis* Extract in High-Fat Diet-Induced Obese Mice. Biosci. Biotechnol. Biochem. 2012;76(4):1-7.

Kang SI, Shin HS, Kim HM, Hong YS, Yoon SA, Kang SW, Kim JH, Kim MH, Ko HC, Kim SJ. Immature *Citrus sunki* Peel Extract Exhibits Antiobesity Effects by β-Oxidation and Lipolysis in High-Fat Diet-Induced Obese Mice. Biol. Pharm. Bull. 2012;35(2):223-230.

Kang SI, Shin HS, Kim HM, Yoon SA, Kang SW, Kim JH, Ko HC, Kim SJ. Petalonia binghamiae extract and its constituent fucoxanthin ameliorate high-fat diet-induced obesity by activating AMP-activated protein kinase. J Agric Food Chem 2012 Apr 4;60(13):3389-95.

Kang YJ, Kim J, Kim D, Lee HS, Kwon O, Kim MK. Effect of Dried Garlic Flesh and Dried Garlic Juice on Body Fat and Lipid Metabolism in 9-month-old Rats with Diet-induced Obesity. Food Sci. Biotechnol. 2010;19(3):589-594.

Kang YR, Lee HY, Kim JH, Moon DI, Seo MY, Park SH, Choi KH, Kim CR, Kim SH, Oh JH, Cho SW, Kim SY, Kim MG, Chae SW, Kim O, Oh HG. Anti-obesity and anti-diabetic effects of Yerba Mate *(Ilex paraguariensis)* in C57BL/6J mice fed a high-fat diet. Lab Anim Res 2012;28(1):23-29.

Kanamoto Y, Yamashita Y, Nanba F, Yoshida T, Tsuda T, Fukuda I, Nakamura-Tsuruta S, Ashida H. A Black Soybean Seed Coat Extract Prevents Obesity and Glucose Intolerance by Up-regulating Uncoupling Proteins and Down-regulating inflammatory Cytokinesis in High-Fat Diet-Fed Mice. J. Agric. Food Chem. 2011;59:8985-8993.

Kanyonga MP, Faouzi MYA, Zellou A, Essassi M, Cherrah Y. Effects of methanolic extract of *Crataegus oxyacantha* on blood homeostasis in rat. J. Chem. Pharm. Res. 2011;3(3):713-717.

Karnick CR. Clinical evaluation of Cyperus rotundus Linn. (motha) on obesity: a randomized double blind placebo controlled trial on Indian patients. Indian Medicine 1992;4(2).

Karstoft K, Winding K, Knudsen SH, Nielsen JS, Thomsen C, Pedersen BK, Solomon TP. The Effects of Free-Living Interval-Walking Training on Glycemic Control, Body Composition, and Physical Fitness in Type 2 Diabetes Patients: A randomized, controlled trial. Diabetes Care 2012 Sep 21.

Kasai M, Nosaka N, Maki H, Negishi S, Aoyama T, Nakamura M, Suzuki Y, Tsuji H, Uto H, OkazakiM, KondoK. Effect of dietary medium- and long-chain triacylglycerols (MLCT) on accumulation of body fat in healthy humans. Asia Pac J Clin Nutr 2003;12(2):151-60.

Kasaoka S, Tsuboyama-Kasaoka N, Kawahara Y, Inoue S, Tsuji M, Ezaki O, Kato H, Tsuchiya T, Okuda H, Nakajima S. Histidine supplementation suppresses food intake and fat accumulation in rats. Nutrition 2004;20:991-996.

Kaul L, Nidiry J. High-fiber diet in the treatment of obesity and hypercholesterolemia. J Natl Med Assoc 1993;85:231-232.

Kaume L, Gilbert WC, Brownmiller C, Howard LR, Devareddy L. Cyanidin 3-O-β-D-glucoside-rich blackberries modulate hepatic gene expression, and anti-obesity effects in overiectomized rats. Journal of Functional Foods 2012;4:480-488.

Kausar S, Zaheer Z, Saqib M, Zia B. Role of Crataegus (Hawthorn) Extract on Obesity in Hyperlipidemic Albino Rats. Pakistan Journal of Medicinal and Health Sciences Jan - Mar 2012;6(1).

Kawabata F, Inou N, Yazawa S, Kawada T, Inou K, Fushiki T. Effects of CH-19 Sweet, a Non-Pungent Cultivar of Red Pepper, in Decreasing the Body Weight and Suppressing Body Fat Accumulation by Sympathetic Nerve Activation in Humans. Biosci. Biotechnol. Biochem. 2006;70(12):2824-2835.

Kawada T, Hagihara K, Iwai K. Effects of capsaicin on lipid metabolism in rats fed a high fat diet. J Nutr 1986 Jul;116(7):1272-8.

Kayashita J, Shimaoka I, Nakajoh M, Arachi Y, Kato N. Feeding of Buckwheat Protein Extract Reduces Body Fat Content in Rats. Current Advances in Buckwheat Research 1995:935-940.

Kayashita J, Shimaoka I, Nakajoh M, Kato N. Feeding of buckwheat protein extract reduces hepatic triglyceride concentraton, adipose tissue weight, and hepatic lipogenesis in rats. Nutritional Biochemistry 1996;7:555-559.

Kenney JL, Carlberg KA. The effect of choline and myo-inositol on liver and carcass fat levels in aerobically trained rats. Int J Sports Med. 1995 Feb;16(2):114-6.

Key T, Davey G. Prevalence of obesity is low in people who do not eat meat. BMJ 1996 Sep 28;313(7060):816-7.

Khairunnuur FA, Zulkhairi A, Hairuszah I, Azrina A, Nursakinah I, Fazali F, Kamal MNH, Zamree MS, Kamilah KAK. Hypolipemic and Weight Reducing Properties from *Tamarindus indica* L. Pulp Extract in Diet-Induced Obese Rats. International Journal of Pharmacology 2010;6(3):216-223.

Khanal RC, Howard LR, Wilkes SE, Rogers TJ, Prior RL. Effect of Dietary Blueberry Pomace on Selected Metabolic Factors Associated with High Fructose Feeding in Growing Sprague-Dawley Rats. J Med Food. 2012 Aug 2.

Kil DY, Ryu SN, Piao LG, Kong CS, Han SJ, Kim YY. Effect of Feeding Cyanidin 3-glucoside (C3G) High Black Rice Bran on Nutrient Digestibility, Blood Measurements, Growth Performance and Pork Quality of Pigs. Asian-Aust. J. Anim. Sci. 2006 Dec;19(12):1790-1798.

Kilic M. Baltaci AK, Gunay M, Gökbel H, Okudan N, Cicioglu I. The effect of exhaustion exercise on thyroid hormones and testosterone levels of elite athletes receiving oral zinc. Neuro Endocrinol Lett 2006 Feb-Apr;27(1-2):247-52.

Kilic M. Effect of fatiguing bicycle exercise on thyroid hormone and testosterone levels in sedentary males supplemented with oral zinc. Neuro Endocrinol Lett 2007 Oct;28(5):681-5.

Kim AR, Lee II, Lee YM, Jung HO, Lee MY. Cholesterol-lowering and Anti-obesity Effects of Polymnia Sonchifolia Poepp. Ad Endl. Powder in Rats Fed a High Fat-High Cholesterol Diet. Journal of The Korean Society of Food Science and Nutrition 2010 Feb;39(2):210-218.

Kim AY, Jeong YJ, Park YB, Lee MK, Jeon SM, McGregor RA, Choi MS. Dose dependent effects of lycopene enriched tomato-wine on liver and adipose tissue in high-fat diet fed rats. Food Chemistry 2012;130:42-48.

Kim CK, Kim M, Oh SD, Lee SM, Sun B, Choi GS, Kim SK, Bae H, Kang C, Min BI. Effect of *Atractylodes macrocephala Koidzumi* rhizome on 3T3-L1 adipogenesis and an animal model of obesity. Journal of Ethnopharmacology 2011;137:396-402.

Kim DY, Kim MS, Sa BK, Kim MB. Hwang JK. *Boesenbergia pandurata* Attenuates Diet-Induced Obesity by Activating AMP-Activated Protein Kinase and Regulating Lipid Metabolism. Int. J. Mol. Sci. 2012;13:994-1005.

Kim EY, Jung EY, Lim HS, Heo YR. The Effects of the Sasa Borealis Leaves Extract on Plasma Adiponectin, Resistin, C-Reactive Protein and Homocysteine Levels in High Fat Diet-Induced Obese C57/BL6J Mice. Korean J Nutr. 2007 Jun;40(4):303-311.

Kim EY, Baek IH, Rhyu MR. Cardioprotective effects of aqueous *Schizandra chinensis* fruit extract on ovariectomized and balloon-induced carotid artery injury rat models: Effects on serum lipid profiles and blood pressure. Journal of Ethnopharmacology 2011;134:668-675.

Kim EY, An SY, Lee MS, Kim TH, Lee HK, Hwang WS, Choe SJ, Kim TY, Han SJ, Kim HJ, Kim DJ, Lee KW. Fermented kimchi reduces body weight and improves metabolic parameters in overweight and obese patients. Nutrition Research 2011;31:436-443.

Kim H, Bartley GE, Rimando AM, Yokoyama W. Hepatic gene expression related to lower plasma cholesterol in hamsters fed high-fat diets supplemented with blueberry peels and peel extract. J Agric Food Chem. 2010 Apr 14;58(7):3984-91.

Kim HJ, Park JM, Kim JA, Ko BP. Effect of Herbal *Ephedra sinica* and *Evodia rutaecarpa* on Body Composition and Resting Metabolic Rate: A Randomized, Double-blind Clinical Trial in Korea Premenopausal Women. J Acupunct Meridian Stud 2008;1(2):128-138.

Kim HJ, Kang HJ, Seo JY, Lee CH, Kim YS, Kim JS. Antiobesity Effect of Oil Extract of Ginseng. Journal of Medicinal Food 2011 Jun;14(6):573-583.

Kim HJ, Ko J, Storni C, Song HJ, Cho YG. Effect of green mate in overweight volunteers: A randomized placebo-controlled human study. Journal of Functional Foods 2012;4:287-293.

Kim HJ, Han JS, Han ES, Song YO. Effect of kimchi intake on lipid profiles and blood pressure. Kidney Research and Clinical Practice 2012 Jun;31(2):91.

Kim HK, Cho DW, Hahm YT. The Effects of Coix Bran on Lipid Metabolism and Glucose Challenge in Hyperlipidemic and

Diabetic Rats. J Korean Soc Food Sci Nutr 2000;29(1):140-14.

Kim HK, Nelson-Dooley C, Della-Fera MA, Yang JY, Zhang W, Duan J, Hartzell DL, Hamrick MW, Baile CA. Genistein decreases food intake, body weight, and fat pad weight and causes adipose tissue apoptosis in ovariectomized female mice. J Nutr. 2006 Feb;136(2):409-14.

Kim HK, Kim JN, Han SN, Nam JH, Na HN, Ha TJ. Black soybean anthocyanins inhibit adipocyte differentation in 3T3-L1 cells. Nutrition Research 2012.

Kim HT, Kim JW, Jin TW, Kim JE, Lim MK, Yeo SG, Jang KH, Oh TH, Lee KW. Effects of Blood Biochemistry and Tumors' Weights of *Artemisia capillaris* Methanol Extract in Mice Bearing Cancer Cells. J Vet Clin 2007;24(3):372-378.

Kim HT, Kim DD, Ku SK, Kim JW, Jang KH, Oh TH, Lee KW. Anti-Obestic Effects of *Artemisiae Capillaris* Herba, *Artemisia Capillaris* Stem Aqueous Extracts on the High Fat Diet Supplied Mice. J Vet Clin 2010;27(4):348-365.

Kim I, Kim JY, Hwang YJ, Hwang KA, Om AS, Kim JH, Cho KJ. The beneficial effects of aged black garlic extract on obesity and hyperlipidemia in rats fed a high-fat diet. Journal Medicinal Plants Research 2011 Jul;5(14):3159-3168.

Kim J, Jang DS, Kim H, Kim JS. Anti-lipase and lipolytic activities of ursolic acid isolated from the roots of Actinidia arguta. Arch Pharm Res. 2009 Jul;32(7):983-7.

Kim J, Lee YS, Kim CS, Kim JS. Betulinic acid has an inhibitory effect on pancreatic lipase and induces adipocyte lipolysis. Phytother Res. 2012 Jul;26(7):1103-6.

Kim JE, Nam SH, Choi SI, Hwang IS, Lee HR, Jang MJ, Lee CY, Soon HJ, Lee HS, Kim HS, Kang BC, Hong JT, Hwang DY. Aqueous Extracts of *Liriope platyphylla* Are Tightly-Regulated by Insulin Secretion from Pancreatic Islets and by Increased Glucose Uptake through Glucose Transporters Expressed in Liver Hepatocytes. Biomol Ther 2011;19(3):348-356.

Kim JE, Hwang IS, Choi SI, Lee HR, Lee YJ, Goo JS, Lee HS, Son HJ, Jang MJ, Lee SH, Kang BC, Hwang DY. Aqueous extract of *Liriope platyphylla*, a traditional Chinese medicine, significantly inhibits abdominal fat accumulation and improves glucose regulation in OLETF type II diabetes model rats. Lab Anim Res 2012;28(3):181-191.

Kim JE, Hwang IS, Goo JS, Nam SH, Choi SI, Lee HR, Lee YJ, Kim YH, Park SJ, Kim NS, Choi YH, Hwang DY. LP9M80-H Isolated from *Liriope platyphylla* Could Help Alleviate Diabetic Symptoms via the Regulation of Glucose and Lipid Concentration. Journal of Life Science 2012;22(5):634-641.

Kim JH, Mun YJ, Im SJ, Han JH, Lee HS, Woo WH. Effects of the aqueous extract of Epimedii Herba on the antibody responses in mice. International Immunopharmacology 2001;1:935-944.

Kim JH, Kim MK. Effect of Different Part of Mandarin Intake on Antioxidative Capacity in 15-month-old Rats. Korean J Nutr. 2003 Jul;36(6):559-569.

Kim JH, Kim J, Park Y. Trans-10, cis-12 conjugated linoleic acid enhances endurance capacity by increasing fatty acid oxidation and reducing glycogen utilization in mice. Lipids 2012 Sep;47(9):855-63.

Kim JK, Kim MK. Effect of Lysine -Limited Diets Containing Different Levels of L-Carnitine on Body Weight and Lipid Metabolism in Obesity-Induced Adult Rats. Korean J Nutr 2007 Mar;40(2):118-129.

Kim JK, So H, Youn MJ, Kim HJ, Kim Y, Park C, Kim SJ, Ha YA, Chai KY, Kim SM, Kim KY, Park R. *Hibiscus sabdariffa* L. water extract inhibits the adipocyte differentiation through the PI3-K and MAPK pathway. Journal of Ethnopharmacology 2007;114:260-267.

Kim JR, Ryu HH, Chung HJ, Lee JH, Kim SW, Kwun WH, Baek SH, Kim JH. Association of anti-obesity activity of N-acetylcysteine with metallothionein-II down-regulation. Experimental and Molecular Medicine 2006 Apr;38(2):162-172.

Kim JW, Kim SD, Youn KS. Effects of Chicken Treated with *Hwangki-Beni Koji* Sauces on Body Weight, Serum and Hepatic Lipid Profiles of Rats Fed High Fat and High Cholesterol Diets. J Korean Soc Food Sci Nutr 2010;39(9):1270-1278.

Kim JY, Kim JH, Lee DH, Kim SH, Lee SS. Meal replacement with mixed rice is more effective than white rice in weight control, while improving antioxidant enzyme activity in obese women. Nutrition Research 2008;28:66-71.

Kim JY, Moon KD, Seo KI, Park KW, Choi MS, Do GM, Jeong YK, Cho YS, Lee MK. Supplementation of SK1 from Platycodi radix ameliorates obesity and glucose intolerance in mice fed a high-fat diet. J Med Food 2009 Jun;12(3):629-36.

Kim JY, Choi BG, Jung MJ, Wee JH, Chung KH, Kwon O. Mulberry Leaf Water Extract Ameliorates Insuln Sensitivity in High Fat or High Sucrose Diet Induced Overweight Rats. J Korean Soc. Appl. Biol. Chem. 2011;54(4):612-618.

Kim JY, Son BK, Lee SS. Effects of adlay, buckwheat, and barley on transit time and the antioxidative system in obesity induced rats. Nutrition Research and Practice 2012;6(3):208-212.

Kim K, Kim H, Kwon J, Lee S, Kong H, Im SA, Lee YH, Lee YR, Oh ST, Jo TH, Park YI, Lee CK, Kim K. Hypoglycemic and hypolipidemic effects of processed Aloe vera gel in a mouse model of non-insulin-dependent diabetes mellitus. Phytomedicine 2009 Sep;16(9):856-63.

Kim KJ, Lee MS, Jo K, Hwang JK. Piperidine alkaloids from *Piper retrofractum* Vahl. protect against high-fat diet-induced obesity by regulating lipid metabolism and activating AMP-activated protein kinase. Biochemical and Biophysical Research Communications 2011;411:219-225.

Kim KS, Seo EK, Lee YC, Lee TK, Cho YW. Ezaki O, Kim CH. Effect of dietary *Platycodon grandiflorum* on the improvement of insulin resistance in obese Zucker rats. J Nutr. Biochem. 2000;11:420-424.

Kim KY, Lee HN, Kim YJ, Park T. *Garcinia cambogia* Extract Ameliorates Visceral Adiposity in C57BL/6J Mice Fed on a High-Fat Diet. Biosci. Biotechnol. Biochem. 2008;72(7):1772-1780.

Kim MH, Kim SH, Park HW, Kim WG, Lee YS. Effects of Calcium and Genistein on Body Fat and Lipid Metabolism in High Fat-induced Obese Mice. Korean J Nutr 2006 Dec;39(8):733-741.

Kim MJ, Park MH, Jeong MK, Yeo J, Cho WI, Pchang PS, Chung JH, Lee JH. Radcal Scavenging Activity and Anti-obesity Effects in 3T3-L1 Preadipocyte Differentation of *Ssuk (Artemisia princeps* Pamp.) Extract. Food Sci. Biotechnol. 2010;19(2):535-540.

Kim MJ, Kim HK. Effect of garlic on high fat induced obesity. Acta Biol Hung 2011 Sep;62(3):244-54.

Kim MK, Cho SW, Park YK. Long-term vegetarians have low oxidative stress, body fat, and cholesterol levels. Nutrition Research and Practice (*Nutr Res Pract*) 2012;6(2):155-161.

Kim MS, Chun SS, Kim SH, Choi JH. Effect of Tumeric *(Curcuma longa)* on Bile Acid and UDP-glucuronyl Transferase Activity in Rats Fed a High-fat and -cholesterol Diet. Journal of Life Science 2012;22(8):1064-1070.

248

Kim MS, Kim JK, Kim HJ, Moon SR, Shin BC, Park KW, Yang HO, Kim SM, Park R. Hibiscus extract inhibits the lipid droplet accumulation and adipogenic transcription factors expression of 3T3-L1 preadipocytes. J Altern Complement Med 2003 Aug;9(4):499-504.

Kim MS, Park JY, Namkoong C, Jang PG, Ryu JW, Song HS, Yun JY, Namgoong IS, Ha J, Park IS, Lee IK, Viollet B, Youn JH, Lee HK, Lee KU. Anti-obesity effects of α-lipoic acid mediated by suppression of hypothalamic AMP-activated protein kinase. Nature Medicine 2004 Jul;10(7):727-733.

Kim MY, Kang KS, Lee YS. The inhibitory effect of genistein on hepatic steatosis is linked to visceral adipocyte metabolism in mice with diet-induced non-alcoholic fatty liver disease. British Journal of Nutrition 2010;104:1333-1342.

Kim MY, Kim EJ, Kim YN, Choi C, Lee BH. Effects of α-lipoic acid and L-carnosine supplementation on antioxidant activities and lipid profiles in rats. Nutrition Research and *Practice (Nutr Res Pract)* 2011;5(5):421-428.

Kim OY, Lee SM, Do H, Moon J, Lee KH, Cha YJ, Shin MJ. Influence of quercetin-rich onion peel extracts on adipokine expression in the visceral adipose tissue of rats. Phytother Res 2012 Mar;26(3):432-7.

Kim S, Jin Y, Choi Y, Park T. Resveratrol exerts anti-obesity effects via mechanisms involving down-regulation of adipogenic and inflammatory processes in mice. Biochemical Pharmacology 2011;81:1343-1351.

Kim SJ, Lee SJ, Lee S, Chae S, Han MD, Mar W, Nam KW. Rutecarpine ameliorates bodyweight gain through the inhibition of orexigenic neuropeptides NPY and AgRP in mice. Biochemical and Biophysical Research Communications 2009;389:437-442.

Kim SJ, Lee YH, Han MD, Mar W, Kim WK,Nam KW. Resveratrol, purified from the stemof Vitis coignetiae Pulliat, inhibits food intake in C57BL/6J Mice. Arch Pharm Res. 2010 May;33(5):775-80.

Kim SK, Kim MK. Effect of Dried Powders or Ethanol Extracts of Onion Flesh and Peel on Lipid Metabolism, Antioxidative and Antithrombogenic Capacities in 16-Month-Old Rats. Korean J Nutr 2004 Oct;37(8):623-632.

Kim SO, Yun SJ, Jung B, Lee EH, Hahm DH, Shim I, Lee HJ. Hypolipidemic effects of crude extract of adlay seed *(Coix lachrymajobi var. mayuen)* in obesity rat fed high fat diet: Relations of TNF-α and leptin mRNA expressions and serum lipid levels. Life Sciences 2004;75:1391-1404.

Kim SO, Yun SJ, Lee EH. The Water Extract of Adlay Seed (*Coix lachrymajobi var. mayuen*) Exhibits Anti-Obesity Effects Through Neuroendocrine Modulation. The American Journal of Chinese Medicine 2007;35(2):297-308.

Kim SO. Ginseng Saponin-Re and *Coix lachrymajobi var. mayuen* Regulate Obesity Related Genes Expressions, TNF-alpha, Leptin, Lipoprotein Lipase and Resistin in 3T3-L1 Adipocytes. Journal of Life Science 2007;17(11):1523-1532.

Kim SS, Park HY, Byun YH, Hwang BG, Lee JH, Shim YJ, Park CK, Park MH, Yang JW. The Effects on the Blood Lipid Profiles and Body Fat by Long Term Administration of Red Ginseng Product. J. Ginseng Res 2002;26(2):67-73.

Kim SS, Kim JD, Kim H, Shin MS, Park CK, Park MH, Yang JW. The Effects of Red Ginseng Product and Combined Exercise on Blood Lipids and Body Composition of Obese Women in Their Twenties. J. Ginseng. Res. 2002;26(2):59-66.

Kim TG, Kim SH, Kang SY, Jung KK, Choi DH, Park YB, Ryu JH, Han HM. Antiatherogenic Effect of the Extract of *Allium victorialis* on the Experimental Atherosclerosis in the Rabbit and Transgenic Mouse. Kor. J. Pharmacogn. 2000;31(2):149-156.

Kim WS, Lee YS, Cha SH, Jeong HW, Choe SS, Lee MR, Oh GT, Park HS, Lee KU, Lane MD, Kim JB. Berberine improves lipid dysregulation in obesity by controlling central and peripheral AMPK activity. Am J Physiol Endocrinol Metab 2009 Jan 27;296: 812-819.

Kim YH, Yoo JY, Lee EG, Kim KB, Jo DH, Hwang JY. Effects of a Dietary Supplement Consisting of *Phaseolus vulgaris* and *Garcinia cambogia* (HCA) on the Lipid Level and Body Weight. J Korean Soc Food Sci Nutr 2004;33(3):518-522.

Kim YN, Ku KH, Kang SK, Choi JH. Effect of Enzyme-Treated Radish Leaves on Lipid Metabolism in Rats Fed a High-Fat Diet. J. Food Sci. Nutr. 2011;16:1-7.

Kim YS, Lee Y, Kim J, Sohn E, Kim CS, Lee YM, Jo K, Shin S, Song Y, Kim JH, Kim JS. Inhibitory Activities of *Cudrania tricuspidata* Leaves on Pancreatic Lipase *In Vitro* and Lipolysis *In Vivo*. Evidence-Based Complementary and Alternative Medicine 2012:1-8.

Kimura Y, Ohminami H, Arichi H, Okuda H, Baba K, Kozawa M, Arichi S. Effects of Various Coumarins from Roots of Angelica dahurica on Actions of Adrenaline, ACTH and Insulin in Fat Cells. Planta Med. 1982 Jul;45(7):183-7.

Kirk EP, Donnelly JE, Smith BK, Honas J, LeCheminant JD, Bailey BW, Jacobsen DJ, Washburn RA. Minimal resistance training improves daily energy expenditure and fat oxidation. Med Sci Sports Exerc. 2009 May;41(5):1122-1129.

Kishino E, Ito T, Fujita K, Kiuchi Y. A mixture of *Salacia reticulata* (Kotala himbutu) aqueous extract and cyclodextrin reduces body weight gain, viscera fat accumulation, and total cholesterol and insuling increases in male Wistar fatty rats. Nutrition Researcg 2009;29:55-63.

Kitano-Okada T, Ito A, Koide A, Nakamura Y, Han KH, Shimada K, Sasaki K, Ohba K, Silbayama S, Fukushima M. Anti-obesity role of adzuki bean extract containing polyphenols: in vivo and in vitro effects. J Sci Food Agric 2012 Oct;92(13):26444-51.

Kizelsztein P, Govorko D, Komarnytsky S, Evans A, Wang Z, Cefalu WT, Raskin I. 20-Hydroxyecdysone decreases weight and hyperglycemia in a diet-induced obesity mice model. Am J Physiol Endocrinol Metab 2009;296:433-439.

Kobayashi Y, Nakano Y, Kizaki M, Hoshikuma K, Yokoo Y, Kamiya T. Capsaicin-like anti-obese activities of evodiamine from fruits of *Evodia rutaecarpa*, a vanilloid receptor agonist. Planta Med 2001;67:628-33.

Kobayashi Y, Hiroi T, Araki M, Hirokawa T, Miyazawa M, Aoki N, Kojima T, Ohsawa T. Facilitative effects of Eucommia ulmoides on fatty acid oxidation in hypertriglyceridaemic rats. J Sci Food Agric 2012 Jan 30;92(2):358-65.

Kobori M, Masumoto S, Akimoto Y, Oike H. Chronic dietary intake of quercetin alleviates hepatic fat accumulation associated with consumption of a Western-style diet in C57/BL6J mice. Mol Nutr Food Res. 2010 Dec 15.

Koh-Banerjee PK, Ferreira MP, Greenwood M, Bowden RG, Cowan PN, Almada AL, Kreider RB. Effects of calcium pyruvate supplementation during trainin on body composition, exercise capacity, and metabolic responses to exercise. Nutrition 2005;21: 312-319.

Koh EH, Lee WJ, Lee SA, Kim EH, Cho EH, Jeong E, Kim DW, Kim MS, Park JY, Park KG, Lee HJ, Lee IK, Lim S, Jang HC, Lee KH, Lee KU. Effects of Alpha-Lipoic Acid on Body Weight in Obese Subjects. The American Journal of Medicine 2011;124.

Koh GY, McCutcheon K, Zhang F, Liu D, Cartwright CA, Martin R, Yang P, Liu Z. Improvement of obesity phenotype by Chinese sweet leaf tea (Rubus suavissimus) components in high-fat diet-induced obese rats. J Agric Food Chem 2011 Jan 12;59(1):98-104.

Koh JB, Lee CU. Effects of *Pleurotus eryngii* on Lipid Metabolism in Rats Fed High Fat Diet. J Korean Soc Food Sci Nutr 2005;34(5):626-631.

Kohima K, Shimada T, Nagareda Y, Watanabe M, Ishizaki J, Sai Y, Miyamoto KI, Aburada M. Preventive Effect of Geniposide on Metabolic Disease Status in Spontaneously Obese Type 2 Diabetic Mice and Free Fatty Acid-Treated HepG2 Cells. Biol. Pharm. Bull. 2011;34(10):1613-1618.

Kojima Y, Kimura T, Nakagawa K, Asai A, Hasumi K, Oikawa S, Miyazawa T. Effects of mulberry leaf extract rich in 1-deoxynojirimycin on blood lipid profiles in humans. J Clin Biochem Nutr. 2010 Sep;47(2):155-61.

Kolawole OT, Kolawole SO, Ayankunle AA, Olaniran IO. Methanol Leaf Extract of *Persea americana* Protects Rats against Cholesterol-Induced Hyperlipidemia. British Journal of Medicine & Medical Research 2012;2(2):235-242.

Komal S, Maheep B. Antiobesity activity of ethanolic extract of *Asparagus racemosus* willd. Roots in female rats. Journal of Herbal Medicine and Toxicology 2012;6(1):95-99.

Kondo T, Kishi M, Fushimi T, Kaga T. Acetic acid upregulates the expression of genes for fatty acid oxidation enzymes in liver to suppress body fat accumulation. J Agric Food Chem. 2009 Jul 8;57(13):5982-6.

Kondo T, Kishi M, Fushimi T, Ugajin S, Kaga T. Vinegar Intake Reduces Body Weight, Body Fat Mass, and Serum Triglyceride Levels in Obese Japanese Subjects. Biosci. Biotechnol. Biochem. 2009;73(8):1837-1843.

Kong YH, Cheigh HS, Song YK, Jo YO, Choi SY. Anti-Obesity Effects of Kimchi Tablet Composition in Rats Fed High-Fat Diet. J. Korean Soc. Food Sci. Nutr. 2007;36(12):1529-1536.

Konukoglu D, Turhan MS, Ercan M, Serin O. Relationship between plasma leptin and zinc levels and the effect of insulin and oxidative stress on leptin levels in obese diabetic patients. Journal of Nutritional Biochemistry 2004;15:757-760.

Koppeschaar HP, Meinders AE, Schwarz F. The effect of low-calorie diet alone and in combination with triiodothyronine therapy on weight loss and hypophyseal thyroid function in obesity. Int J Obes. 1983;7(2):123-31.

Koyama T, Miyata M, Nishimura T, Yazawa K. Suppressive Effects by Leaves of the *Dypsis lutescens* Palm on Fat Accumulation in 3T3-L1 Cells and Fat Absorption in Mice. Biosci. Biotechnol. Biochem. 2012;76(1):189-192.

Koya-Miyata S, Arai N, Mizote A, Taniguchi Y, Ushio S, Iwaki K, Fukuda S. Propolis Prevents Diet-Induced Hyperlipidemia and Mitigates Weight Gain in Diet-Induced Obesity in Mice. Biol. Pharm. Bull. 2009;32(12):2022-2028.

Kreider RB, Miller GW, Williams MH, Somma CT, Nasser TA. Effects of phosphate loading on oxygen uptake, ventilatory anaerobic threshold, and run performance. Med Sci Sports Exerc 1990 Apr;22(2):250-6.

Kreider RB, Miller GW, Schenck D, Cortes CW, Miriel V, Somma CT, Rowland P, Turner C, Hill D. Effects of phosphate loading on metabolic and myocardial responses to maximal and endurance exercise. Int J Sport Nutr 1992 Mar;2(1):20-47.

Kristensen M, Toubro S, Jensen MG, Ross AB, Riboldi G, Petronio M, Bügel S, Tetens I, Astrup A. Whole grain compared with refined wheat decreases the percentage of body fat following a 12-week, energy-restricted dietary intervention in postmenopausal women. J Nutr 2012 Apr;142(4):710-6.

Kroboth PD, Amico JA, Stone RA, Folan M, Frye RF, Kroboth FJ, Bigos KL, Fabian TJ, Linares AM, Pollock BG, Hakala C. Influence of DHEA administration on 24-hour cortisol concentrations. J Clin Psychopharmacol 2003 Feb;23(1):96-9.

Krotkiewski M. Effect of guar gum on body-weight, hunger ratings and metabolism in obese subjects. British Journal of Nutrition 1984;52:97-105.

Ku SK, Chung IK, Cheon WH, Kim JW. *Allium victorialis* Leaf Extract Prevents High Fat Diet Induced Obesity in Mice. J Vet Clin 2011;28(3):280-286.

Kuate D, Etoundi BC, Ngondi JL, Oben JE. Effects of *Dichrostachys glomerata* spice on cardiovascular diseases risk factors in normoglycemic and type 2 diabetic obese volunteers. Food Research International 2011;44:1197-1202.

Kubo K, Nanba H. Anti-hyperliposis Effect of Maitake Fruit Body *(Grifola frondosa)*. Biol. Pharm. Bull. 1997;20(7):781-785.

Kumar A, Vimalavathini R. Possible anorectic effect of methanol extract of *Benincasa hispida* (Thunb). Cogn, fruit. Indian J Pharmacol 2004 Dec;36(6):348-350.

Kumar DS, Muthu AK, Smith AA, Manavalan R. Hypolipidemic Effect of Various Extract of Whole Plant of *Mucuna pruriens* (Linn) in Rat Fed with High Fat Diet. European Journal of Biological Sciences 2010;2(2):32-38.

Kumar DS, Muthu AK. Evaluation of hypolipidemic activity of various extracts from whole plant of *Ionidium suffruticosum* (Ging.) (Family: Violaceae) in rat fed with high fat diet. International Journal of Pharmacy and Pharmaceutical Sciences 2012;4(4):69-73.

Kumar S, Alagawadi KR. Influence of *Alpinia galanga* rhizomes on cafeteria diet induced obesity in rats. Pharmacologyonline 2010;3:84-91.

Kumar S, Alagawadi KR, Rao MR. Effect of *Argyreia speciosa* root extract on cafeteria diet-induced obesity in rats. Indian J Pharmacol 2011 Apr;43(2):163-167.

Kumarnsit E, Keawpradub N, Nuankaew W. Acute and long-term effects of alkaloid extract of *Mitragyna speciosa* on food and water intake and body weight in rats. Fitoterapia 2006;77:339-345.

Kunkel SD, Suneja M, Ebert SM, Bongers KS, Fox DK, Malmberg SE, Alipour F, Shields RK, Adams CM. MRNA Expression Signatures of Human Skeletal Muscle Atrophy Identify a Natural Compound that Increases Muscle Mass. Cell Metabolism 2011 Jun;13:627-638.

Kunkel SD, Elmore CJ, Bongers KS, Ebert SM, Fox DK, Dyle MC, Bullard SA, Adams CM. Ursolic Acid Increases Skeletal Muscle and Brown Fat and Decreases Diet-Induced Obesity, Glucose Intolerance and Fatty Liver Disease. PloS ONE 2012 Jun;7(6):1-7.

Kuo DH, Yeh CH, Shieh PC, Cheng KC, Chen FA, Cheng JT. Effect of ShanZha, a Chinese herbal product, on obesity and dyslipidemia in hamsters receiving high-fat diet. Journal of Ethnopharmacology 2009;124:544-550.

Kuo DH, Hung MC, Hung CM, Liu LM, Chen FA, Shie PC, Ho CT, Way TD. Body weight management effect of burdock *(Arctium lappa* L.) root is associated with the activation of AMP-activated protein kinase in human HepG2 cells. Food Chemistry 2012;134:1320-1326.

Kuo JJ, Chang HH, Tsai TH, Lee TY. Positive effect of curcumin on inflammation and mitochondrial dysfunction in obese mice with liver steatosis. Int J Mol Med. 2012 Sep;30(3):673-9.

Kuo KL, Weng MS, Chiang CT, Tsai YJ, Lin-Shiau SY, Lin JK. Comparative studies on the hypolipidemic and growth suppressive effects of oolong, black, pu-erh, and green tea leaves in rats. J Agric Food Chem 2005 Jan 26;53(2):480-9.

Kuriyan R, Raj T, Srinivas SK, Vaz M, Rajendran R, Kurpad AV. Effect of Caralluma Fimbriata extract on appetite, food intake and anthropometry in adult Indian men and women. Appetite 2007;48:338-344.

Kusano S, Abe H. Antidiabetic Activity of White Skinned Sweet Potato *(Ipomoea batatas* L.) in Obese Zucker Fatty Rats. Biol. Pharm. Bull. 2000;23(1):23-26.

Kushiro M, Masaoka T, Hageshita S, Takahashi Y, Ide T, Sugano M. Comparative effect of sesamin and episesamin on the activity and gene expression of enzymes in fatty acid oxidation and synthesis in rat liver. Journal of Nutritional Biochemistry 2002;13: 289-295.

Kwak JH, Ahn CW, Park SH, Jung SU, Min BJ, Kim OY, Lee JH. Weight reduction effects of a black soy peptide supplement in overweight and obese subjects: Double blind, randomized controlled study. Food Funct 2012 Jun 28.

Kwon CS, Sohn HY, Kim SH, Kim JH, Son KH, Lee JS, Lim JK, Kim JS. Anti-obesity Effect of *Dioscorea nipponica* Makino with Lipase-inhibitory Activity in Rodents. Biosci. Biotechnol. Biochem. 2003;67(7):1451-1456.

Kwon CS, Sohn KH, Kim JS. Effect of *Lonicera japonica* Flower on Body Weight Gain and Glucose Tolerance in Rodents. Food Sci. Biotechnol. 2004;13(6):768-771.

Kwon JY, Cheigh HS, Song YO. Weight Reduction and Lipid Lowering Effects of Kimchi Lactic Acid Powder in Rats Fed High Fat Diets. Korean J Food Sci. Technol. 2004;36(6):1014-1019.

Kwon JY, Ann IS, Park KY, Cheigh HS, Song YO. The Beneficial Effects of Pectin on Obesity *in vitro* and *in vivo*. J Korean Soc Food Sci Nutr 2005;34(1):13-20.

Kwon SH, Ahn IS, Kim SO, Kong CS, Chung HY, Do MS, Park KY. Anti-obesity and hypolipidemic effects of black soybean anthocyanins. J Med Food 2007 Sep;10(3):552-6.

Lacaria MT, Preziosa I, Leo SD, Canelli A, Molfino A, Muscaritoli M, Fanelli FR, Laviano A. PP198-Su Glutamine supplementation and body weight loss in obese, non-dieting, non-diabetic female patients: a pilot study. Clinical Nutrition Supplements 2011;6(1):98.

Lai CS, Tsai ML, Badmaev V, Jimenez M, Ho CT, Pan MH. Xanthigen suppresses preadipocyte differentiation and adipogenesis through down-regulation of PPARγ and C/EBPs and modulation of SIRT-1, AMPK, and FoxO pathways. J Agric Food Chem 2012 Feb;60(4):1094-101.

Lappalainen R, Mennen L, van Weert L, Mykkänen H. Drinking water with a meal: a simple method of coping with feelings of hunger, satiety and desire to eat. Eur J Clin Nutr. 1993 Nov;47(11):815-9.

Latha BP, Reddy RM, Vijaya T, Rao SD, Ismail SM, Girish BP. Effect of saponin rich extract of *Achyranthes aspera* on high fat diet fed male wistar rats. Journal of Pharmacy Research 2011;4(9):3190-3193.

Latha BP, Vijaya T, Reddy IRM, Ismail M, Rao SD. Therapeutic efficacy of *Achyranthes aspera* saponin extract in high fat diet induced hyperlipidaemia in male wistar rats. Journal of Biotechnology 2011 Nov;10(74):17038-17042.

Latiffah AL, Saadat P, Mohd NG, Parichehr H, Mohammad AD, Syed TSH. Therapeutic effects of *Nigella sativa* (Black seed) on menopauseassociated metabolic syndrome: A crossover study. 1st World Congress on Healthy Ageing, Kuala Lumpur, Malaysia, 2012.

Lau FC, Golakoti T, Krishnaraju AV, Sengupta K, Bachi D. Efficacy and tolerability of Merastin- A randomized, double-blind, placebo-controlled study. FASEB J. April 2011; 25: (Meeting Abstract Supplement) 601:9. Presented at Experimental Biology 2011. Washington, DC. April 10, 2011. Program No. 601.9, Poster No. A278.

Lê KA, Faeh D, Stettler R, Ith M, Kreis R, Vermathen P, Boesch C, Ravussin E, Tappy L. A 4-wk high-fructose diet alters lipid metabolism without affecting insulin sensitivity or ectopic lipids in healthy humans. AmJ Clin Nutr. 2006 Dec;84(6):1374-9.

Lê KA, Ith M, Kreis R, Faeh D, Bortolotti M, Tran C, Boesch C, Tappy L. Fructose overconsumption causes dyslipidemia and ectopic lipid deposition in healthy subjects with and without a family history of type 2 diabetes. Am J Clin Nutr 2009 Jun;89(6):1760-5.

Lee CM, Lee TJ, Kim BH. Improving Effect of Cudrania Tricuspidata Ethanol Extract on Lipid Profile and Blood Glucose in HFD-induced Obese Mice. Journal of Investigative Cosmetology 2011;7(3):309-318.

Lee CM, Kim BH. The Anti-obesity Effect of *Cudrania Tricuspidata* Ethanol Extract by Focusing on the Changes of Hepatic and Adipose Tissue in HFD-induced Obese Mice. J. Kor. Soc. Cosm. 2012;18:677-687.

Lee EJ, Joo EJ, Hong YN, Kim YS. Inhibition of Adipocyte Differentiation by MeOH Extract from *Carduus crispus* through ERK and p38 MAPK Pathways. Natural Product Sciences 2011;17(4):273-278.

Lee GW, Yoon HC, Byun SY. Inhibitory effect of *Eucommia ulmoides* Oliver on adipogenic differentiation through proteome analysis. Enzyme and Microbial Technology 2004;35:632-638.

Lee HI, Kim MS, Lee KM, Park SK, Seo KI, Kim HJ, Kim MJ, Choi MS, Lee MK. Anti-visceral obesity and antioxidant effects of powdered sea buckthorn *(Hippophae rhamnoides* L) leaf tea in diet-induced obese mice. Food and Chemical Toxicology ' 2011;49:2370-2376.

Lee HJ, Lee KH, Park E, Chung HK. Effect of Onion Extract on Serum Cholesterol in Borderline Hypercholesterolemic Participants. J Korean Soc. Food Sci. Nutr. 2010;39(12):1783-1789.

Lee HM, Paik IY, Park TS. Effects of Dietary Supplementation of Taurine, Carnitine or Glutamine on Endurance Exercise Performance and Fatigue Parameters in Athletes. Korean J Nutr. 2003 Sep;36(7):711-719.

Lee HS, Park HJ, Kim MK. Effect of *Chlorella vulgaris* on lipid metabolism in Wistar rats fed high fat diet. Nutrition Research and Practice 2008;2(4):204-210.

Lee HY, Kim JH, Jeung HW, Lee CU, Kim DS, Li B, Lee GH, Sung MS, Ha KC, Back HI, Kim SY, Park SH, Oh MR, Kim MG, Jeon JY, Im YJ, Hwang MH, So BO, Shin SJ, Yoo WH, Kim HR, Chae HJ, Chae SW. Effects of *Ficus carica* paste on loperamide-induced constipation in rats. Food and Chemical Toxicology 2012;50:895-902.

Lee IA, Lee JH, Baek NI, Kim DH. Antihyperlipidemic Effect of Crocin Isolated from the Fructus of *Gardenia jasminoides* and Its Metabolite Crocetin. Biol. Pharm. Bull. 2005;28(11):2106-2110.

Lee J, Chae K, Ha J, Park BY, Lee HS, Jeong S, Kim MY, Yoon M. Regulation of obesity and lipid disorders by herbal extracts from *Morus alba, Melissa officinalis,* and *Artemisia capillaris* in high-fat diet-induced obese mice. Journal of Ethnopharmacology

2008;115:263-270.

Lee J, Jung E, Lee J, Kim S, Huh S, Kim Y, Kim Y, Byun SY, Kim YS, Park D. Isorhamnetin Represses Adipogenesis in 3T3-L1 Cells. Obesity 2009;17(2):226-232.

Lee J, Jeong JY, Cho YS, Park SK, Kim K, Kim MJ, Lee MK. Effect of Young *Phragmites communis* Leaves Powder on Lipid Metabolism and Erythrocyte Antioxidant Enzyme Activities in High-Fat Diet Fed Mice. J Korean Soc Food Sci Nutr 2010;39(5):677-683.

Lee J, Lee J, Jung E, Hwang W, Kim YS, Park D. Isorhamnetin-induced anti-adipogenesis is mediated by stabilization of β-catenin protein. Life Sciences 2010;86:416-423.

Lee JH, Son CW, Kim MY, Kim MH, Kim HR, Kwak ES, Kim S, Kim MR. Red beet *(Beta vulgaris* L.) leaf supplementation improves antioxidant status in C57BL/6J mice fed high fat high cholesterol diet. Nutrition Research and Practice 2009;3(2): 114-121.

Lee JJ, Shin HD, Lee YM, Kim AR, Lee MY. Effect of Broccoli Sprouts on Cholesterol-lowering and Anti-obesity Effects in Rats Fed High Fat Diet. J Korean Soc Food Sci Nutr 2009;38(3):309-318.

Lee JR, Shin JH, Byun SH, Park SJ, Jo MJ, Park SM, Ku SK, Kim SC. Anti-obese and Hypolipemic Effects of the Aqueous Extracts of Raphani Semen in Mice Fed High Fat Diet. J. Korean. Soc. Appl. Biol. Chem. 2009;52(1):50-57.

Lee JS, Lee MK, Ha TY, Bok SH, Park HM, Jeong KS, Woo MN, Do GM, Yeo JY, Choi MS. Supplementation of whole persimmon leaf improves lipid profiles and suppresses body weight gain in rats fed high-fat diet. Food and Chemical Toxicology 2006;44: 1875-1883.

Lee KH, Kim Y, Park E, Hwang HJ. Effect of Onion Powder Supplementation on Lipid Metabolism in High Fat-cholesterol Fed SD Rats. J Food Sci. Nutr 2008;13:71-76.

Lee KH, Park E, Lee HJ, Kim MO, Cha YJ, Kim JM, Lee H, Shin MJ. Effects of daily quercetin-rich supplementation on cardiometabolic risks in male smokers. Nutrition Research and Practice *(Nutr Res Pract)* 2011;5(1):28-33.

Lee MG, Park KS, Kim DU, Choi SM, Kim HJ. Effects of high-intensity exercise training on body composition, abdominal fat loss, and cardiorespiratory fitness in middle-aged Korean females. Appl Physiol Nutr Metab 2012 Dec;37(6):1019-27.

Lee MS, Lee HJ, Lee HS, Kim Y. L-carnitine stimulates lipolysis via induction of the lipolytic gene expression and suppression of the adipogenic gene expression in 3T3-L1 adipocytes. J Med Food 2006 Winter;9(4):468-73.

Lee OH, Kwon YI, Apostolidis E, Shetty K, Kim YC. Rhodiola-induced inhibition of adipogenesis involves antioxidant enzyme response associated with pentose phosphate pathway. Phytother Res. 2011 Jan;25(1):106-15.

Lee S, You Y, Yoon HG, Kim K, Park J, Kim S, Ho JN, Lee J, Shm S, Jun W. Fatigue-Alleviating Effect on Mice of an Ethanolic Extract from *Rubus coreanus*. Biosci. Biotechnol. Biochem. 2011;75(2):349-351.

Lee SH, Lim SW, Mihn NV, Hur JM, Song BJ, Lee YM, Lee HS, Kim DK. Administration of *Triticum aestivum* Sprout Water Extracts Reduce the Level of Blood Glucose and Cholesterol in Leptin Deficient *ob/ob* Mice. J. Korean Soc Food Sci Nutr 2011;40(3):401-408.

Lee SI, Kim JW, Lee YK, Yang SH, lee IA, Suh JW, Kim SD. Anti-obesity Effect of *Monascus pilosus* Mycelial Extract in High Fat Diet-induced Obese Rats. J. Appl. Biol. Chem. 2011;54(3):197-205.

Lee SJ, Kim CW, Jang HJ, Cho SY, Choi JW. Anti-hyperlipidemia and Anti-arteriosclerosis Effects of *Laminaria japonica* in Sprague-Dawley Rats. Fish Aquat Sci 2011;14(4):235-241.

Lee YS, Cha BY, Yamaguchi K, Choi SS, Yonezawa T, Teruya T, Nagai K, Woo JT. Effects of Korean white ginseng extracts on obesity in high-fat diet-induced obese mice. Cytotechnology 2010;62:367-376.

Lee YS, Cha BY, Saito K, Choi SS, Wang XX, Choi BK, Yonezawa T, Teruya T, Nagai K, Woo JT. Effects of a *Citrus depressa Hayata* (shiikuwasa) extract on obesity in high-fat diet-induced obese mice. Phytomedicine 2011;18:648-654.

Lee YS, Cha BY, Choi SS, Choi BK, Yonezawa T, Teurya T, Nagai K, Woo JT. Nobiletin improves obesity and isulin resistance in high-fat diet-induced obese mice. Journal of Nutritional Biochemistry 2012.

Legette LL, Luna AYM, Reed RL, Miranda CL, Bobe G, Proteau RR, Stevens JF. Xanthoumol lowers body weight and fasting plasma glucose in obese male Zucker fa/fa rats. Phytochemistry 2012.

Lemaure B, Touché A, Zbinden I, Moulin J, Courtois D, Macé K, Darimont C. Administration of Cyperus rotundus tubers extract prevents weight gain in obese Zucker rats. Phytother Res. 2007 Aug;21(8):724-30.

Lemhadri A, Eddouks M, Sulpice T, Burcelin R. Anti-hyperglycaemic and Anti-obesity Effects of *Capparis spinosa* and *Chamaemelum nobile* Aqueous Extracts in HFD Mice. American Journal of Pharmacology and Toxicology 2007;2(3):106-110.

Lemhadri A, Hajji L, Michel J-B, Eddouks M. Cholesterol and triglycerides lowering activities of caraway fruits in normal and streptozotocin diabetic rats. Journal of Ethnopharmacology 2006;106:321-326.

Li F, Tang H, Xiao F, Gong J, Peng Y, Meng X. Protective effect of salidroside from Rhodiolae Radix on diabetes-induced oxidative stress in mice. Molecules 2011 Dec 1;16(12):9912-24.

Li J, Kaneko T, Qin LQ, Wang J, Wang Y. Effects of Barley Intake on Glucose Tolerance, Lipid Metabolism, and Bowel Function in Women. Nutrition 2003;19:926-929.

Li J, Fu YM, Zhu WJ, Zhang SM, Yan YX, Yan L. Effects of *Retinervus luffae fructus* on serum lipid level in experimental hyperliidemia rats. Chin J Pathophysiol 2004;20(7):1264-1266.

Li JL, Wang W, Zeng CZ, Liu ZM, Li ZH. Effects of Kumquat Flavonoid Extracts on the Blood Lipid Reduction Of Obese Rats with Hyperlipidemia. Journal of Central South University of Forestry & Technology 2008.

Li JX, Wang N, Wang HJ, Zhou XH, Li MJ, Xie XH, Li ZL. Effects of Apple Polyphenols on Weight Losing and Lipid Lowing of Mice. Food Science 2008.

Li MH, Tang CF, Ouyang JQ. Influence of salidroside from Rhodiola Sachalinensis A. Bor on some related indexes of free radical and energy metabolism after exercise in mice. Zhongguo Ying Yong Sheng Li Xue Za Zhi 2012 Jan;28(1):53-6.

Li MR, Yu YR, Deng G. Astragalus membranaceus improves endothelial-dependent vasodilator function in obese rats. Nan Fang Yi Ke Da Xue Xue Bao 2010 Jan;30(1):7-10.

Li SY, Chang CQ, Ma FY, Yu CL. Modulating Effects of Chlorogenic Acid on Lipids and Glucose Metabolism and Expression of Hepatic Peroxisome Proliferator-activated Receptor-α in Golden Hamsters Fed on High Fat Diet. Biomedical and Environmental

Sciences 2009;22:122-129.

Li Y, Kang Z, Li S, Kong T, Liu X, Sun C. Ursolic acid stimulates lipolysis in primary-cultured rat adipocytes. Mol Nutr Food Res 2010 Nov;54(11):1609-17.

Lien DN, Quynh NT, Quang NH, Phuc DV, Ngan NTT. Anti-Obesity and Body Weight Reducing Effect of *Fortunella japonica* Peel Extract Fractions in Experimentally Obese Mice. KKU Sci. J. 2009;37:96-104.

Lien DN, Quynh NTH, Quang NH, Phuc DV, Phong VC, Huong PT. Effect of pomelo *(citrus grandis* (l). osbeck) peel extract on lipid-carbohydrate metabolic enzymes and blood lipid, glucose parameters in experimental obese and diabetic mice. VNU Journal of Sciences, Natural Sciences and Technology 2010;26:224-232.

Lim K, Ryu S, Ohishi Y, Watanabe I, Tomi H, Suh H, Lee WK, Kwon T. Short-term (-)-hydroxycitrate ingestion increases fat oxidation during exercise in athletes. J Nutr Sci Vitaminol (Tokyo) 2002 Apr;48(2):128-33.

Lim K, Ryu S, Nho HS, Choi SK, Kwon T, Suh H, So J, Tomita K, Okuhara Y, Shigematsu N. (-)-Hydroxycitric acid ingestion increases fat utilization during exercise in untrained women. J Nutr Sci Vitaminol (Tokyo) 2003 Jun;49(3):163-7.

Lim SH, Park YH, Kwon CJ, Ham HJ, Jeong HN, Kim KH, Ahn YS. Anti-diabetic and Hypoglycemic Effects of *Eleutherococcus* spp.. J Korean Soc Food Sci Nutr 2010;39(12):1761-1768.

Lin CC, Yin MC, Hsu CC, Lin MP. Effects of five cysteine-containing compounds on three lipogenic enzymes in Balb/cA mice consuming a high saturated fat diet. Lipids 2004 Sep;39(9):843-8.

Lin CC, Yin MC. Effects of cysteine-containing compounds on biosynthesis of triacylglycerol and cholesterol and anti-oxidative protection in liver from mice consuming a high-fat diet. British Journal of Nutrition 2008;99:37-43.

Lin GP, Jiang T, Hu XB, Qiao XH, Tuo QH. Effect of *Siraitia grosvenorii* Polysaccharide on Glucose and Lipid of Diabetic Rabbits Induced by Feeding High Fat/High Sucrose Chow. Experimental Diabetes Research 2007.

Lin MC, Hsu PC, Yin MC. Protective effects of Houttuynia cordata aqueous extract in mice consuming high saturated fat diet.. Food Funct. 2012.

Little JP, Safdar A, Wilkin GP, Tarnopolsky MA, Gibala MJ. A practical model of low-volume high-intensity interval training induces mitochondrial biogenesis in human skeletal muscle: a potential mechanisms. J Physiol 2010;588(6):1011-1022.

Liu IM, Tzeng TF, Liou SS, Chang CJ. Regulation of obesity and lipid disorders by extracts from Angelica acutiloba root in high-fat diet-induced obese rats. Phytother Res. 2012 Feb;26(2):223-30.

Liu JW, DeMichele SJ, Palombo J, Chuang LT, Hastilow C, Bobik E Jr, Huang YS. Effect of long-tem dietary supplementation of high-gamma-linolenic canola oil versus borage oil on growth, hematology, serum biochemistry, and N-6 fatty acid metabolism in rats. J Agric Food Chem. 2004 Jun 16;52(12):3960-6.

Liu Q, Hong IP, Ahn MJ, Yoo HS, Han SB, Hwang BY, Lee MK. Anti-adipogenic activity of Cordyceps militaris in 3T3-L1 cells. Nat Prod Commun 2011 Dec;6(12):1839-41.

Liu W, Zheng Y, Han L, Wang H, Saito M, Ling M, Kimura Y, Feng Y. Saponins (Ginsenosides) from stems and leaves of *Panax quinquefolium* prevented high-fat diet-induced obesity in mice. Phytomedicine 2008;15:1140-1145.

Liu XG, Zhang J, Lu JL, Liu TC. Laser Acupuncture Reduces Body Fat in Obese Female Undergraduate Students. International Journal of Photoenergy 2012:1-4.

Liu Y, Fukuwatari Y, Okumura K, Takeda K, Ishibashi KI, Furukawa M, Ohno N, Mori K, Gao M, Motoi M. Immunomodulating Activity of *Agaricus brasiliensis* KA21 in Mice and in Human Volunteers. ECAM 2008;5(2):205-219.

Liu Y, Wang J, Zhang R, Zhang Y, Xu Q, Zhang J, Zhang Y, Zheng Z, Yu X, Jing H, Nosaka N, Kasai M, Aoyama T, Wu J, Xue C. A good response to oil with medium- and long-chain fatty acids in body fat and blood lipid profiles of male hypertriglyceridemic subjects. Asia Pac J Clin Nutr 2009;18(3):351-358.

Liu ZG, Zhang R, Li C, Ma X, Liu L, Wang JP, Mei QB. The osteoprotective effect of Radix Dipsaci extract in ovariectomized rats. Journal of Ethnopharmacology 2009;123:74-81.

Loan NTT, Tan HTM, Tam VTH, Luan CL, Huong LM, Lien DN. Anti-obesity and body weight reducing effect of *Docynia indica* (Wall.) Decne fruit extract fractions in experimentally obese mice. VNU Journal of Science, Natural Sciences and Technology 2011;27:125-133.

Lokesh D, Amitsankar D. Evaluation of mechanism for antihypertensive action of Clerodendrum colebrookianum Walp., used by folklore healers in nort-east India. J Ethnopharmacol 2012 Aug 30;143(1):207-12.

Longquan Y, Shirai N, Suzuki H. Effects of Some Chinese Spices on Body Weights, Plasma Lipids, Lipid Peroxides, and Glucose, and Liver Lipids in Mice. Food Sci. Technol. Res. 2007;13(2):155-161.

Lou Y, Peng Q, Nolan B, C.Wagner G, Lu Y. Oral administration of caffeine during voluntary exercise markedly decreases tissue fat and stimulates apoptosis and cyclin B1 in UVB-treated skin of hairless p53-knockout mice. Carcinogenesis 2010;31(4):671-678.

Lourenco S, Oliveira A, Lopes C. The effect of current and lifetime alcohol consumption on overall and central obesity. Eur J Clin Nutr. 2012 Jul;66(7):813-8.

Lu J, He T, Putheti R. Compounds of *Purslane* extracts and effects of anti-kinetic fatigue. Journal of Medicinal Plants Research 2009 Jul;3(7):506-510.

Lucas EA, Li W, Peterson SK, Brown A, Kuvibidila S, Perkins-Veazie P, Clarke SL, Smith BJ. Mango modulates body fat and plasma glucose and lipids in mice fed a high-fat diet. Br J Nutr. 2011 Nov;106(10):1495-505.

Lucotti P, Setola E, Monti LD, Galluccio E, Costa S, Sandoli EP, Fermo I, Rabaiotti G, Gatti R, Piatti PM. Beneficial effects of a long-term oral L-arginine treatment added to a hypocaloric diet and exercise training program in obese, insulin-resistant tye 2 diabetic patients. Am J Physiol Endocrinol Metab 2006;291:906-912.

Ludvik B, Neuffer B, Pacini G. Efficacy of *Ipomoea batatas* (Caiapo) on Diabetes Control in Type 2 Diabetic Subjects Treated With Diet. Diabetes Care 2004 Feb;27(2):436-440.

Ludvik B, Hanefeld M, Pacini G. Improved metabolic control by Ipomoea batatas (Caiapo) is associated with incresed adiponectin and decreased fibrinogen levels in type 2 diabetic subjects. Diabetes Obes Metab 2008 Jul;10(7):586-92.

Luo H, Kashiwagi A, Shibahara T, Yamada K. Decreased bodyweight without rebound and regulated lipoprotein metabolism by gymnemate in genetic multifactor syndrome animal. Mol Cell Biochem. 2007 May;299(1-2):93-8.

Macarulla MT, Medina C, De Diego MA, Chávarri M, Zulet MA, Martinez JA, Nöel-Suberville C, Higueret P, Portillo MP. Effect of the whole seed and protein isolate of faba bean (*Vicia faba*) on the cholesterol metabolism of hypercholesterolaemic rats. British Journal of Nutrition 2001;85:607-614.

Macarulla MT, Alberdi G, Gómez S, Tueros I, Bald C, Rodriguez VM, MartinezJA, Portillo MP. Effects of different doses of resveratrol on body fat and serum parameters in rats fed a hypercaloric diet. J Physiol Biochem. 2009 Dec;65(4):369-76.

MacEwen EG, Kurzman ID. Obesity in the dog: role of the adrenal steroid dehydroepiandrosterone (DHEA). J Nutr 1991 Nov;121(11):51-5.

Mae T, Kishida H, Nishiyama T, Tsukagawa M, Konishi E, Kuroda M, Mimaki Y, Sashida Y, Takahashi K, Kawada T, Nakagawa K, Kitahara M. A licorice ethanolic extract with peroxisome proliferator-activated receptor-gamma ligand-binding activity affects diabetes in KK-Ay mice, abdominal obesity in diet-induced obese C57BL mice and hypertension in spontaneously hypertensive rats. J Nutr 2003 Nov;133(11):3369-77.

Maeda H, Hosokawa M, Sashima T, Funayama K, Miyashita K. Fucoxanthin from edible seaweed, *Undaria pinnatifida*, shows antiobesity efect through UCP1 expression in white adipose tissues. Biochemical and Bophysical Research Communication 2005;332:392-397.

Maeda H, Hosokawa M, Sashima T, Miyashita K. Dietary combinaton of fucoxanthin and fish oil attenuates the weight gain of white adipose tissue and decreases blood glucose in obese/diabetic KK-Ay mice. J Agric Food Chem. 2007 Sep;55(19):7701-6.

Maeda H, Hosokawa M, Sashima T, Funayama K, Miyashita K. Effect of Medium-chain Triacylglycerols on Anti-obesity Effect of Fucoxanthin. Journal of Oleo Science 2007;56(12):615-621.

Maeda H, Hosokawa M, Sashima T, Murakami-Funayama K, Miyashita K. Anti-obesity and anti-diabetic effects of fucoxanthin on diet-induced obesity conditions in a murine model. Molecular medicine reports 2009;2:897-902.

Major GC, Alarie FP, Doré J, Tremblay A. Calcium plus vitamin D supplementation and fat mass loss in female very low-calcium consumers: potential link with a calcium-specific appetite control. Br J Nutr. 2009 Mar;101(5):659-63.

Maki KC, Rains TM, Kaden VN, Raneri KR, Davidson MH. Effects of a reduced-glycemic-load diet on body weight, body composition, and cardiovascular disease risk markers in overweight and obese adults. Am J Clin Nutr 2007 Mar;85(3):724-34.

Maki KC, Galant R, Samuel P, Tesser J, Witchger MS, Ribaya-Mercado JD, Blumberg JB, Geohas J. Effects of consuming foods containing oat β-glucan on blood pressure, carbohydrate metabolism and biomarkers of oxidative stress in men and women with elevated blood pressure. European Journal of Clinical Nutrition 2007;61:786-795.

Malaguarnera M, Cammalleri L, Gargante MP, Vacante M, Colonna V, Motta M. L-Carnitine treatment reduces severity of physical and mental fatigue and increases cognitive functions in centenarians: a randomized and controlled clinical trial. Am J Clin Nutr. 2007 Dec;86(6):1738-44.

Malarvili T, Veerappan RM, Begum VH. Effect of *Achyranthes aspera* seeds on lipid profiles in selected tissues of rats fed with high doses of fructose. Journal of Pharmacy Research 2011;4(6):1769-1771.

Malik VS, Schulze MB, Hu FB. Intake of sugar-sweetened beverages and weight gain: a systematic review. Am J Client Nutr. 2006 Aug;84(2):274-88.

Malik ZA, Sharma PL. An ethanolic extract from licore *(glycyrrhiza glabra)* exhibits anti-obesity effects by decreasing dietary fat absorption in a high-fat diet-induced obesity rat model. International Journal of Pharmaceutical Science and Research 2011;2(11):3010-3018.

Malik ZA, Sharma PL. Attenuation of High-fat Diet Induced Body Weight Gain, Adiposity and Biochemical Anomalies after Chronic Administration of Ginger *(Zingiber officinale)* in Wistar Rats. International Journal of Pharmacology 2011;7(8):801-812.

Mangal A, Sharma MC. Evaluation of certain medicinal plants for antiobesity properties. Indian Journal of Traditional Knowledge Oct 2009;8(4):602-605.

Manish K, Aditi K, Renu A, Gajraj S, Poonam M. Anti-obesity property of hexane extract from the leaves of *Gymnema sylvestre* in high fed cafeteria diet induced obesity rats. International Research Journal of Pharmacy 2011;2(8):112-116.

Manuela PGML, Eva MRK, Margriet SWP. Effect of capsaicin on substrate oxidation and weight maintenance after modest body-weight loss in human subjects. British Journal of Nutrition 2003;90:651-659.

Mao XQ, Yu F, Wang N, Wu Y, Zou F, Wu K, Liu M, Ouyang JP. Hypoglycemic effect of polysaccharide enriched extract of *Astragalus membranaceus* in diet induced insulin resistant C57BL/6J mice and its potential mechanism. Phytomedicine 2009;16:416-425.

Marinangeli CP, Jones PJ. Chronic intake of fractionated yellow pea flour reduces postprandial energy expenditure and carbohydrate oxidation. J Med Food 2011 Dec;14(12):1654-62.

Marinangeli CP, Krause D, Harding SV, Rideout TC, Zhu F, Jones PJ. Whole and fractionated yellow pea flours modulate insulin, glucose, oxygen consumption, and the caecal microbiome in Golden Syrian hamsters. Appl Physiol Nutr Metab. 2011 Dec;36(6):811-20.

Marinangeli CPF, Jones PJH. Whole and fractionated yellow pea flours reduce fasting insulin and insulin resistance in hypercholesterolaemic and overweight human subjects. British Journal of Nutrition 2011;105:110-117.

Marková M, Adámeková E, Bojková B, Kubatka P, Kassayová M, Ahlersová E, Ahlers I. Effect of Low-dose Chronic Melatonin Administration on Metabolic and Hormonal Variables in Young Laboratory Rats. ACTA VET. BRNO 2004;73:445-453.

Marotte C, Weisstaub A, Bryk G, Olguin MC, Posadas M, Lucero D Schreier L, Pita Martin de Portela ML, Zeni SN. Effect of dietary calcium (Ca) on body composition and Ca metabolism during growth in genetically obese (β) male rats. Eur J Nutr 2012 Mar 29.

Martin J, Wang ZQ, Zhang XH, Wachtel D, Volaufova J, Matthews DE, Cefalu WT. Chromium picolinate supplementation attenuates body weight gain and increases insulin sensitivity in subjects with type 2 diabetes. Diabetes Care 2006 Aug;29(8): 1826-32.

Martinez JA, Marcos R, Macarulla MT, Larralde J. Growth, hormonal status and protein turnover in rats fed on a diet containing peas (Pisum sativum L.) as the source of protein. Plant Foods Hum. Nutr. 1995 Apr;47(3):211-20.

Martins JM, Riottot M, de Abreu MC, Lanca MJ, Viegas-Crespo AM, Almeida JA, Freire JB, Bento OP. Dietary raw peas (*Pisum sativum* L.) reduce plasma total and LDL cholesterol and hepatic esterified cholesterol in intact and ileorectal anastomosed pigs fed cholesterol-rich diets. J Nutr 2004 Dec;134(12):3305-12.

Maruyama C, Araki R, Kawamura M, Kondo N, Kigawa M, Kawai Y, Takanami Y, Miyashita K, Shimomitsu T. Azuki Bean Juice Lowers Serum Triglyceride Concentrations in Healthy Young Women. J. Clin. Biochem. Nutr. 2008 Jul;43:19-25.

Mathern JR, Raatz SK, Thomas W, Slavin JL. Effect of fenugreek fiber on satiety, blood glucose and insulin response and energy intake in obese subjects. Phytother Res. 2009 Nov;23(11):1543-8.

Matsuda Y, Kobayshi M, Yamauchi R, Ojika M, Hiramitsu M, Inoue T, Katagiri T, Murai A, Horio F. Coffee and Caffeine Improve Insulin Sensitivity and Glucose Tolerance in C57BL/6J Mice Fed a High-Fat Diet. Biosci. Biotechnol. Biochem. 2011;75(12): 2309-2315.

Matsumoto Y, Ono A. Effect of Dietary Adzuki Bean *(Phaseolus angularis)* on Serum Lipid Concentrations in Adult Rats. Kawasaki Journal of Medical Welfare 2002;8(2):49-55.

Matsui N, Ito R, Nishimura E, Yoshikawa M, Kato M, Kamei M, Shibata H, Matsumoto I, Abe K, Hashizume S. Ingested cocoa can prevent high-fat diet-induced obesity by regulating the expression of genes for fatty acid metabolism. Nutrition 2005;21:594-601.

Matsumara T, Bohgaki T, Watarai M, Suzuki H, Ohashi K, Shibuya H. Antihypertensive actions of methylripariochromene A from Orthosiphon aristatus, an Indonesian traditional medicinal plant. Biol. Pharm Bull. 1999 Oct;22(10):1083-8.

Matsumoto K, Yokoyama SI, Gato N. Hypolipidemic Effect of Young Persimmon Fruit in C57BL/6.KOR-*ApoE*^{shl} Mice. Biosci. Biotechnol. Biochem. 2008;72(10):2651-2659.

Matsumoto K, Koba T, Hamada K, Tsujimoto H, Mitsuzono R. Branched-Chain Amino Acid Supplementation Increases the Lactate Threshold during an Incremental Exercise Test in Trained Individuals. J Nutr Sci Vitaminol 2009;55:52-58.

McAnuff MA, Harding WW, Omoruyi FO, Jacobs H, Morrison EY, Asemota HN. Hypoglycemic effects of steroidal sapogenins isolated from Jamaican bitter yam, *Dioscorea polygonoides*. Food and Chemical Toxicology 2005;43:1667-1672.

McIntosh M, Bao H, Lee C. Opposing actions of dehydroepiandrosterone and corticosterone in rats. Proc Soc Exp Biol Med 1999 Jul;221(3):198-206.

McKnight JR, Satterfield MC, Jobgen WS, Smith SB, Spencer TE, Meininger CJ, McNeal CJ, Wu G. Beneficial effects of L-arginine on reducing obesity: potential mechanisms and important implications for human health. Amino Acids 2010 Jul;39(2): 349-57.

Meckel Y, Nemet D, Bar-Sela S, Radom-Aizik S, Cooper DM, Sagiv M, Eliakim A. Hormonal and inflammatory responses to different types of sprint interval training. J Strength Cond Res. 2011 Aug;25(8):2161-9 .

Meckling KA, Sherfey R. A randomized trial of a hypocaloric high-protein diet, with and without exercise, on weight loss, fitness, and markers of the Metabolic Syndrome in overweight and obese women. Appl Physiol Nutr Metab 2007 Aug;32(4):743-52.

Megalli S, Aktan F, Davies NM, Roufogalis BD. Phytopreventative Anti-Hyperlipidemic Effects Of Gynostemma Pentaphyllum in Rats. J Pharm Pharmaceut Sci 2005;8(3):507-515.

Megalli S, Davies NM, Roufogalis BD. Anti-Hyperlipidemic and Hypoglycemic Effects of Gynostemma pentaphyllum in the Zucker Fatty Rat. J Pharm Pharmaceut Sci 2006;9(3):281-291.

Mehra R, Prasad M, Lavekar GS. An approach of *Ashwagandha + Guggulu* in Atheromatous CHD associated with Obesity. Ayu 2009;30(2):121-125.

Mehta LK, Balaraman R, Amin AH, Bafna PA, Gulati OD. Effect of fruits of *Moringa oleifera* on the lipid profile of normal and hypercholesterolaemic rabbits. Journal of Ethnopharmacology 2003;86:191-195.

Meirelles CM, Gomes PSC. Acute effects of resistance exercise on energy expenditure: revisiting the impact of the training variables. Rev Bras Med Esporte 2004;10(2):131-138.

Melo CL, Queiroz MGR, Fonseca SGC, Bizerra AMC, Lemos TLG, Melo TS, Santos FA, Rao VS. Oleanolic acid, a natural triterpenoid improves blood glucose tolerance in normal mice and ameliorates visceral obesity in mice fed a high-fat diet. Chemico-Biological Interactions 2010;185:59-65.

Meneguetti QA, Brenzan MA, Batista MR, Bazotte RB, Silva DR, Garcia Cortez DA. Biological effects of hydrolyzed quinoa extract from seeds of Chenopodium quinoa Willd. J Med Food 2011 Jun;14(6):653-7.

Meng R, Zhu DL, Bi Y, Yang DH, Wang YP. Apocynin Improves Insulin Resistance through Suppressing Inflammation in High-Fat Diet-Induced Obese Mice. Mediators of Inflammation 2010:1-9.

Mesallamy HOE, El-Demerdash E, Hammad LN, Magdoub HME. Effect of taurine supplementation on hyperhomocysteinemia and markers of oxidative stress in high fructose diet induced insulin resistance. Diabetology & Syndrome 2010;2(46):1-11.

Michelle LA, Angela LC, Leigh EN, Rachel MC, Michael BS, Szu-Yu T, Jason CH, Martha AB. Time-dependent effects of safflower oil to improve glycemia, inflammation and blood lipids in obese, post-menopausal women with type 2 diabetes: A randomized, double-masked, crossover study. Clinical Nutrition 2011;30:443-449.

Michishita T, Kobayashi S, Katsuy T, Ogihara T, Kawabuchi K. Evaluation of the Antiobesity Effects of an Amno Acid Mixture and Conjugated Linoleic Acid on Exercising Healthy Overweight Humans: a Randomized, Double-blind, Placebo-controlled Trial. The Journal of International Medical Research 2010;38:844-859.

Mifflin MD, St Jeor ST, Hill LA, Scott BJ, Daugherty SA, Koh YO. A new predictive equation for resting energy expenditure in healthy individuals. Am J Clin Nutr. 1990 Feb;51(2):241-7.

Mikami N, Hosokawa M, Miyashita K. Dietary Combination of Fish Oil and Taurine Decreases Fat Accumulation and Ameliorates Blood Glucose Levels in Type 2 Diabetic/Obese KK-A(y) Mice. J Food Sci. 2012 Jun;77(6):114-20.

Miller WC, Niederpruem MG, Wallace JP, Lindeman AK. Dietary fat, sugar, and fiber predict body fat content. J Am Diet Assoc. 1994 Jun;94(6):612-5.

Miller WC, Koceja DM, Hamilton EJ. A meta-analysis of the past 25 years of weight loss research using diet, exercise or diet plus exercise intervention. International Journal of Obesity 1997;21:941-947.

Mingorance C, del Pozo MG, Herrera MD, de Sotomayor MA. Oral supplementation of propionyl-L-carnitine reduces body weight and hyperinsulinaemia in obese Zucker rats. British Journal of Nutrition 2009;102:1145-1153.

Mingorance C, Duluc L, Chalopin M, Simard G, Ducluzeau PH, Herrera MD, Alvarez de Sotomayor M, Andriantsitohaina R. Propionyl-L-carnitine corrects metabolic and cardiovascular alterations in diet-induced obese mice and improves liver respiratory chain activity. PloS One 2012;7(3):1-10.

Misawa E, Tanaka M, Nomaguchi K, Yamada M, Toida T, Takase M, Iwatsuki K, Kawada T. Administration of phytosterols isolated from Aloe vera gel reduce visceral fat mass and improve hyperglycemia in Zucker diabetic fatty (ZDF) rats. Obesity Research & Clinical Practice 2008;2:239-245.

Misawa E, Tanaka M, Nomaguchi K. Oral Ingestion of *Aloe vera* Phytosterols Alters Hepatic Gene Expression Profiles and Ameliorates Obesity-Associated Metabolic Disorders in Zucker Diabetic Fatty Rats. J. Agric. Food Chem. 2012;60(11):2799-2806.

Mishra S, Singh RB. Effect of Mushroom on the Lipid Profile, Lipid Peroxidation and Liver Functions of Aging Swiss Albino Rats. The Open Nutraceuticals Journal 2010;3:248-253.

Mitra A. Effects of Fenugreek in Type 2 Diabetes and Dyslipidaemia. Indian Journal for the Practising 2006;3(2):5-6.

Miura T, Iwamoto N, Kato M, Ichiki H, Kubo M, Komatsu Y, Ishida T, Okada M, Tanigawa K. The Suppressive Effect of Mangiferin with Exercise on Blood Lipids in Type 2 Diabetes. Biol. Pharm. Bull. 2001;24(9):1091-1092.

Miyata M, Koyama T, Kamitani T. Anti-Obesity Effect on Rodents of the Traditional Japanese Food, Tororokombu, Shaved *Laminaria*. Biosci. Biotechnol. Biochem. 2009;73(10):2326-2328.

Miyata M, Koyama T, Yazawa K. Water Extract of *Houttuynia cordata* Thunb. Leaves Exerts Anti-Obesity Effects by Inhibiting Fatty Acid and Glycerol Absorption. J Nutr Sci Vitaminol 2010;56:150-156.

Mizoguchi T, Takehara I, Masuzawa T, Saito T, Naoki Y. Nutrigenomic Studies of Effects of *Chlorella* on Subjects with High-Risk Factors for Lifestyle-Related Disease. Journal of Medicinal Food 2008;11(3):395-404.

Mizutani K, Ikeda K, Kawai Y, Yamori Y. Extract of Wine Phenolics Improves Aortic Biomechanical Properties in Stroke-Prone Spontaneously Hypertensive Rats (SHRSP). J Nutr Sci Vitaminol 1999;45:95-106.

Mnafgui K, Hamden K, Salah HB, Kchaou M, Nasri M, Slama S, Derbali F, Allouche N, Elfeki A. Inhibitory Activities of *Zygophyllum album:* A Natural Weight-Lowering Plant on Key Enzymes in High-Fat Diet-Fed Rats. Evidence-Based Complementary and Alternative Medicine 2012:1-9.

Moghadasi M, Mohebbi H, Rahmani-Nia F, Hassan-Nia S, Noroozi H, Pirooznia N. High-intensity endurance training improves adiponectin mRNA and plasma concentrations. Eur J Appl Physiol 2012 Apr;112(4):1207-14.

Moghe SS, Juma S, Imrhan V, Vijayagopal P. Effect of Blueberry Polyphenols on 3T3-F442A Preadipocyte Differentiation. Journal of Medicinal Food May 2012;15(5):448-452.

Molan AL, Lila MA, Mawson J. Satiety in rats following blueberry extract consumption induced by appetite-suppressing mechanisms unrelated to *in vitro* or *in vivo* antioxidant capacity. Food Chemistry 2008;107:1039-1044.

Mong MC, Chao CY, Yin MC. Histidine and carnosine alleviated hepatic steatosis in mie consumed high saturated fat diet. European Journal of Pharmacology 2011;653:82-88.

Montagut G, Bladé I, Blay M, Fernández-Larrea J, Pujadas G, Salvadó MJ, Arola L, Pinent M, Ardévol A. Effects of a grapeseed procyanidin extract (GSPE) on insulin resistance. Journal of Nutritional Biochemistry 2010;21:961-967.

Monteiro R, Soares R, Guerreiro S, Pestana D, Calhau C, Azevedo I. Red wine increases adipose tissue aromatase expression and regulates body weight and adipocyte size. Nutrition 2009;25:699-705.

Moon MK, Ahn J, Lee H, Ha TY. Anti-obesity and hypolipidemic effects of chufa *(Cyperus esculentus* L.) in mice fed a high-fat diet. Food Science and Biotechnology 2012 Apr;21(2):317-322.

Moon YJ, Choi DS, Oh SH, Song YS, Cha YS. Effects of Persimmon-vinegar on Lipid and Carnitine Profiles in Mice. Food Sci. Biotechnol. 2010;19(2):343-348.

Moore R, Grant AM, Howard AN, Mills IH. Treatment of obesity with triiodothyronine and a very-low-calorie liquid formula diet. Lancet 1980 Feb 2;1(8162):223-6.

Moore R, Mehrishi JN, Verdoorn C, Mills IH. The role of T3 and its receptor in efficient metabolisers receiving very-low-calorie diets. Int J Obes. 1981;5(3):283-6.

Morales AJ, Nolan JJ, Nelson JC, Yen SS. Effects of replacement dose of dehydroepiandrosterone in men and women of advancing age. J Clin Endocrinol Metab 1994 Jun;78(6):1360-7.

Morales AJ, Haubrich RH, Hwang JY, Asakura H, Yen SS. The effect of six months treatment with a 100 mg daily dose of dehydroepiandrosterone (DHEA) on circulating sex steroids, body composition and muscle strength in age-advanced men and women. Clin Endocrinol (Oxf) 1998 Oct;49(4):421-32.

Moreno DA, Ilic N, Poulev A, Brasaemle DL, Fried SK, Raskin I. Inhibitory Effects of Grape Seed Extract on Lipases. Nutrition 2003;19:876-879.

Moreno DA, Ripoli C, Ilic N, Poulev A, Aubin C, Raskin I. Inhibition of lipid metabolic enzymes using *Mangifera indica* extracts. Journal: Food, Agriculture & Environment (JFAE) 2006;4(1):21-26.

Mori S, Satou M, Kanazawa S, Yoshizuka N, Hase T, Tokimitsu I, Takema Y, Nishizawa Y, Yada T. Body fat mass reduction and up-regulation of uncoupling protein by novel lipolysis-promoting plant extract. Int J Biol. Sci. 2009;5(4):311-8.

Morimoto C, Satoh Y, Hara M, Inoue S, Tsujita T, Okuda H. Anti-obese action of raspberry ketone. Life Sciences 2005;77:194-204.

Morise A, Mourot J, Riottot M, Weill P, Fénart E, Hermier D. Dose effect of alpha-linolenic acid on lipid metabolism in the hamster. Reprod. Nutr. Dev. 2005;45:405-418.

Morsi RMY, EL-Tahan NR, El-Hadad AMA. Effect of Aqueous Extract Mangifera Indica Leaves, as Functional Foods. Journal of Applied Sciences Research 2010;6(6):712-721.

Morteza P, Shahin MAS, Oryan S. The effects of anethum on plasma lipid and lipoprotein in normal and diabetic rats fed high fat diets. Shahrekord university of medical sciences journal winter 2010;11(4):15-25.

Motawea HM, Hashem FA, El-Shabrawl AE, El-Sherbini SM. Brassica Oleracea L. var Italica: A Nutritional Supplement for Weight Loss. Australian Journal of Medicinal Herbalism 2010;22(4):127-131.

Mourier A, Bigard AX, de Kerviler E, Roger B, Legrand H, Guezennec CY. Combined effects of caloric restriction and branched-chain amino acid supplementation on body composition and exercise performance in elite wrestlers. Int J Sports Med 1997 Jan;18(1):47-55.

Mukai Y, Sun Y, Sato S. Azuki bean polyphenols intake during lactation upregulate AMPK in male rat offspring exposed to fetal malnutrition. Nutrition 2012:1-7.

Mukai Y, Sun Y, Sato S. Azuki bean polyphenols intake during lactation upregulate AMPK in male rat offspring exposed to fetal malnutrition. Nutrition 2012:1-7.

Mulvihill EE, Assini JM, Lee JK, Allister EM, Sutherland SG, Koppes JB, Sawyez CG, Edwards JY, Telford DE, Charbonneau A, St-Pierre P, Marette A, Huff MW. Nobiletin attenuates VLDL overproduction, dyslipidemia, and atherosclerosis in mice with diet-induced insulin resistance. Diabetes 2011 May;60(5):1446-57.

Mun EG, Soh JR, Cha YS. L-Carnitine Reduces Obesity Caused by High-Fat Diet in C57BL/6J Mice. Food Science and Biotechnology 2007;16(2):228-233.

Mundada S, Shivhare R. Pharmacology of *Tridax procumbens* a Weed: Review. International Journal of PharmTech Research 2010 Apr-Jun;2(2):1391-1394.

Muraki E, Matsuoka C, Oikawa R, Sato S, Chiba H, Tsunoda N, Kasono K. Fenugreek Attenuates Lipid Accumulation in Normal Rats. J. Jpn Soc Nutr Food Sci 2011;64:99-106.

Muraki E, Chiba H, Taketani K, Hoshino S, Tsuge N, Tsunoda N, Kasono K. Fenugreek with reduced bitterness prevents dietinduced metabolic disorders in rats. Lipids in Health and Disease 2012;11:58.

Murase T, Haramizu S, Shimotoyodome A, Tokimitsu I, Hase T. Green tea extract improves running endurance in mice by stimulating lipid utilization during exercise. Am J Physiol Regul Integr Comp Physiol 2006 Jun;290(6):1550-6.

Murase T, Haramizu S, Shimotoyodome A, Tokimitsu I. Reduction of diet-induced obesity by a combination of tea-catechin intake and regular swimming. International Journal of Obesity 2006;30:561-568.

Murase T, Misawa K, Minegishi Y, Aoki M, Ominami H, Suzuki Y, Shibuya Y, Hase T. Coffee polyphenols suppress diet-induced body fat accumulation by downregulating SREBP-1c and molecules in C57BL/6J mice. Am J Physiol Endocrinol Metab 2011;300:122-133.

Murata M, Sano Y, Ishihara K, Uchida M. Dietary fish oil and Undaria pinnatifida (wakame) synergistically decrease rat serum and liver triacylglycerol. J Nutr. 2002 Apr;132(4):742-7.

Muruganandan S, Srinivasan K, Gupta S, Gupta PK, Lal J. Effect of mangiferin on hyperglycemia and atherogenicity in streptozotocin diabetic rats. J Ethnopharmacol 2005 Mar 21;97(3):497-501.

Muthu AK, Sethupathy S, Manavalan R, Karar PK. Hypolipidemic effect of of methanolic extract of Dolichos biflorus Linn. In high fat diet fed rats. Indian J Exp. Biol. 2005 Jun;43(6):522-5.

Muthu AK, Sethupathy S, Manavalan R, Karar PK. Antioxidant potential of methanolic extract of *Dolichos biflorus* Linn in high fat diet fed rabbits. Indian Journal of Pharmacology 2006;38(2):131-132.

Muthu K, Alagumanivasagam G, Satheesh Kumar D, Manavalan R. Effect of Methanolic Extract of Tuberous Root of *Ipomoea Digitata* (Linn) on Hyperlipidemia induced by rat fed with high fat diet. Research Journal of Pharmaceutical Biological and Chemical Sciences 2011;2(3):183-191.

Mustajoki P, Pekkarinen T. Very low energy diets in the treatment of obesity. The International Association for the Study of Obesity, obesity reviews 2001;2:61-72.

Myoung HJ, Kim G, Nam KW. Apigenin isolated from the seeds of *Perilla frutescens* britton var *crispa* (Benth.) inhibits food intake in C57BL/6J mice. Archives of Pharmacal Research 2010;33(11):1741-1746.

Na M, Hung TM, Oh WK, Min BS, Lee SH, Bae K. Fatty acid synthase inhibitory activity of dibenzocyclooctadiene lignans isolated from Schisandra chinensis. Phytother Res. 2010 Jun;24(2):225-8.

Naaz A, Yellayi S, Zakroczymski MA, Bunick D, Doerge DR, Lubahn DB, Helferich WG, Cooke PS. The Soy Isoflavone Genistein Decreases Adipose Deposition in Mice. Endocrinology 2003;144(8):3315-3320.

Nadeem S, Dhore P, Quazi M, Pawar S, Raji N. *Lagenaria siceraria* fruit extract ameliorate fat amassment and serum TNF − α in high-fat diet-induced obese rats. Asian Pacific Journal of Tropical Medicine 2012:698-702.

Nagao T, Komine Y, Soga S, Meguro S, Hase T, Tanaka Y, Tokimitsu I. Ingestion of a tea rich in catechins leads to a reduction in body fat and malondialdehyde-modified LDL in men. Am J Clin Nutr 2005 Jan;81(1):122-9.

Nagao T, Hase T, Tokimitsu I. A green tea extract high in catechins reduces body fat and cardiovascular risks in humans. Obesity (Silver Spring) 2007 Jun;15(6):1473-83.

Nagasako-Akazome Y, Kanda T, Ohtake Y, Shimasaki H, Kobayashi T. Apple Polyphenols Influence Cholesterol Metabolism in Healthy Subjects with Relatively High Body Mass Index. Journal of Oleo Science 2007;56(8):417-428.

Nagata E, Ichi I, Kataoka R, Matsushima M, Adachi N, Kitamura Y, Sasaki T, Kojo S. Effect of Nobiletin on Lipid Metabolism in Rats. Journal of Health Science 2010;56(6):705-711.

Nainwal P, Nanda D, Tripathi S. Reduction in Blood Cholesterol Level Using the Hydroalcoholic Extract of Fruits of *Lagenaria* siceraria. International Journal of Research in Pharmaceutical and Biomedical Sciences 2011;2(1):110-113.

Najmi A, Haque SF, Khan RA, Nasiruddin M. Therapeutic Effect Of Nigella Sativa Oil On Different Clinical And Biochemical Parameters In Metabolic Syndrome. The Internet Journal of Pharmacology 2008;5(2).

Nakagawa K, Kishida H, Arai N, Nishiyama T, Mae T. Licorice Flavonoids Suppress Abdominal Fat Accumulation and Increase in Blood Glucose Level in Obese Diabetic KK-A^y Mice. Biol. Pharm. Bull. 2004;27(11):1775-1778.

Nakamura Y, Tonogai Y. Effects of Grape Seed Polyphenols on Serum and Hepatic Lipid Contents and Fecal Steroid Excretion in Normal and Hypercholesterolemic Rats. Journal of Health Science 2002;48(6):570-578.

Nakamura Y, Natsume M, Yasuda A, Ishizaka M, Kawahata K, Koga J. Fructooligosaccharides suppress high-fat diet-induced fat accumulation in C57BL/6J mice. Biofactors 2011 Jun 14.

Nakatani T, Kim HJ, Kaburagi Y, Yasuda K, Ezaki O. A low fish oil inhibits SREBP-1 proteolytic cascade, while a high-fish-oil feeding decreases SREBP-1 mRNA in mice liver: relationship to anti-obesity. Journal of Lipid Research 2003;44:369-379.

Nakaya Y, Minami A, Harada N, Sakamoto S, Niwa Y, Ohnaka M. Taurine imroves insulin sensitivity in the Otsuka Long-Evans Tokushima Fatty rat, a model of spontaneous type 2 diabetes. Am J Clin Nutr 2000;71:54-8.

Nakazato K, Song H, Waga T. Effects of Dietary Apple Polyphenol on Adipose Tissues Weights in Wistar Rats. Exp. Anim. 2006;55(2):383-389.

Nam J, Choi H. Effect of butanol fraction from *Cassia tora L.* seeds on glycemic control and insulin secretion in diabetic rats. Nutrition Research and Practice 2008;2(4):240-246.

Nam KH, Baik HW, Choi TY, Yoon SG, Park SW, Joung H. Effects of Ethanol Extract of Onion on the Lipid Profiles in Patients with Hypercholesterolemia. Korean J Nutr. 2007 Apr;40(3):242-248.

Nammi S, Sreemantula S, Roufogalis BD. Protective effects of ethanolic extract of Zingiber officinale rhizome on the development of metabolic syndrome in high-fat diet-fed rats. Basic Clin Pharmacol Toxicol 2009 May;104(5):366-73.

Naowaboot J, Chung CH, Pannangpetch P, Choi R, Kim BH, Lee MY, Kukongviriyapan U. Mulberry leaf extract increases adiponectin in murine 3T3-L1 adipocytes. Nutrition Research 2012;32:39-44.

Narayanswamy VB, Setty MM, Malini S, Shirwaikar A. Preliminary aphrodisiac activity of hybanthus enneaspermus in rats. Pharmacologyonline 2007;1:152-161.

Nardelli TR, Ribeiro RA, Balbo SL, Vanzel EC, Carneiro EM, Boschero AC, Bonfleur ML. Taurine prevents fat deposition and ameliorates plasma lipid profile in monosodium glutamate-obese rats. Amino Acids 2011 Oct;41(4):901-8.

Naylor GJ, Grant L, Smith C. A double blind placebo controlled trial of ascorbic acid in obesity. Nutr Health 1985;4(1):25-8.

Nazar K, Kaciuba-Uscilko H, Szczepanik J, Zemba AW, Kruk B, Chwalbinska-Moneta J, Titow-Stupnicka E, Bicz B, Krotkiewski M. Phosphate supplementation prevents a decrease of triiodothyronine and increases resting metabolic rate during low energy diet. J Physiol Pharmacol 1996 Jun;47(2):373-83.

Nazari A, Delfan B, Shirkhani Y, Kiyani A. Effect of Satureja Khuzestanica on blood coagulation activity in rats. The Journal of Qazvin University of Medical Sciences 2006;9(4):15-18.

Nduhirabandi F, Du Toit EF, Blackhurst D, Marais D, Lochner A. Chronic melatonin consumption prevents obesity-related metabolic abnormalities and protects the heart against myocardial ischemia and reperfusion injury in a prediabetic model of diet-induced obesity. J Pineal Res. 2011 Mar;50(2):171-82.

Nehal MAE. Hepatoprotective effect of feeding celery leaves mixed with chicory leaves and barley grains to hypercholesterolemic rats. Pharmacognosy Magazine 2011;7(26):151-156.

Nemoseck TM, Carmody EG, Furchner-Evanson A, Gleason M, Li A, Potter H, Rezende LM, Lane KJ, Kern M. Honey promotes lower weight gain, adiposity, and triglycerides than sucrose in rats. Nutrition Research 2011;31:55-60.

Nestel PJ, Chronopulous A, Cehun M. Dairy fat in cheese raises LDL cholesterol less than that in butter in mildly hypercholesterolaemic subjects. Eur J Clin Nutr. 2005 Sep;59(9):1059-63.

Nestler JE, Barlascini CO, Clore JN, Blackward WG. Dehydroepiandrosterone reduces serum low density lipoprotein levels and body fat but does not alter insulin sensitivity in normal men. J Clin Endocrinol Metab 1988 Jan;66(1):57-61.

Neyestani TR, Shariat-Zadeh N, Gharavi A, Kalayi A, Khalaji N. The Opposite Associations of Lycopene and Body Fat Mass wtth Humoral Immunity in Type 2 Diabetes Mellitus: A Possible Role in Atherogenesis. Iran J Allergy Asthma Immunol 2007 June;6(2):79-87.

Ngondi JL, Oben JE, Minka SR. The effect *of Irvingia gabonensis* seeds on body weight and blood lipids of obese subjects in Cameroon. Lipids in Health and Disease 2005;4:12.

Ngondi JL, Etoundi BC, Nyangono CB, Mbofung CM, Oben JE. IGOB131, a novel seed extract of the West African plant Irvingia gabonensis, significantly reduces body weight and improves metabolic parameters in overweight humans in a randomized double-blind placebo controlled investigation. Lipids Health and Disease 2009 Mar 2;8:7.

Ninomiya K, Matsuda H, Kubo M, Morikawa T, Nishida N, Yoshikawa M. Potent anti-obese principle from *Rosa canina*: Structural requirements and mode of action of *trans*-tiliroside. Bioorganic & Medicinal Chemistry Letters 2007;17:3059-3064.

Nishi S, Saito Y, Koaze H, Hironaka K, Kojima M. Anti-obesity Effects of Seaberry *(Hippophae rhamnoides)* Leaf Polyphenols (SBLPP) in Male Mice Fed a High-fat Diet. Nippon Shokuhin Kagaku Kogaku Kaishi 2007;54(11):477-481.

Nishibe S, Yamaguchi S, Hasegawa M, Oba K, Fujikawa T. Anti-obesity effect of Forsythia leaf extract containing polyphenolic compounds and its mechanism. Journal of Traditional Medicines 2012 Aug 15;29(3):149-155.

Nishida H, Kuriyama Y, Kawakami K, Takei Y, Chiba T, Masuda H, Kazama K, Ohtsuka A, Sato S, Konishi T. Anti-obesitic Effect of Petit Vert on Mice Fed a High-fat Diet. J Jpn Soc Nutr Food Sci 2011;64:169-175.

Nishida S, Segawa T, Murai I, Nakagawa S. Long-term melatonin administration reduces hyperinsulinemia and improves the altered fatty-acid compositions in type 2 diabetic rats via the restoration of Δ-5 desaturase activity. J. Pineal Res. 2002;32:26-33.

Nissen SL, Abumrad NN. Nutritional role of the leucine metabolite β-hydroxy .β-methylbutyrate (HMB). Nutritional Biochemistry 1997;8:300-311.

Niu C, Chen C, Chen L, Cheng K, Yeh C, Cheng J. Decrease of blood lipids induced by Shan-Zha (fruit of Crataegus pinnatifida) is mainly related to an increase of PPARα in liver of mice fed high-fat diet. Horm Metab Res Aug 2011;43(9):625-30.

Niwano Y, Beppu F, Shimada T, Kyan R, Yasura K, Tamaki M, Nishino M, Midorikawa Y, Hamada H. Extensive Screening for Plant Foodstufs in Okinawa, Japan with Anti-Obese Activity on Adipocytes *In Vitro*. Plant Foods Hum Nutr 2009;64:6-10.

Noakes M, Keogh JB, Foster PR, Clifton PM. Effect of an energy-restricted, high-protein, low-fat diet relative to a conventional high-carbohydrate, low-fat diet on weight loss, body composition, nutritional status, and markers of cardiovascular health in obese women. Am J Clin Nutr 2005;81:1298-306.

Nomaguchi K, Tanaka M, Misawa E, Yamada M, Toida T, Iwatsuki K, Goto T, Kawada T. Aloe vera phytosterols act as ligands for PPAR and improve the expression levels of PPAR target genes in the livers of mice with diet-induced obesity. Obesity Research & Clinica Practice 2011;5:190-201.

Norazmir MN, Ayub MY, Ummi MMA. Enzyme Activities and Histology Study on High Fat Diet-induced Obese Rats by Pink Guave Puree. Pakistan Journal of Nutrition 2010;9(11):1100-1106.

Noreen EE, Sass MJ, Crowe ML, Pabon VA, Brandauer J, Averill LK. Effects of supplemental fish oil on resting metabolic rate, body composition, and salivary cortisol in healthy adults. Journal of the International Society of Sports Nutrition 2010;7:31.

Norris LE, Collene AL, Asp ML, Hsu JC, Liu LF, Richardson JR, Li D, Bell D, Osei K, Jackson RD, Belury MA. Comparison of dietary conjugated linoleic acid with safflower oil on body composition in obese postmenopausal women with type 2 diabetes mellitus. Am J Clin Nutr. 2009 Sep;90(3):468-76.

Nosaka N, Maki H, Suzuki Y, Haruna H, Ohara A, Kasai M, Tsuji H, Aoyama T, Okazaki M, Igarashi O, Kondo K. Effects of margarine containing medium-chain triacylglycerols on body fat reduction in humans. J Atheroscler Thromb 2003;10(5):290-8.

Novelli ELB, Santos PP, Assalin HB, Souza G, Rocha K, Ebaid GX, Seiva FRF, Mani F, Fernandes AA. N-acetylcysteine in high-sucrose diet-induced obesity: Energy expenditure and metabolic shifting for cardiac health. Pharmacological Research 2009;59:74-79.

Nugroho A, Bachri MS, Choi J, Choi JS, Kim WB, Lee BI, Kim JD, Park HJ. The Inhibitory Effect of Caffeoylquinic acid-Rich Extract of *Ligularia stenocephala* Leaves on Obesity in th High Fat Diet-Induced Rat. Natural Product Sciences 2010;16(2):80-87.

Nurrochmad A, Leviana F, Wulancarsari CG, Lukitaningsih E. Phytoestrogens of *Pachyrhizus erosus* prevent Bone Loss in an Ovariectomized Rat Model of Osteoporosis. International Journal of Phytomedicine 2010;2:363-372.

Nwaoguikpe RN, Braide W. The effect of aqueus seed extract of *persea americana* (avocado pear) on serum lipid and cholesterol levels in rabbits. Africn Journal of Pharmacy and Pharmacology Research 2011 Apr;1(2):23-29.

Nwozo SO, Orojobi BF, Adaramoye OA. Hypolipidemic and antioxidant potentials of Xylopia aethiopica seed extract in hypercholesterolemic rats. J Med Food 2011;14(1-2):114-9.

Nyarko AK, Asare-Anane H, Ofosuhene M, Addy ME. Extract of *Ocimum canum* lowers blood glucose and facilitates insulin release by isolated pancreatic β-islet cells. Phytomedicine 2002;9:346-351.

Nyarko AK, Asare-Anane H, Ofosuhene M, Addy ME, Teye K, Addo P. Aqueous extract of *Ocimum canum* decreases levels of fasting blood glucose and free radicals and increases antiatherogenic lipid levels in mice. Vascular Pharmacology 2003;39:273-279.

Nybo L, Sundstrup E, Jakobsen MD, Mohr M, Hornstrup T, Simonsen L, Bülow J, Randers MB, Nielsen JJ, Aagaard P, Krustrup P. High-intensity training versus traditional exercise interventions for promoting health. Med Sci Sports Exerc 2010 Oct;42(10):1951- 8.

Obara K, Mizutani M, Hitomi Y, Yajima H, Kondo K. Isohumulones, the bitter component of beer, improve hyperglycemia and decrease body fat in Japanese subjects with prediabetes. Clinical Nutrition 2009;28:278-284.

Oben J, Kuate D, Agbor G, Momo C, Talla X. The use of *a Cissus quadrangularis* formulation in the management of weight loss and metabolic syndrome. Lipids in Health and Disease 2006;5:24.

Oben J, Enonchong E, Kothari S, Chambliss W, Garrison R, Dolnick D. *Phellodendron* and *Citrus* extracts benefit cardiovascular health in osteoarthritis patients: a double-blind, placebo-controlled pilot study. Nutrition Journal 2008;7:16.

Oben J, Enonchong E, Kothari S, Chambliss W, Garrison R, Dolnick D. Phellodendron and Citrus extracts benefit joint health in osteoarthritis patients: a pilot, double-blind, placebo-controlled study. Nutr J. 2009 Aug 14;8:38.

Oben JE, Ngondi JL, Momo CN, Agbor GA, Sobgui CSM. The use of *a Cissus quadrangularis/Irvingia gabonensis* combination in the management of weight loss: a double-blind placebo-controlled study. Lipids in Health and Disease 2008;7:12.

O'Dea K. Marked improvement in carbohydrated and lipid metabolism in diabetic Australian aborigines after temporary reversion to traditional lifestyle. Diabetes 1984 Jun;33(6):596-603.

Odetola AA, Iranloye YO, Akinloye O. Hypolipidaemic Potentials of *Solanum melongena* and *Solanum gilo* on Hypercholesterolemic Rabbits. Pakistan Journal of Nutrition 2004;3(3):180-187.

Oh J, Min OJ, Kim HA, Kim YJ, Baek HY, Rhyu DY. Effect of *Eriobotrya japonica* on Adipogenesis and Body Weight. J Korean Soc. Appl. Biol. Chem. 2011;54(3):382-387.

Oh JK, Shin YO, Jung HJ, Lee JE. Effect of Rhodiola Sachalinensis Administration and Endurance Exercise on Insulin Sensitivity and Expression of Proteins Related with Glucose Transport in Skeletal Muscle of Obese Zucker Rat. Korean J Nutr 2006 Jun;39(4):323-330.

Oh KS, Ryu SY, Lee S, Seo HW, Oh BK, Kim YS, Lee BH. Melanin-concentrating hormone-1 receptor antagonism and anti-obesity effects of ethanolic extract from *Morus alba* leaves in diet-induced obese mice. Journal of Ethnopharmacology 2009;122:216-220.

Oh SH, Moon YJ, Soh JR, Cha YS. Effect of Water Extract of Germinated Brown Rice on Adiposity and Obesity Indices in Mice Fed a High Fat Diet. J Food Sci Nutr 2005;10:251-256.

Oh TW, Ohta F. Capsaicin increases endurance capacity and spares tissue glycogen through lipolytic function in swimming rats. J Nutr Sci Vitaminol (Tokyo) 2003 Apr;49(2):107-11.

Ohara K, Kiyotani Y, Uchida A, Nagasaka R, Maehara H, Kanemoto S, Hori M, Ushio H. Oral administration of γ-aminobutyric acid and γ-oryzanol prevents stress-induced hypoadiponectinemia. Phytomedicine 2011;18:655-660.

Ohashi K, Bohgaki T, Shibuya H. Antihypertensive substance in the leaves of kumis kucing (Orthosiphon aristatus) in Java Island. Yakugaku Zasshi 2000 May;120(5):474-82.

Ohkoshi E, Miyazaki H, Shindo K, Watanabe H, Yoshida A, Yajima H. Constituents from the leaves of Nelumbo nucifera stimulate lipolysis in the white adipose tissue of mice. Planta Med 2007 Oct;73(12):1255-9.

Ohnogi H, Hayami S, Kudo Y, Enoki T. Efficacy and Safety of *Ashitaba (Angelica keiskei)* on the Patients and Candidates with Metabolic Syndrome: A Pilot Study. Japanese Journal of Complementary and Alternative Medicine 2012 March;9(1):49-55.

Ohnuki K, Niwa S, Maeda S, Inoue N, Yazawa S, Fushiki T. CH-19 Sweet, a Non-Pungent Cultivar of Red Pepper, Increased Body Temperature and Oxygen Consumption in Humans. Biosci. Biotechnol. Biochem. 2001;65(9):2033-2036.

Ohta Y, Sami M, Kanda T, Saito K, Osada K, Kato H. Gene Expression Analysis of the Anti-obesity Effect by Apple Polyphenols in Rats Fed a High Fat Diet or a Normal Diet. Journal of Oleo Science 2006;55(6):305-314.

Ohtsuki M, Umeshita K, Kokean Y, Nishii T, Sakakura H, Yanagita T, Hisamatsu M, Furuichi Y. Suppressive Effects of Bunashimeji (*Hypsizigus marmoreus*) on Triacylglycerol Accumulation in C57BL/6J Mice. Nippon Shokuhin Kagaku Kogaku Kaishi 2007;54(4):167-172.

Ohyama K, Furuta C, Nogusa Y, Nomura K, Miwa T, Suzuki K. Catechin-rich grape seed extract supplementation attenuates diet-induced obesity in C57BL/6J mice. Ann Nutr Metab 2011;58(3):250-8.

Oi-Kano Y, Kawada T, Watanabe T, Koyama F, Watanabe K, Senbongi R, Iwai K. Oleuropein, a Phenolic Compound in Extra Virgin Olive Oil, Increases Uncoupling Protein 1 Content in Brown Adipose Tissue and Enhances Noradrenaline and Adrenaline Secretions in Rats. J Nutr Sci Vitaminol 2008;54:363-370.

Oi-Kano Y, Kawada T, Watanabe T, Koyama F, Watanabe K, Senbongi R, Iwai K. Oleuropein supplementation increases urinary noradrenaline and testicular testosterone levels and decreases plasma corticosterone level in rats fed high-protein diet. Journal of Nutritional Biochemistry 2012.

Oi Y, Kawada T, Shishido C, Wada K, Kominato Y, Nishimura S, Ariga T, Iwai K. Allyl-containing sulfides in garlic increase uncoupling protein content in brown adipose tissue, and noradrenaline and adrenaline secretion in rats. J Nutr. 1999 Feb;129(2):336-42.

Oi Y, Hou IC, Fujita H, Yazawa K. Antiobesity effects of Chinese black tea (Pu-erh tea) extract and gallic acid. Phytother Res 2012

Apr;26(4):475-81.

Ojewole J, Kamadyaapa DR, Gondwe MM, Moodley K, Musabayane CT. Cardiovascular effects of *Persea americana* Mill (Lauraceae) (avocado) aqueous leaf extract in experimental animals. Cardiovascular Journal of South Africa 2007 Apr;18(2):69-76.

Okada T, Mizuno Y, Sibayama S, Hosokawa M, Miyashita K. Antiobesity effects of Undaria lipid capsules prepared with scallop phospholipids. J Food Sci. 2011 Jan-Feb;76(1):2-6.

Okada Y, Okada M, Sagesaka Y. Screening of dried plant seed extracts for adiponectin production activity and tumor necrosis factor-alpha inhibitory activity on 3T3-L1 adipocytes. Plant Food Hum Nutr. 2010 Sep;65(3):225-32.

Okuda H, Morimoto C, Tsujita T. Relationship between cyclic AMP production and lipolysis induced by forskolin in rat fat cells. J Lipid Res. 1992 Feb;33(2):225-31.

Okumura Y, Narukawa M, Watanabe T. Adiposity Suppression Effect in Mice Due to Black Pepper and Its Main Pungent Component, Piperine. Biosci. Biotechnol. Biochem. 2010;74(8):1545-1549.

Olorunnisola OS, Bradley G, Afolayan AJ. Protective Effect of *Tulbaghia violacea* Harv. on Aortic Pathology, Tissue Antioxidant Enzymes and Liver Damage in Diet-Induced Atherosclerotic Rats. Int. J. Mol. Sci. 2012;13:12747-12760.

Oluremi OIA, Okafor FN, Adenkola AY, Orayaga KT. Effect of Fermentation of Sweet Orange *(Citrus sinensis)* Fruit Peel on its Phytonutrients and the Performance of Broiler Starter. International Journal of Poultry Science 2010;9(6):546-549.

Onakpoya I, Terry R, Ernst E. The Use of Green Coffee Extract as a Weight Loss Supplement. A Systematic Review and Meta-Analysis of Randomized Clinical Trials. Hindawi Publishing Corporation Gastroenterology Research and Practice Volume 2011;1-6.

Onderoglu S, Sozer S, Erbil KM, Ortac R, Lermioglu F. The evaluation of long-term effects of cinnamon bark and olive leaf on toxicity inducedd by streptozotocin administration to rats. J Pharm Pharmacol 1999 Nov;51(11):1305-12.

Ong KW, Hsu A, Song L, Huang D, Tan BKH. Polyphenols-rich *Vernonia amygdalina* shows anti-diabetic effects in streptozotocin-induced diabetic rats. Journal of Ethnopharmacology 2011;133:598-607.

Ono T, Morishita S, Fujisaki C, Ohdera M, Murakoshi M, Iida N, Kato H, Miyashita K, Iigo M, Yoshida T, Sugiyama K, Nishino H. Effects of pepsin and trypsin on the anti-adipogenic actio of lactoferrin against pre-adipocytes derived from rat mesenteric fat. British Journal of Nutrition 2011;105:200-211.

Ono T, Murakoshi M, Suzuki N, Iida N, Ohdera M, Iigo M, Yoshida T, Sugiyama K, Nishino H. Potent anti-obesity effect of enteric-coated lactoferrin: decrease in visceral fat accumulation in Japanese men and women with abdominal obesity after 8-week administration of enteric-coated lactoferrin tablets. British Journal of Nutrition 2010;104:1688-1695.

Ono Y, Hattori E, Fukaya Y, Imai S, Ohizumi Y. Anti-obesity effect of *Nelumbo nucifera* leaves extract in mice and rats. Journal of Ethnopharmacology 2006;106:238-244.

Opara EC, Petro A, Tevrizian A, Feinglos MN, Surwit RS. L-glutamine supplementation of a high fat diet reduces body weight and attenuates hyperglycemia and hyperinsuliemia in C57BL/6J mice. J Nutr 1996 Jan;126(1):273-9.

Oscai LB, Miller WC, Arnall DA. Effects of dietary sugar and of dietary fat on food intake and body fat content in rats. Growth 1987 Spring;51(1):64-73.

Osterdahl M, Kocturk T, Koochek A, Wändell PE. Effects of a short-term intervention with a paleolithic diet in healthy volunteers. Eur J Clin Nutr 2008 May;62(5):682-5.

Ostojic SM. Yohimbine: the effects on body composition and exercise performance in soccer players. Res Sports Med. 2006 Oct-Dec;14(4):289-99.

Ostojic SM, Calleja J, Jourkesh M. Effects of Short-Term Dehydroepiandrosterone Supplementation on Body Composition in Young Athletes. Chinese Journal of Physiology 2010;53(1):19-25.

Ota N, Soga S, Murase T, Shimotoyodome A, Hase T. Consumption of Coffee Polyphenols Increases Fat Utilization in Humans. Journal of Health Science 2010;56(6):745-751.

Ou TT, Hsu MJ, Chan KC, Huang CN, Ho HH, Wang CJ. Mulberry extract inhibits oleic acid-induced lipid accumulation via reduction of lipogenesis and promotion of hepatic lipid clearance. J Sci Food Agric 2011 Dec;91(15):2740-8.

Oulmouden F, Saïle R, Gnaoui NE, Benomar H, Lkhider M, Amrani S, Ghalim N. Hypolipidemic and Anti-Atherogenic Effect of Aqueous Extract of Fennel *(Foeniculum Vulgare)* Extract in an Experimental Model of Atherosclerosis Induced by Triton WR-1339. European Journal of Scientific Research 2011;52(1):91-99.

Pahua-Ramos ME, Ortiz-Moreno A, Chamorro-Cevallos G, Hernández-Navarro MD, Garduño-Siciliano L, Necoechea-Mondragón H, Hernández-Ortega M. Hypolipidemic Effect of Avocado (*Persea americana* Mill) Seed in a Hypercholesterolemic Mouse Model. Plant Foods Hum Nutr 2012;67:10-16.

Paiva-Martins F, Barbosa S, Pinheiro V, Mourão JL, Outor-Monteiro D. The effect of olive leaves supplementation on the feed digestibility, growth performance of pigs and quality of pork meat. Meat Science 2009;82:438-443.

Pal S, Khossousi A, Binns C, Dhaliwal S, Ellis V. The effect of a fibre supplement compared to a healthy diet on body composition, lipids, glucose, insulin and other metabolic syndrome risk factors in overweight and obese individuals. British Journal of Nutrition 2011;105:90-100.

Panchal SK, Wong WY, Kauter K, Ward LC, Brown L. Caffeine attenuates metabolic syndrome in diet-induced obese rats. Nutrition 2012:1-8.

Panchal SK, Poudyal H, Waanders J, Brown L. Coffee extract attenuates changes in cardiovascular and hepatic structure and function without decreasing obesity in high-carbohydrate, high-fat diet-fed male rats. Nutrition 2012 Apr;142(4):690-7.

Panchal SK, Ward L, Brown L. Ellagic acid attenuates high-carbohydrate, high-fat diet-induced metabolic syndrome in rats. Eur J Nutr. 2012 Apr 27.

Panchal SK, Poudyal H, Brown L. Quercetin ameliorates cardiovascular, hepatic, and metabolic changes in diet-induced metabolic syndrome in rats. J Nutr 2012 Jun;142(6):1026-32.

Panchal SK, Poudyal H, Arumugam TV, Brown L. Rutin attenuates metabolic changes, nonalcoholic steatohepatitis, and cardiovascular remodeling in high-carbohydrate, high-fat diet-fed rats. J Nutr 2011 Jun;141(6):1062-9.

Pande S, Srinivasan K. Potentiation of Hypolipidemic and Weight Reducing Influence of Dietary Tender Cluster Bean (Cyamopsis tetragonoloba) when combined with Capsaicin in High-fat fed Rats. J Agric Food Chem. 2012 Jul 27

Pande VV, Dubey S. Antihyperlipidemic activity of *Sphaeranthus indicus* on atherogenic diet induced hyperlipidemia in rats.

Indian Journal of Green Pharmacy 2009;3(2):159-161.

Pandey D, Pandey S, Hemalatha S. Hypolipidemic Activity of Aqueous Extract of *Melothria Maderaspatana*. Pharmacologyonline 2010;3:76-83.

Panton LB, Rathmacher JA, Baier S, Nissen S. Nutritional Supplementation of the Leucine Metabolite β-Hydroxy-β-Methylbutyrate (HMB) During Resistance Training. Nutrition 2000;16:734-739.

Paoli A, Pacelli F, Bargossi AM, Marcolin G, Guzzinati S, Neri M, Bianco A, Palma A. Effect of three distinct protocols of fitness training on body composition, strength and blood lactate. J Sports Med Phys Fitness 2010 Mar;50(1):43-51.

Paoli A, Cenci L, Grimaldi KA. Effect of ketogenic Mediterranean diet with phytoextracts and low carbohydrates/high-protein meals on weight, cardiovascular risk factors, body composition and diet compliance in Italian council employees. Nutr J 2011 Oct 12;10:112.

Paranjpe P, Patki P, Patwardhan B. Ayurvedic treatment of obesity: A randomised double-blind, placebo-controlled clinical trial. Journal of Ethnopharmacology 1990;29:1-11.

Parhizkar S, Latiff LA, Sabariah AR, Mohammad AD. Preventive effect of *Nigella sativa* on metabolic sydrome in menopause induced rats. Journal of Medicinal Plants Research 2011 Apr;5(8):1478-1484.

Park CH, Cho EJ, Yokozawa T. Protection against hypercholesterolemia by Corni fructus extract and its related protective mechanism. J Med Food 2009 Oct;12(5):973-81.

Park HJ, Lee MK, Park YB, Shin YC, Choi MS. Beneficial effects of *Undaria pinnatifida* ethanol extract on diet-induced-insulin resistance in C57BL/6J mice. Food and Chemical Toxicology 2011;49:727-733.

Park HJ, Cho JY, Kim MK, Koh PO, Cho KW, Kim CH, Lee KS, Chung BY, Kim GS, Cho JH. Anti-obesity effect of *Schisandra chinensis* in 3T3-L1 cells and high fat diet-induced obese rats. Food Chemistry 2012;134:227-234.

Park HJ, Jung UJ, Cho SJ, Jung HK, Shim S, Choi MS. Citrus unshiu peel extract ameliorates hyperglycemia and hepatic steatosis by altering inflammation and hepatic glucose- and lipid-regulation enzymes in *db/db* mice. Journal of Nutritional Biochemistry 2012.

Park HW, Yang MS, Lee JH, Shin ES, Kim Y, Chun JY, Lee TR, Lee SJ. Long Term Feeding with Soy Isoflavone and L-Carnitine Synergistically Suppresses Body Weight Gain and Adiposity in High-Fat Diet Induced Obese Mice. Nutritional Sciences 2006 Aug;9(3):179-189.

Park JA, Ha SK, Kang TH, Oh MS, Cho MH, Lee SY, Park JH, Kim SY. Protective effect of apigenin on ovariectomy-induced bone loss in rats. Life Sciences 2008;82:1217-1223.

Park JA, Tirupathi Pichiah PB, Yu JJ, Oh SH, Daily JW 3rd, Cha YS. Anti-obesity effect of kimchi fermented with Weissella koreensis OK1-6 as starter in high-fat diet-induced obese C57BL/J mice. J Appl Microbiol. 2012 Sep 15.

Park JB, Velasquez MT. Potential effects of lignan-enriched flaxseed powder on bodyweight, visceral fat, lipid profile, and blood pressure in rats. Fitoterapia 2012;83:941-946.

Park JE, Cha YS. *Stevia rebaudiana* Bertoni extract supplementation improves lipid and carnitine profiles in C57BL/6J mice fed a high-fat diet. J Sci Food Agric 2010;90:1099-1105.

Park JH, Lee KW, Sung KS, Kim SS, Cho KD, Lee BH, Han CK. Effect of Diets with Job's Tears and *Cudrania tricuspidata* Leaf Mixed-powder Supplements on Body Fat and Serum Lipid Levels in Rats Fed a High-Fat Diet. J Korean Soc. Food Sci. Nutr. 2012;41(7):943-949.

Park JY, Kim MK. Effect of Feeding Garcinia Cambogia Extract (HCA) and/or L-Carnitine and Exercise on Body Weight in Rats. Korean J Nutr. 2005 Oct;38(8):637-648.

Park KW, Lee JE, Park KM. Diets containing *Sophora japonica* L. prevent weight gain in high-fat diet-induced obese mice. Nutrition Research 2009;29:819-824.

Park MY, Seo DW, Lee JY, Sung MK, Lee YM, Jang HH, Choi HY, Kim JH, Park DS. Effects of *Panicum milliaceum* L. extract on adipogenic transcription factors and fatty acid accumulation in 3T3-L1 adipocytes. Nutrition Research and Practice *(Nutr Res. Pract)* 2011;5(3):192-197.

Park MY, Jang HH, Kim JB, Yoon HN, Lee JY, Lee YM, Kim JH, Park DS. Hog millet *(Panicum milliaceum* L.)-supplemented diet ameliorates hyperlipidemia and hepatic lipid accumulation in C57BL/6J-*ob/ob* mice. Nutrition Research and Practice *(Nutr Res. Pract)* 2011;5(6):511-519.

Park MY, Jang HH, Lee JY, Lee YM, Kim JH, Park JH, Park DS. Effect of Hog Millet Supplementation on Hepatic Steatosis and Insulin Resistance in Mice Fed a High-fat Diet. J. Korean Soc Food Sci. Nutr. 2012;41(4):501-509.

Park SA, Choi MS, Kim MJ, Jung UJ, Kim HJ, Park KK, Noh HJ, Park HM, Park YB, Lee JS, Lee MK. Hypoglycemic and hypolipidemic action of Du-zhong *(Eucommia ulmoides* Oliver) leaves water extract in C57BL/KsJ-*db/db* mice. Journal of Ethnopharmacology 2006;107:412-417.

Park SH, Ko SK, Chung SH. *Euonymus alatus* prevents the hyperglycemia and hyperlipidemia induced by high-fat diet in ICR mice. Journal of Ethnopharmacology 2005;102:326-335.

Park SH, Ko SK, Choi JG, Chung SH. Salicornia herbacea prevents high fat diet-induced hyperglycemia and hyperlipidemia in ICR mice. Arch Pharm Res 2006 Mar;29(3):256-64.

Park SH, Park TS, Cha YS. Grape seed extract *(Vitis vinifera)* partially reverses high fat diet-induced obesity in C57BL/6J mice. Nutrition Research and Practice 2008;2(4):227-233.

Park UH, Jeong JC, Jang JS, Sung MR, Youn H, Lee SJ, Kim EJ, Um SJ. Negative Regulation of Adipogenesis by Kaempferol, a Component of Rhizoma Polygonati falcatum in 3T3-L1 Cells. Biol. Pharm. Bull. 2012;35(9):1525-33.

Park Y, Suzuki H, Lee YS, Hayakawa S, Wada S. Effect of coix on plasma, liver, and fecal lipid components in the rat fed on lard- or soybean oil-cholesterol diet. Biochem Med Metab Biol. 1988 Feb;39(1):11-7.

Park YH, Kim HY, Lim SH, Kim KH, Lee JH, Kim YG, Ahn YS. Effects of Ethanol Extract from Leaves of *Eleuterococcus senticosu* on Hyperlipidemia in Rats. J Korean Soc. Food Sci. Nutr 2012;41(3):333-338.

Park YS, Cha MH, Yoon YS, Ahn HS. Effect of Low Calorie Diet on *Platycodon Grandiflorum* Extract on Fatty Acid Binding Protein Expression in Rats with Diet-induced Obesity. Nutritional Sciences 2005 Feb;8(1):3-9.

Park YS, Yoon Y, Ahn HS. *Platycodon grandiflorum* extract represses up-regulated adipocyte fatty acid binding protein triggered by a high fat feeding in obese rats. World J Gastroenterol 2007 July;13(25):3493-3499.

Park YS, Kang JS. Korean Red Ginseng Extract Suppresses the Progression of Alcoholic Fatty Liver in a Rat Model. Journal of Health Science 2011;57(6):512-520.

Parmar HS, Kar A. Possible amelioration of atherogenic diet induced dyslipidemia, hypothyroidism and hyperglycemia by the peel extracts of Mangifera indica, Cucumis melo ad Citrullus vulgaris fruits in rats. Biofactors 2008;33(1):13-24.

Parmar HS, Kar A. Protective role of Mangifera indica, Cucumis melo and Citrullus vulgaris peel extracts in chemically induced hypothyroidism. Chem Biol Interact 2009 Feb 12;177(3):254-8.

Parra P, Bruni G, Palou A, Serra F. Dietary calcium attenuation of body fat gain during high-fat feeding in mice. Journal of Nutritional Biochemistry 2008;19:109-117.

Partida-Hernández G, Arreola F, Fenton B, Cabeza M, Román-Ramos R, Revilla-Monsalve MC. Effect of zinc replacement on lipids and lipoproteins in type 2-diabetic patients. Biomedicine & Pharmacotherapy 2006;60:161-168.

Patel DK, Patel KA, Patel UK, Thounaojam MC, Jadeja RN, Ansarullah, Padate GS, Salunke SP, Devkar RV, Ramachandran AV. Assessment of lipid lowering effect of *Sida rhomboidea Roxb* methanolic extract in experimentally induced hyperlipidemia. Pharmacology 2009;1(3):233-238.

Patel DK, Desai SN, Devkar RV, Ramachandran AV. *Coriandrum sativum* L. aqueous extract mitigates high fat diet induced insulin resistance by controlling visceral adiposity in C57BL/6J mice. Boletin Latinoamericano y del Caribe de Plantas Medicinales y Aromátics 2011;10(2):127-135.

Patil RH, Prakash K, Maheshwari VL. Hypolipidemic Effect of *Celastrus paniculatus* in Experimentally Induced Hypercholesterolemic Wistar Rats. Ind J Clin Biochem 2010 Oct-Decd;25(4):405-410.

Patil RH, Prakash K, Maheshwari VL. Hypolipidemic effect of *Terminalia arjuna* (L.) in experimentally induced hypercholesteremic rats. Acta Biologica Szegediensis 2011;55(2):289-293.

Patil YR, Sawant RS. Evaluation of efficacy of karshaniya yavagu (an ayurvedic preparation) in management of obesity. IJRAP 2012 Mar - Apr;3(2):295-298.

Pecháňová O, Zicha J, Kojšová S, Dobešová Z, Jendeková L, Kuneš J. Effect of chronic N-acetylcysteine treatment on the development of spontaneous hypertension. Clinical Science 2006;110:235-242.

Peng CH, Chang HC, Yang MY, Huang CN, Wang SJ, Wang CJ. Oat attenuate non-alcoholic fatty liver and obesity via inhibiting lipogenesis in high fat-fed rat. Journal of Functional Foods 2012.

Pérez YY, Jiménez-Ferrer E, Zamilpa A, Hernández-Valencia M, Alarcón-Aguilar FJ, Tortoriello J, Román-Ramos R. Effect of a Polyphenol-Rich Extract from *Aloe vera* Gel on Experimentally Induced Insulin Resistance in Mice. The American Journal of Chinese Medicine 2007;35(6):1037-1046.

Perez-Guisado J, Muñoz-Serrano A, Alonso-Moraga A. Spanish Ketogenic Mediterranean Diet: a healthy cardiovascular diet for weight loss. Nutr J. 2008 Oct 26;7:30.

Petrofsky J, Batt J, Morris A. Weight Loss and Cardiovascular Fitness During a 1-Week Diet and Exercise Program. The Journal of Applied Research 2006;6(1):51-61.

Petrofsky JS, Bonacci J, Bonilla T, Jorritsma R, Morris A, Hanson A, Somers R, Laymon M, Hill J. Effect of a 1-Week Dietand Exercise Program on Weight and Limb Girth. The Journal of Applied Research 2004;4(2):369-379.

Pfeuffer M, Auinger A, Bley U, Kraus-Stojanowic I, Laue C, Winkler P, Rüfer CE, Frank J, Bösch-Saadatmandi C, Rimbach G, Schrezenmeir J. Effect of quercetin on traits of the metabolic syndrome, endothelial function and inflammatory parameters in men with different *APOE* isoforms. Nutrition, Metabolism & Cardiovascular Diseases 2011:1-7.

Phachonpai W, Muchimapura S, Wattanathorn J, Wannanon P, Thukhammee W, Thipkaew C, Tong-Un T. The 100-Days Oral Toxicity of Tomato Pomace in Healthy Mice. American Journal of Pharmacology and Toxicology 2012;7(1):27-32.

Phinney SD, Tang AB, Thumond DC, Nakamura MT, Stern JS. Abnormal Polyunsaturated Lipid Metabolism in the Obese Zucker Rat, With Partial Metabolic Correction by γ-Linolenic Acid Administration. Metabolism 1993;42(9):1127-1140.

Pierro FD, Menghi AB, Barreca A, Lucarelli M, Calandrelli A. GreenSelect® Phytosome as an Adjunct to a Low-Calorie Diet for Treatment of Obesity: A Clinical Trial. Alternative Medicine Review 2009;14(2):154-160.

Piers LS, Walker KZ, Stoney RM, Soares MJ, O'Dea K. The influence of the type of dietary fat on postprandial fat oxidation rates: monounsaturated (olive oil) *vs* saturated fat (cream). International Journal of Obesity 2002;26:814-821.

Piers LS, Walker KZ, Stoney RM, Soares MJ, O'Dea K. Substitution of saturated with monounsaturated fat in a 4-week diet affects body weight and composition of overweight and obese men. British Journal of Nutrition 2003;90:717-727.

Pilon G, Ruzzin J, Rioux LE, Lavigne C, White PJ, Frøyland L, Jacques H, Bryl P, Beaulieu L, Marette A. Differential effects of various fish proteins in altering body weight, adiposity, inflammatory status, and insulin sensitivity in high-fat-fed rats. Metabolism Clinical and Experimental 2011;60:1122-1130.

Pittas AG, Das SK, Hajduk CL, Golden J, Saltzman E, Stark PC, Greenberg AS, Roberts SB. A low-glycemic load diet facilitates greater weight loss in overweight adults with high insulin secretion but not in overweight adults with low insulin secretion in the CALERIE Trial. Diabetes Care 2005 Dec;28(12):2939-41.

Pilvi TK, Korpela R, Huttunen M, Vapaatalo H, Mervaala EM. High-calcium diet with whey protein attenuates body-weight gain in high-fat-fed C57Bl/J mice. British Journal of Nutrition 2007;98:900-907.

Pilvi TK, Harala S, Korpela R, Mervaala EM. Effects of high-calcium diets with different whey proteins on weight loss and regain in high-fat-fed C57BL/6J mice. British Journal of Nutrition 2009;102:337-341.

Piña-Zentella G, de la Rosa-Cuevas G, Vázquez-Meza H, Piña E, de Piña MZ. Taurine in adipocytes prevents insulin-mediated H(2)o(2) generation and activates Pka and lipolysis. Amino Acids 2012 May;42(5):1927-35.

Piyachaturawat P, Teeratagolpisal N, Toskulkao C, Suksamrarn A. Hypolipidemic effect of Curcuma comosa in mice. Artery 1997;22(5):233-41.

Piyachaturawat P, Charoenpiboonsin J, Toskulkao C, Suksamrarn A. Reduction of plasma cholesterol by Curcuma comosa extract in hypercholesterolaemic hamsters. J Ethnopharmacol 1999 Aug;66(2):199-204.

Poduri A, Rateri DL, Saha SK, Saha S, Daugherty A. *Citrullus lanatus* 'sentinel' (watermelon) extract reduces atherosclerosis in LDL receptor-deficient mice. Journal of Nutritional Biochemistry 2012.

Polak J, Klimcakova E, Moro C, Viguerie N, Berlan M, Hejnova J, Richterova B, Kraus I, Langin D, Stich V. Effect of aerobic training on plasma levels and subcutaneous abdominal adipose tissue gene expression of adiponectin, leptin, interleukin 6, and tumor necrosis factor alpha in obese women. Metabolism 2006 Oct;55(10):1375-81.

Popkin BM, Barclay DV, Nielsen SJ. Water and food consumption patterns of U.S. Adults from 1999 to 2001. Obes Res. 2005 Dec;13(12):2146-52.

Poole C, Bushey B, Foster C, Campbell B, Willoughby D, Kreider R, Taylor L, Wilborn C. The effects of a commercially available botanical supplement on strength, body composition, power output, and hormonal profiles in resistance-trained males. Journal of the International Society of Sports Nutrition 2010;7:34.

Poudyal H, Panchal S, Brown L. Comparison of purle carrot juice and β-carotene in a high-carbohydrate, high-fat diet-fed rat model of the metabolic syndrome. British Journal of Nutrition 2010;104:1322-1332.

Poudyal H, Campbell F, Brown L. Olive leaf extract attenuates cardiac, hepatic, and metabolic changes in high carbohydrate-, high fat-fed rats. J Nutr. 2010 May;140(5):946-53.

Pourkabir M, Shomali T, Asadi F. Alternations in serum lipid, lipoprotein and visceral abdominal fat pad parameters of hypercholestrolemic guinea pigs in response to short term garlic consumption. African Journal of Biotechnology 2010 Nov;9(46):7930-7933.

Prabhu TP, Selvakumari S, Murali K, Sureh R, Shantha A, Kishore PVM. Hypolipidemic effect of alcoholic extract of *Alpinia Calcarata* Rosc rhizomes in experimenta animals. Journal of Pharmacy Research 2010;3(8):1703-1705.

Prada PO, Hirabara SM, Souza de CT, Schenka AA, Zecchin HG, Vassallo J, Velloso LA, Carneiro E, Carvalheira JBC, Curi R, Saad MJ. L-glutamine supplementation induces insulin resistance in adipose tissue and improves insulin signalling in liver and muscle of rats with diet-induced obesity. Diabetologia 2007;50:1949-1959.

Prasannarong M, Saengsirisuwan V, Piyachaturawat P, Suksamrarn A. Improvements of insulin resistance in ovariectomized rats by a novel phytoestrogen from *Curcuma comosa* Roxb. BMC Complementary & Alternative Medicine 2012;12(28):1-11.

Pratley R, Nicklas B, Rubin M, Miller J, Smith A, Smith M, Hurley B, Goldberg A. Strength training increases resting metabolic rate and norepinephrine levels in healthy 50- to 65-yr-old men. J Appl Physiol 1994 Jan;76(1):133-7.

Preuss HG, Rao C, Garis R, Bramble JD, Ohia SE, Bagchi M, Bagchi D. An overview of the safety and efficacy of a novel, natural(-)-hydroxycitric acid extract (HCA-SX) for weight management. J Med. 2004;35(1-6):33-48.

Prieto-Hontoria PL, Pérez-Matute P, Fernández-Galilea M, Barber A, Martinez JA, Moreno-Aliaga MJ. Lipoic acid prevents body weight gain induced by a high fat diet in rats: effects on intestinal sugar transport. J Physiol Biochem 2009 Mar;65(1):43-50.

Prieto-Hontoria PL, Pérez-Matute P, Fernández-Galilea M, Barber A, Martinez JA, Moreno-Aliaga MJ. Effects of lipoic acid on AMPK and adiponectin in adipose tissue of low- and high-fat-fed rats. Eur J Nutr. 2012 Jun 5.

Prior RL, Wilkes SE, Rogers TR, Khanal RC, Wu X, Howard LR. Purified Blueberry Anthocyanins and Blueberry Juice Alter Development of Obesity in Mice Fed an Obesogenic High-Fat Diet. J Agric Food Chem 2010;58:3970-3976.

Prunet-Marcassus B, Desbazeille M, Bros A, Louche K, Delagrange P, Renard P, Casteilla L, Pénicaud L. Melatonin Reduces Body Weight Gain in Sprague Dawley Rats with Diet-Induced Obesity. Endocrinology 2003;144(12):5347-5352.

Przygodda F, Martins ZN, Castaldelli APA, Minella TV, Vieira LP, Cantelli K, Fronza J, Padoin MJ. Effect of erva-mate *(Ilex paraguariensis* A. St.-Hil., Aquifoliaceae*)* on serum cholesterol, triacylglycerides and glucose in Wistar rats fed a diet supplemented with fat and sugar. Revista Brasileira de Farmacognosia Brazilian Journal of Pharmacognosy 2010 Dez: 20(6):956-961.

Pu P, Wang XA, Salim M, Zhu LH, Wang L, Chen KJ, Xiao JF, Deng W, Shi HW, Jiang H, Li HL. Baicalein, a natural product, selectively activating AMPKα$_2$ and ameliorates metabolic disorder in diet-induced mice . Molecular and Cellular Endocrinology 2012.

Puchalski SS, Green JN, Rasmussen DD. Melatonin Effect on Rat Body Weight Regulation in Response to High-Fat Diet at Middle Age. Endocrine 2003;21(2):163-167.

Pulbutr P, Thunchomnang K, Lawa K, Mangkhalathon A, Saenubol P. Lipolytic Effects of Zingerone in Adipocytes Isolated from Normal Diet-Fed Rats and High Fat Diet-Fed Rats. International Journal of Pharmacology 2011;7(5):629-634.

Puska P. Fat and heart disease: yes we can make a change-the case of North Karelia (Finland). Ann Nutr Metab 2009;54(1):33-8.

Qi XY, Chen WJ, Zhang LQ, Xie BJ. Mogrosides extract from Siraitia grosvenori scavenges free radicals in vitro and lowers oxidative stress, serum glucose, and lipid levels in alloxan-induced diabetic mice. Nutr Res. 2008 Apr;28(4):278-84.

Qi Z, Xue J, Zhang Y, Wang H, Xie M. Osthole ameliorates insulin resistance by increment of adiponectin release in high-fat and high-sucrose-induced fatty liver rats. Planta Med 2011 Feb;77(3):231-5.

Qin B, Anderson RA. An extract of chokeberry attenuates weight gain and modulates insulin, adipogenic and inflammatory signalling pathways in epididymal adipose tissue of rats fed a fructose-rich diet. Br J Nutr 2012 Aug;108(4):581-7.

Qingfu S. A Survey of the treatment of obesity by traditional Chinese medicina. Journal of Traditional Chinese Medicine 1993;13(2):124-128.

Quinn TJ, Klooster JR, Kenefick RW. Two short, daily activity bouts vs. one long bout: are health and fitness improvements similar over twelve and twenty-four weeks?. Jstrength Cond Res. 2006 Feb;20(1):130-5.

Qunli W, Zhicheng L. Acupuncture treatment of simple obesity. J Tradit Chin Med 2005 Jun;25(2):90-4.

Rabøl R, Svendsen PF, Skovbro M, Boushel R, Haugaar SB, Schjerling P, Schrauwen P, Hesselink MKC, Nilas L, Madsbad S, Dela F. Reduced skeletal muscle mitochondrial respiration and improved glucose metabolism in nondiabetic obese women during a very low calorie dietary intervention leadingto rapid weight loss. Metabolism Clinical and Experimental 2009;58:1145-1152.

Racine NM, Watras AC, Carrel AL, Allen DB, McVean JJ, Clark RR, O'Brien AR, O'Shea M, Scott CE, Schoeller DA. Effect of conjugated linoleic acid on body fat accretion in overweight or obese children. Am J Clin Nutr 2010 May;91(5):1157-64.

Raff M, Tholstrup T, Toubro S, Bruun JM, Lund P, Straarup EM,Christensen R,Sandberg MB, Mandrup S. Conjugated linoleic acids reduce body fat in healthy postmenopausal. J Nutr. 2009 Jul;139(7):1347-52.

Rafieian-Kopaei M, Asgary S, Adelnia A, Setorki M, Khazaei M, Kazemi S, Shamsi F. The effects of cornelian cherry on atherosclerosis and atherogenic factors in hypercholesterolemic rabbits. Journal of Medicinal Plants Research 2011 Jul;5(13): 2670-2676.

Rahimi R, Qaderi M, Faraji H, Boroujerdi SS. Effects of very short rest periods on hormonal responses to resistance exercise in men.

J Strength Cond Res. 2010 Jul;24(7):1851-9.

Raj N, Nadeem S, Jain S, Raj C, Nandi KCP. Ameliorative effects of *Alpinia calcarata* in alloxan-induced diabetic rats. Digest Journal of Nanomaterials and Biostructures 2011 Jul - Sep;6(3):991-997.

Raja B, Kaviarasan K, Arjunan MM, Pugalendi KV. Effect of *Melothria maderaspatana* Leaf-Tea Consumption on Blood Pressure, Lipid Profile, Anthropometry, Fibrinogen, Bilirubin, and Albumin Levels in Patients with Hypertension. The Journal of Alternative and Complementary Medicine 2007;13(3):349-354.

Rajashekar V, Hucklebridge F, Kennedy O, Cunliffe A. Metabolic effects of long-term oral ingestion of L-histidine in overweight and obese men. Proceedings of the Nutrition Society 2008;67(8):380.

Rajashekar V, Hucklebridge F, Kennedy O, Cunliffe A. Possible histaminergic modulation of energy expenditure and blood glucose regulation in man. Proceedings of the Nutrition Society 2008;67(8):424.

Ramadan G, Nadia ME, Hanaa FAE. Anti-metabolic syndrome and immunostimulant activities of Egyptian fenugreek seeds in diabetic/obese and immunosuppressive rat models. British Journal of Nutrition 2011;105:995-1004.

Ramchandran L, Shah NP. Yogurt can beneficially affect blood contributors of cardiovascular health status in hypertensive rats. J Food Sci 2011 May;76(4):131-6.

Ramgopal M, Attitalla IH, Avinash P, Balaji M. Evaluation of Antilipidemic and Anti Obesity Efficacy of *Bauhinia purpurea* Bark Extract on Rats Fed with High Fat Diet. Academic Journal of Plant Sciences 2010;3(3):104-107.

Ramos AT, Cunha MAL, Sabaa-Srur AUO, Pires VCF, Cardoso MAA, Diniz MFM, Medeiros CCM. Uso de *Passiflora edulis f. flavicarpa* na reducão do colesterol. Brazilian Journal of Pharmacognosy 2007;17(4):592-597.

Rani N, Sharma SK, Vasudeva N. Assessment of Antiobesity Potential of *Achyranthes aspera* Linn. Seed. Evidence-Based Complementary and Alternative Medicine 2012.

Rankin JW, Goldman LP, Puglisi MJ, Nickols-Richardson SM, Earthman CP, Gwazdauskas FC. Effect of post-exercise supplement consumption on adaptations to resistance training. J Am Coll Nutr 2004 Aug;23(4):322-30.

Rao VS, de Melo CL, Queiroz MG, Lemos TL, Menezes DB, Melo TS, Santos FA. Ursolic acid, a pentacyclic triterpene from Sambucus australis, prevents abdominal adiposity in mice fed a high-fat diet. J Med Food 2011 Nov;14(11):1375-82.

Rasineni K, Desireddy S. Preventive effect of *Catharanthus roseus* (Linn.) against high-fructose diet-induced insulin resitance and oxidative stress in male Wistar rats. Journal of Diabetes Mellitus 2011;1(3):63-70.

Rasmussen DD, Boldt BM, Wilkinson CW, Yellow SM, Matsumoto AM. Daily melatonin administration at middle age suppresses ale fat visceral fat, plasma leptin, and plasma insulin to youthful levels. Endocrinology 1999 Feb;140(2):1009-12.

Ratamess NA, Hoffman JR, Ross R, Shanklin M, Faigenbaum AD, Kang J. Effects of an amino acid/creatine energy supplement on the acute hormonal response to resistance exercise. Int J Sports Nutr Exerc Metab 2007 Dec;17(6):608-23.

Ravussin E, Burnand B, Schutz Y, Jéquier E. Energy expenditure before and during energy restriction in obese patients. Am J Clin Nutr. 1985 Apr;41(4):753-9.

Razquin C, Martinez JA, Martinez-Gonzalez MA, Mitjavila MT, Estruch R, Marti A. A 3 years follow-up of a Mediterranean diet rich in virgin olive oil is associated with high plasma antioxidant capacity and reduced body weight gain. Eur J Clin. Nutr. 2009 Dec;63(12):1387-93.

Reddy RM, Latha PB, Vijaya T, Rao DS. The saponin-rich fraction of a Gymnema sylvestre R. Br. Aqueous leaf extract reduces cafeteria and high-fat diet-induced obesity. Z Naturforsch C. 2012 Jan-Feb;67(1-2):39-46.

Refaie FM, Esmat AY, Daba AS, Taha SM. Characterization of polysaccaropeptides from *Pleurotus ostreatus* mycelium: Assessment of toxicity and immunomodulation *in vivo*. Micologia Aplicada International 2009;21(2):67-75.

Reinbach HC, Smeets A, Martinussen T, Møller P, Westerterp-Plantenga MS. Effects of capsaicin, green tea and CH-19 sweet pepper on appetite and energy intake in humans in negative and positive energy balance. Clinical Nutrition 2009;28:260-265.

Rendón-Huerta JA, Juárez-Flores B, Pinos-Rodriguez JM, Aguirre-Rivera JR, Delgado-Portales RE. Effects of different sources of fructans on body weight, blood metabolites and fecal bacteria in normal and obese non-diabetic and diabetic rats. Plant Foods Hum Nutr. 2012 Mar;67(1):64-70.

Rerksuppaphol L, Rerksuppaphol S. Efficacy of electro-acupuncture at the main acupoints for weight reduction in Thai obese women. Asian Biomedicine 2010 Dec;4(6):943-947.

Reyna NY, Cano C, Bermúdez VJ, Medina MT, Souki AJ, Ambard M, Nuñez M, Ferrer MA, Inglett GE. Sweeteners and beta-glucans improve metabolic and anthropometrics variables in well controlled type 2 diabetic patients. Am J Ther 2003 Nov - Dec;10(6):438-43.

Reyna-Villasmil NY, Bermúdez-Pirela V, Mengual-Moreno E, Arias N, Cano-Ponce C, Leal-Gonzalez E, Souki A, Inglett GE, Israili ZH, Hernández-Hernández R, Valasco M, Arraiz N. Oat-derived beta-glucan significantly improves HDLC and diminishes LDLC and non-HDL cholesterol in overweight individuals with mild hypercholesterolemia. Am J Ther 2007 Mar - Apr;14(2):203-12.

Rhee SJ, Ahn JM, Ku KH, Choi JH. Effects of Radish Leaves Powder on Hepatic Antioxidative System in Rats Fed High-Cholesterol Diet. J. Korean Soc. Food Sci. Nutr. 2005;34(8):1157-1163.

Rhee YH, Lee EO, Park SY, Lee HJ, Yoon BS, Kim JH, Kim SH. Effect of Brassica rapa L. extracts and β-sitosterol on hyperlipidemic rats. Korean J. Oriental Physiology & Pathology 2005;19(6):1528-1533.

Ribeiro PFA, Santos VS, Machado AR, Fernandes CG, Silva JA, Rodrigues RS. Benefits of blackberry nectar (Rubus spp.) relative to hypercholesterolemia and lipid peroxidation. Nutr Hosp. 2011;26(5):984-990.

Richards D, Marley J. Stimulation of auricular acupuncture points in weight loss. Aust Fam Physician 1998 Jul;27(2):73-7.

Rigamonti E, Parolini C, Marchesi M, Diani E, Brambilla S, Sirtori CR, Chiesa G. Hypolipidemic effect of dietary pea proteins: Impact on genes regulating hepatic lipid metabolism. Mol Nutr Food Res. 2010 May;54(1):24-30.

Rios-Lugo MJ, Cano P, Jiménez-Ortega V, Fernández-Mateos MP, Scacchi PA, Cardinali DP, Esquifino AI. Melatonin effect on plasma adiponectin, leptin, insulin, glucose, triglycerides and cholesterol in normal and high fat-fed rats. J Pineal Res. 2010 Nov;49(4):342-8.

Risérus U, Berglund L, Vessby B. Conjugated linoleic acid (CLA) reduced abdominal adipose tissue in obese middle-aged men with signs of the metabolic syndrome: a randomised controlled trial. International Journal of Obesity 2001;25:1129-1135.

Rivera L, Morón R, Sánchez M, Zarzuelo A, Galisteo M. Quercetin ameliorates metabolic syndrome and improves the inflammatory status in obese Zucker rats. Obesity (Silver Spring) 2008 Sep;16(9):2081-7.

Rivera L, Morón R, Zarzuelo A, Galisteo M. Long-term resveratrol administration reduces metabolic disturbances and lowers blood pressure in obese Zucker rats. Biochem Pharmacol 2009 Mar 15;77(6):1053-63.

Roccisano D, Henneberg M. Soy Consumption and Obesity. Food and Nutrition Sciences 2012;3:260-266.

Rock W, Rosenblat M, Borochov-Neori H, Volkova N, Judeinstein S, Elias M, Aviram M. Effects of data (Phoenix dactylifera L., Medjool or Hallawi Variety) consumption by healthy subjects on serum glucose and lipid levels and on serum oxidative status: a pilot study. J Agric Food Chem. 2009 Sep 9;57(17):8010-7.

Roh C, Park MK, Shin HJ, Kim I, Kim JK, Jung U. Anti-Obesity Effect of Nepetae spica Extract in High-Fat Mice. Agriculture 2012;2:204-210.

Roh C, Park MK, Shin HJ, Jung U, Kim JK. *Buddleja officinalis Maximowicz* Extract Inhibits Lipid Accumulation on Adipocyte Differentiation in 3T3-L1 Cells and High-Fat Mice. Molecules 2012;17:8687-8695.

Roh C, Jung U. Screening of Crude Plant Extracts with Anti-Obesity Activity. Int. J. Mol. Sci. 2012;13:1710-1719.

Roesler R. Effect of extracts from araticum *(Annona crassiflora)* on CCl$_4$-induced liver damage in rats. Ciênc. Tecnol. Aliment.Campinas. 2011 Jan-Mar;31(1):93-100.

Rolls BJ, Bell EA, Thorwart ML. Water incorporated into a food but not served with a food decreases energy intake in lean women. Am J Clin Nutr 1999;70:448-55.

Roongpisuthipong C, Kantawan R, Roongpisuthipong W. Reduction of adipose tissue and body weight: effect of water soluble calcium hydroxycitrate in *Garcinia atroviridis* on the short term treatment of obese women in Thailand. Asia Pac J Clin Nutr 2007;16(1):25-29.

Rosén T, Bosaeus I, Tölli J, Lindstedt G, Bengtsson BA. Increased body fat mass and decreased extracellular fluid volume in adults with growth hormone deficiency. Clin Endocrinol (Oxf) 1993 Jan;38(1):63-71.

Rosenblum JL, Castro VM, Moore CE, Kaplan LM. Calcium and vitamin D supplementation is associated with decreased abdominal visceral adipose tissue in overweight and obese adults. Am J Clin Nutr 2012 Jan;95(1):101-8.

Rotella CM, Cresci B, Mannucci E, Rizzello SM, Colzi G, Galli G, Giannini S, Messeri G, Piani F, Vannini R. Short cycles of very low calorie diet in the therapy of obese type II diabetes mellitus. J Endocrinol Invest. 1994 Mar;17(3):171-9.

Rubio LA, Grant G, Bardocz S, Dewey P, Pusztai A. Nutritional response of growing rats to faba beans (*Vicia faba* L., minor) and faba bean fractions. British Journal of Nutrition 1991;66:533-542.

Rutherford JA, Spriet LL, Stellingweff T. The effect of acute taurine ingestion on endurance performance and metabolism in well-trained cyclists. Int J Sport Nutr Exerc Metab 2010 Aug;20(4):322-9.

Ryou SH, Kang MS, Kim KI, Kang YH, Kang JS. Effects of green tea or *Sasa quelpaertensis* bamboo leaves on plasma and liver lipids, erythrocyte Na efflux, and platelet aggregation in ovariectomized rats. Nutrition Research and Practice *(Nutr Res Pract)* 2012;6(2):106-112.

Ryttig KR, Tellnes G, Haegh L, Bøe E, Fagerthun H. A dietary fibre supplement and weight maintenance after weight reduction: a randomized, double-blind, placebo-controlled long-term trial. Int J Obes 1989;13(2):165-71.

Ryu HJ, Um MY, Ahn JY, Jung CH, Huh D, Kim TW, Ha TY. Anti-obesity Effect of *Hypsizigus marmoreus* in High Fat-fed Mice. J Korean Soc Food Sci Nutr 2011;40(12):1708-1714.

Ryu KS, Wang CW, Song GS, Paik SW. Effect of Dietary Supplemental *Astragalus membranaceus* on Performance, Blood Components and Meat Quality of Broiler Chicks. K.J. Poult. Sci. 1998;25(4):185-193.

Rössner S, von Zweigbergk D, Ohlin A, Ryttig K. Weight reduction with dietary fibre supplements. Results of two double-blind randomized studies. Acta Med Scand 1987;222(1):83-8.

Sabaté J, Wien M. Vegetarian diets and childhood obesity prevention. Am J Clin Nutr 2010 May;91(5):1525-1529.

Sachan DS, Hongu N. Increases in VO$_2$ max and metabolic markers of fat oxidation by caffeine, carnitine, and choline supplementation in rats. J. Nutr. Biochem. 2000;11:521-526.

Sae-tan S, Grove KA, Lambert JD. Weight control and prevention of metabolic syndrome by green tea. Pharmacological Research 2011;64:146-154.

Said O, Saad B, Fulder S, Khalil K, Kassis E. Weight Loss in Animals and Humans Treated with "Weighlevel", a Combination of Four Medicinal Plants Used in Traditional Arabic and Islamic Medicine. Evidence-Based Complementary and Alternative Medicine 2011.

Sagwal R, Kansal VK. Synergistic effect of synthetic conjugated linoleic acid & non fat milk on fat deposition & lipid metabolism in mice. Indian J Med Res 2010 Mar;131:449-454.

Sakuramata Y, Kusano S. Screening of Plant Extrats with Potential to Stimulate Lipolysis in 3T3-L1 Cells. J. Jpn. Soc. Nutr. Food Sci. 1998;51:361-364.

Salas-Salvadó J, Farrés X, Luque X, Narejos S, Borrell M, Basora J. Effect of two doses of a mixture of soluble fibres on body weight and metabolic variables in overweight or obese patients: a randomized trial. British Journal of Nutrition 2008;99:1380-1387.

Salehpour A, Hosseinpanah F, Shidfar F, Vafa M, Razaghi M, Dehghani S, Hoshiarrad A, Gohari M. A 12-week double-blind randomized clinical trial of vitamin D3 supplementation on body fat mass in healthy overweight and obese women. Nutr J 2012 Sep 22;11(1):78.

Salimeh A, Mohammadi M, Mohaddes G, Badalzadeh R. Protective Effect of Diosgenin and Exercise Training on Biochemical and ECG Alteration in Isoproterenol- Induced Myocardial Infarction in Rats. Iranian Journal of Basic Medical Sciences 2011 May-Jun 2011;14(3):264-274.

Sambaiah K, Satyanarayana MN. Influence of red pepper and capsaicin on body composition and lipogenesis in rats. J Biosci. 1982 Dec;4(4):425-430.

Sampathkumar MT, Kasetti RB, Nabi SA, Sudarshan PR, Swapna S, Apparao C. Antihyperlipidemic and antiatherogenic activities of *Terminalia pallida* Linn. Fruits in high fat diet-induced hyperlipidemic rats. J Pharm Bioallied Sci. 2011 Jul-Sep;3(3):449-452.

Sánchez D, Moulay ML, Hernández R,Miguel M, Aleixandre A. Highly Methoxylated Pectin Improves Insulin Resistance and Other Cardiometabolic Risk Factors in Zucker Fatty Rats. J Agric Food Chem 2008;56:3574-3581.

Sánchez J, Pérez-Heredia F, Priego T, Portillo MP, Zamora S, Garaulet M, Palou A. Dehydroepiandrosterone prevents age-associated alterations, increasing insulin sensitivity. Journal of Nutritional Biochemistry 2008;19:809-818.

Sanchez-Mateos S, Alonso-Gonzales C, Gonzales A, Martinez-Campa CM, Mediavilla MD, Cos S, Sanchez-Barcelo EJ. Melatonin and estradiol effects on food intake, body weight, and leptin in ovariectomized rats. Maturitas 2007;58:91-101.

Sankar D, Rao MR, Sambandam G, Pugalendi KV. A pilot study of open label sesame oil in hypertensive diabetics. J Med Food. 2006;9(3):408-12.

Sankar D, Ramakrishna R, Sambandam G, Pugalendi KV. Effect of Sesame Oil on Diuretics or β-blockers in the Modulation of Blood Pressure, Anthropometry, Lipid Profile, and Redox Status. Yale Journal of Biology and Medicine 2006;79:19-26.

Santiago JVA, Jayachitra J, Shenbagam M, Nalim N. *d*-limonene attenuates blood pressure and improves the lipid and antioxidant status in high fat diet and L-NAME treated rats. J. Pharm. Sci. & Res. 2010;2(11):752-758.

Saraf MN, Sanaye MM, Mengi SA. Antifatigue effect of *Murraya koenigii*. Pharmacologyonline 2011;2:1025-1037.

Saravanan S, Srikumar R, Manikandan S, Parthasarathy NJ, Devi RS. Hypolipidemic Effect of Triphala in Experimentally Induced Hypercholesteremic Rats. Yakugaku Zasshi 2007;127(2):385-388.

Sartor F, Jackson MJ, Squillace C, Shepherd A, Moore JP, Ayer DE, Kubis HP. Adaptive metabolic response to 4 weeks of sugar-sweetened beverage consumption in healthy, lightly active individuals and chronic high glucose availability in primary human myotubes. Eur J Nutr 2012 Jun 26.

Sato M, Uzu K, Yoshida T, Hamad EM, Kawakami H, Matsuyama H, Abd El-Gawad IA, Imaizumi K. Effects of milk fermented by Lactobacillus gasseri SBT2055 on adipocyte size in rats. Br J Nutr. 2008 May;99(5):1013-7.

Saunier EF, Vivar OI, Rubenstein A, Zhao X, Olshansky M, Baggett S, Staub RE, Tagliaferri M, Cohen I, Speed TP, Baxter JD, Leitman DC. Estrogenic Plant Extracts Reverse Weight Gain and Fat Accumulation without Causing Mammary Gland or Uterine Proliferation. PloS ONE 2011 Dec;6(2):1-9.

Schjerve IE, Tyldum GA, Tjønna AE, Stølen T, Loennechen JP, Hansen HE, Haram PM, Heinrich G, Bye A, Najjar SM, Smith GL, Slørdahl SA, Kemi OJ, Wisløff U. Both aerobic endurance and strength training programmes improve cardiovascular health in obese adults. Clin Sci (Lond) 2008 Nov;115(9):283-93.

Schirmer MA, Phinney SD. Gamma-linolenate reduces weight regain in formerly obese humans. J Nutr. 2007 Jun;137(6):1430-5.

Seddeag M, Madawe G, El Badwi SMA, Bakhiet AO. The Effect of Dietary *Alpinia officinarum* (Hance) Supplementation in Bovns-type Chicks. International Journal of Poultry Science 2010;9(5):499-502.

Sedghi M, Golian A, Kermanshahi H, Ahmadi H. Effect of dietary supplementation of licorice extract and a prebiotic on performance and blood metabolites of broilers. South African Journal of Animal Science 2010;40(4):371-380.

Seidlova-Wuttke D, Ehrhardt C, Wuttke W. Metabolic effects of 20-OH-Ecdysone in ovariectomized rats. Journal of Steroid Biochemistry & Molecular Biology 2010;119:121-126.

Seiva FRF, Gustavo L, Chuffa A, Braga CP, Amorim JPA, Fernandes AAH. Quercetin ameliorates glucose and lipid metabolism and improves antioxidant status in postnatally monosodium glutamate-induced metabolic alterations. Food and Chemical Toxicology 2012;50:3556-3561.

Seo DI, Jun TW, Park KS, Chang H, So WY, Song W. 12 weeks of combined exercise is better than aerobic exercise for increasing growth hormone in middle-aged women. Int J Sport Nutr Exerc Metab 2010 Feb;20(1):21-6.

Seo DI, So WY, Ha S, Yoo EJ, Kim D, Singh H, Fahs CA, Rossow L, Bemben DA, Bemben MG, Kim E. Effects of 12 weeks of combined exercise training on visfatin and metabolic syndrome factors in obese middle-aged women. Journal of Sports Science and Medicine 2011;10:222-226.

Seo DY, Lee SR, Kim HK, Baek YH, Kwak YS, Ko TH, Kim N, Rhee BD, Ko KS, Park BJ, Han J. Independent beneficial effects of aged garlic extract intake with regular exercise on cardiovascular risk in postmenopausal women. Nutrition Research and Practice *(Nutr Res Pract)* 2012;6(3):226-231.

Seo HB, Kwak Y, Nam JO, Song YJ, Kim BO, Ryu S. Glasswort Powder Diet Activates Lipid Metabolism in Rat. Journal of Life Science 2012;22(4):478-485.

Seo JB, Choe SS, Jeong HW, Park SW, Shin HJ, Choi SM, Park JY, Choi EW, Kim JB, See DS, Jeong JY, Lee TG. Anti-obesity effects of *Lysimachia foenum-graecum* characterized by decreased adipogenesis and regulated lipid metabolism. Experimental and Molecular Medicine 2011 Apr;43(4):205-215.

Seo JB, Park SW, Choe SS, Jeong HW, Park JY, Choi EW, Seen DS, Jeong JY, Lee TG. Foenumoside B from *Lysimachia foenum-graecum* inhibits adipocyte differentiation and obesity induced by high-fat diet. Biochemical and Biophysical Research Communications 2012;417:800-806.

Seong SH, Ahn EM, Sohn HS, Baik SH, Park HW, Lee SJ, Cha YS. Genistein Combined with Exercise Improves Lipid Profiles and Leptin Levels in C57BL/6J Mice Fed a High Fat Diet. Food Sci. Biotechnol. 2007;16(5):910-917.

Seymour EM, Lewis SK, Urcuyo-Llanes DE, Tanone II, Kirakosyan A, Kaufman PB, Bolling SF. Regular Tart Cherry Intake Alters Abdominal Adiposty, Adipose Gene Transcription, and Inflammation in Obesity-Prone Rats Fed a High Fat Diet. Journal of Medicinal Food 2009;12(5):935-942.

Seymour EM, Tanone II, Urcuyo-Llanes DE, Lewis SK, Kirakosyan A, Kondoleon MG, Kaufman PB, Bolling SF. Blueberry Intake Alters Skeletal Muscle and Adipose Tissue Peroxisome Proliferator-Activated Receptor Activity and Reduces Insulin Resistance in Obese Rats. Journal of Medicinal Food 2011;14(12):1511-1518.

Shah KA, Patel MB, Shah SS, Chauhan KN, Parmar PK, Patel NM. Antihyperlipidemic activity of *Mangifera indica* l. leaf extract on rats fed with high cholesterol diet. Der Pharmacia Sinica 2010;1(2):156-161.

Shah SS, Shah GB, Singh SD, Gohil PV, Chauhan K, Shah KA, Chorawala M. Effect of piperine in the regulartion of obesity-induced dyslipidemia in high-fat diet rats. Indian J Pharmacol 2011;43(3):296-299.

Shahraki MR, Harati M, Shahraki AR. Prevention of high fructose-induced metabolic syndrome in male wistar rats by aqueous extract of Tamarindus indica seed. Acta Med Iran 2011;49(5):277-83.

Shang J, Chen LI, Xiao FX, Sun H, Ding HC, Xiao H. Resveratrol improves non-alcoholic fatty liver disease by activating AMP-activated protein kinase. Acta Pharmacol Sin 2008 Jun;29(6):698-706.

Shao W, Yu Z, Chiang Y, Yang Y, Chai T, Foltz W, Lu H, Fantus IG, Jin T. Curcumin Prevents High Fat Diet Induced Insulin Resistance and Obesity via Attenuating Lipogenesis in Liver and Inflammatory Pathway in Adipocytes. PloS ONE 2012

Jan;7(1):28784.

Shara M, Ohia SE, Yasmin T, Zardetto-Smith A, Kincaid A, Bagchi M, Chatterjee A, Bagchi D, Stohs SJ. Dose- and time-dependent effects of a novel (-)-hydroxycitric acid extract on body weight, hepatic and testicular lipid peroxidation, DNA fragmentation and histopathological data over a period of 90 days. Mol Cell Biochem. 2003 Dec;254(1-2):339-46.

Sharma AK, Bharti S, Bhatia J, Nepal S, Malik S, Ray R, Kumari S, Arya DS. Sesamol alleviates diet-induced cardiometabolic syndrome in rats via up-regulating PPARγ, PPARα and e-NOS. Journal of Nutritional Biochemistry 2012.

Sharma V, Thakur M, Dixit VK. A comparative study of ethanolic extracts of Pedalium murex Linn. Fruits and sildenafil citrate on sexual behaviors and serum testosterone level in male rats during and after treatment. J Ethnopharmacol 2012 Aug 30;143(1):201-6.

Sharma V, Verma RB, Sharma S. Preliminary evaluation of the hepatic protection by pharmacological properties of the aqueous extract of *Asparagus racemosus* in lead loaded swiss albino mice. International Journal of Pharmacy and Pharmaceutical Sciences 2012;4(1):55-62.

Sharmila BG, Kumar G, Rajasekara PM. Cholesterol lowering activity of the aqueous fruit extract of *Trichosanthes dioica* roxb (L.) in normal and streptozotocin diabetic rats. Journal of Clinical and Diagnostic Research 2007;1:561-569.

Shen QW, Jones CS, Kalchayanand N, Zhu MJ, Du K. Effect of dietary alpha-lipoic acid on growth, body composition, muscle pH, and AMP-activated protein kinase phosphorylation in mice. J Anim Sci 2005 Nov;83(11):2611-7.

Shen W, Fan WH, Shi HM. Effects of rhodiola on expression of vascular endothelial cell growth factor and angiogenesis in aortic atherosclerotic plaque of rabbits. Zhongguo Zhong Xi Yi Jie He Za Zhi 2008 Nov;28(11):1022-5.

Sheng L, Qian Z, Shi Y, Yang L, Xi L, Zhao B, Xu X, Ji H. Crocetin improves the insulin resistance induced by high-fat diet in rats. British Journal of Pharmacology 2008;154:1016-1024.

Sheng L, Qian Z, Zheng S, Xi L. Mechanism of hypolipidemic effect of crocin in rats: crocin inhibits pancreatic lipase. Eur J Pharmacol 2006 Aug 14;543(1-3):116-22.

Sheo HJ, Seo YS. The effects of dietary chinese cabbage *kimchi* juice on the lipid metabolism and body weight gain in rats fed high-calories-diet. J Korean Soc. Food Sci. Nutr. 2004;33(1):91-100.

Sheyab FM, Abuharfeil N, Salloum L, Hani RB, Awad DS. The Effect of Rosemary *(Rosmarinus officinalis.* L.) Plant Extracts on the Immune Response and Lipid Profile in Mice. Journal of Biology and Life Science 2012;3(1):37-58.

Shi H, Dirienzo D, Zemel MB. Effects of dietary calcium on adipocyte lipid metabolism and body weight regulation in energy-restricted aP2-agouti transgenic mice. FASEB J. 2001 Feb;15(2):291-3.

Shi J, Finckenberg P, Martonen E, Ahlroos-Lehmus A, Pilvi TK, Korpela R, Mervaala EM. Metabolic effects of a lactoferrin during energy restriction and weight regain in diet-induced obese mice. Journal of Functional Foods 2012;4:66-78.

Shi J, Ahlroos-Lehmus A, Pilvi TK, Korpela R, Tossavainen O, Mervaala EM. Metabolic effects of a novel microfiltered native whey protein in diet-induced obese mice. Journal of Functional Foods 2012;4:440-449.

Shigematsu N, Asano R, Shimosaka M, Okazaki M. Effect of Administration with the Extract of *Gymnema sylvestre* R.Br Leaves on Lipid Metabolism in Rats. Biol. Pharm. Bull. 2001;24(6):713-717.

Shih CC, Wu YW, Lin WC. Ameliorative effects of *Anoectochilus formosanus* extract on osteopenia in ovariectomized rats. Journal of Ethnopharmacology 2001;77:233-238.

Shih CC, Lin CH, Lin WL. Effects of *Momordica charantia* on insulin resistance and visceral obesity in mice on high-fat diet. Diabetes research and clinical practice 2008;81:134-143.

Shih CC, Lin CH, Wu JB. Eriobotrya japonica improves hyperlipidemia and reverses insulin resistance in high-fat-fed mice. Phytother Res 2010 Dec;24(12):1769-80.

Shikov AN, Pozharitskaya ON, Makarova MN, Dorman IIJD, Makarov VG, Hiltunen R, Galambosi B. Adaptogenic effect of black and fermented leaves of *Bergenia crassifolia* L. in mice. Journal of Functional Foods 2010;2:71-76.

Shikov AN, Pozharitskaya ON, Makarova MN, Kovaleva MA, Laakso I, Dorman HJD, Hiltunen R, Makarov VG, Galambosi B. Effect of *Bergenia crassifolia* L. extracts on weight gain and feeding behavior of rats with high-caloric diet-induced obesity. Phytomedicine 2012.

Shim WS, Back H, Seo EK, Lee HT, Shim CK. Long-term administration of an aqueous extract of dried, immature fruit of *Poncirus trifoliata* (L.) Raf. Suppresses body weight gain in rats. Journal of Ethnopharmacology 2009;126:294-299.

Shimada T, Hiramatsu N, Kasai A, Mukai M, Okamura M, Yao J, Huang T, Tamai M, Takahashi S, Nakamura T, Kitamura M. Suppression of adipocyte differentiation by *Cordyceps militaris* through activation of the aryl hydrocarbon receptor. Am J Physiol Endocrinol Metab 2008;295:859-867.

Shimada T, Nagai E, Harasawa Y, Akase T, Aburada T, Iizuka S, Miyamoto K, Aburada M. Metabolic disease prevention and suppression of fat accumulation by Salacia reticulata. J Nat Med. 2010 Jul;64(3):266-74.

Shimada T, Kosugi M, Tokuhara D, Tsubata M, Kamiya T, Sameshima M, Nagamine R, Takagaki K, Miyamoto KI, Aburada M. Preventive Effect of Pine Bark Extract (Flavangenol) on Metabolic Disease in Western Diet-Loaded Tsumura Suzuki Obese Diabetes Mice. Evidence-Based Complementary and Alternative Medicine 2011.

Shimada T, Horikawa T, Ikeya Y, Matsuo H, Kinoshita K, Taguchi T, Ichinose K, Takahashi K, Aburada M. Preventive effect of *Kaempferia parviflora* ethyl acetate extract and its major components polymethoxyflavonoid on metabolic diseases. Fitoterapia 2011;82:1272-1278.

Shimada T, Tokuhara D, Tsubata M, Kamiya T, Kamiya-Sameshima M, Nagamine R, Takagaki K, Sai Y, Miyamoto KI, Aburada M. Flavangenol (pine bark extract) and its major component procyanidin B1 enhance fatty acid oxidation in fat-loaded models. European Journal of Pharmacology 2012;677:147-153.

Shimizu C, Kihara M, Aoe S, Araki S, Ito K, Hayashi K, Watari J, Sakata Y, Ikegami S. Effect of High β-Glucan Barley on Serum Cholesterol Concentrations and Visceral Fat Area in Japanese Men – A Randomized, Double-blinded, Placebo-controlled Trial. Plant Foods Hum Nutr 2008;63:21-25.

Shimoda H, Seki E, Aitani M. Inhibitory effect of green coffee bean extract on fat accumulation and body weight gain in mice. BMC Complement Altern Med. 2006 Mar 17;6:9.

Shimomura Y, Tamura T, Suzuki M. Less body fat accumulation in rats fed a safflower oil diet than in rats fed a beef tallow diet. J Nutr. 1990 Nov;120(11):1291-6.

267

Shimotoyodome A, Haramizu S, Inaba M, Murase T, Tokimitsu I. Exercise and green tea extract stimulate fat oxidation and prevent obesity in mice. Med Sci Sports Exerc 2005 Nov;37(11):1884-92.

Shimura S, Tsuzuki W, Kobayashi S, Suzuki T. Inhibitory Effect on Lipase Activity of Extracts from Medicinal Herbs. Biosci. Biotech. Biochem. 1992;56(9):1478-1479.

Shimura S, Tsuzuki W, Kobayashi S, Suzuki T. Screening of Lipase Inhibitors from Natural Materials. Nippon Shokuhin Kogyo Gakkaishi 1993;40(3):214-217.

Shin JE, Han MJ, Kim DH. 3-Methylethergalangin Isolated from *Alpinia officinarum* Inhibits Pancreatic Lipase. Biol. Pharm. Bull. 2003;26(6):854-857.

Shin SJ, Hong ST. Acanthopanax and Platycodi Independently Prevents the Onset of High Fat Diet Induced Hyperglyceridemia and Obesity in C57BL/6 Mice. Food Sci. Biotechnol 2005;14(6):841-846.

Shinjo S, Asato L, Arakaki S, Kina T, Kohrin T, Mori M, Yamamoto S. Comparative Effect of Casein and Soybean Protein Isolate on Body Fat Accumulation in Adult Rats. J Nutr Sci Vitaminol 1992;38:247-253.

Shirakura Y, Takayanagi K, Mukai K, Tanabe H, Inoue M. B-Cryptoxanthin Suppresses the Adipogenesis of 3T3-L1 Cells vis RAR Activation. J Nutr Sci Vitaminol 2011;57:426-431.

Shittu LAJ, Bankole MA, Ogundipe OA,Falade AK, Shittu RK, Bankole MN, Ahmed TA, Tayo AO, Oladapo AA. Weight reduction with improvement of serum lipid profile and ratios of *Sesamum radiatum* leaves diet in a non-obese Sprague Dawley rats. African Journal of Biotechnology 2007 Nov 5;6(21):2428-2433.

Shuang-kui D, Xiao-ye Z, Zhi-x L. Hepatoprotective, Weight-Reducing and Hypolipidemic Effects of *Hovenia dulcis* Thunb. Fruit Vinegar. Food Science 2012;33(1):235-238.

Sibuyi NRS, Katerere DR, Boboyi T, Madiehe AM. Dietary supplementation with *Aloe ferox* extracts reverses obesity in rats. South African Journal of Botany 2007 Apr;73(2):336.

Siddiqi HS, Mehmood MH, Rehman NU, Gilani AH. Studies on the antihypertensive and antidyslipidemic activities of Viola odorata leaves extract. Lipids Health Dis. 2012 Jan 10;11:6.

Siddiqui SMK, Chang E, Li J, Burlage C, Zou M, Buhman KK, Koser S, Donkin SS, Teegarden D. Dietary intervention with vitamin D, calcium, and whey protein reduced fat mass and increased lean mass in rats.Nutrition Research 2008;28:783-790.

Sidhu LS, Keertisharma, Puri AS, Prakash S. Effect of gum guggul on body weight and subcutaneous tissue folds. J Res Indian Med Yoga Homeo II 1976:16

Siegner R, Heuser S, Holtzmann U, Söhle J, Schepky A, Raschke T, Stäb F, Wenck H, Winnefeld M. Lotus leaf extract and L-carnitine influence different processes during the adipocyte life cycle. Nutrition & Metabolism 2010;7(66):1-10.

Silver HJ, Dietrich MS, Niswender KD. Effects of grapefruit, grapefruit juice and water preloads on energy balance, weight loss, body composition, and cardiometabolic risk in free-living obese adults. Nutr Metab (Lond). 2011 Feb 2;8(1):1-11

Simmen FA, Mercado CP, Zavacki AM, Huang SA, Greenway AD, Kang P, Bowman MT, Prior RL. Soy protein diet alters expression of hepatic genes regulating fatty acid and thyroid hormone metabolism in the male rat. Journal of Nutritional Biochemistry 2010;21:1106-1113.

Singh AK, Pralhad SP, Mitra SK. Evaluation of clinical efficacy of AyurSlim on body weight, body mass index, lipid profile and skin fold thickness: A Phase IV clinical trial. The Antiseptic 2008;105(5):241-243.

Singh J, Handa G, Rao PR, Atal CK. Pangamic acid, a stamina building,antistress and anti-hyperlipidemic principle from *Cicer arietinum* L. Journal of Ethnopharmacology 1983;7:239-242.

Sinnott RA, Maddela RL, Nelson ED, Bae S, Singh KP, Anderson JA. The Modifying Effects of A Calcium-rich Whey Protein Supplement (OsoLean™ Powder) on Weight LOSS and Waist Circumference in Overweight Subjects: A Preliminary Study. The Open Nutraceuticals Journal 2009;2:36-41.

Sirato-Yasumoto S, Katsuta M, Okuyama Y, Takahashi Y, Ide T. Effect of sesame seeds rich in sesamin and sesamolin on fatty acid oxidation in rat liver. J Agric Food Chem 2001 May;49(5):2647-51.

Slanc P, Doljak B, Kreft S, Lunder M, Janes D, Strukelj B. Screening of selected food and medicinal plant extract for pancreatic lipase inhibition. Phytother Res. 2009 Jun;23(6):874-7.

Slavin JL. Dietary fiber and body weight. Nutrition 2005;21:411-418.

Smith AE, Fukuda DH, Kendall KL, Stout JR. The effects of a pre-workout supplement containing caffeine, creatine, and amino acids during three weeks of high-intensity exercise on aerobic and anaerobic performance. J Int Soc Sports Nutr 2010 Feb 15;97(10):1-11.

Snel M, Gastaldelli A, Ouwens DM, Hesselink MK, Schaart G, Buzzigoli E, Frölich M, Romijn JA, Pijl H, Meinders AE, Jazet IM. Effects of adding exercise to a 16-week very long low-calorie diet in obese, insulin-dependent type 2 diabetes mellitus patients. J Clin Endocrinol Metab 2012 Jul;97(7):2512-20.

Snel M, Jonker JT, Hammer S, Kerpershoek G, Lamb HJ, Meinders AE, Pijl H, de Roos A, Romijn JA, Smit JW, Jazet IM. Long-term beneficial effect of a 16-week very low calorie diet on pericardial fat in obese type 2 diabetes mellitus patients. Obesity (Silver Spring) 2012 Aug;20(8):1572-6.

Snitker S, Fujishima Y, Shen H, Ott S, Pi-Sunyer X, Furuhata Y, Sato H, Takahashi M. Effects of novel capsinoid treatment on fatness and energy metabolism in humans: possible pharmacogenetic implications. Am J Clin Nutr. 2009 Jan;89(1):45-50.

Soares MJ, Cummings SJ, Mamo JCL, Kenrick M, Piers LS. The acute effects of olive oil *v.* Cream on postprandial thermogenesis and substrate oxidation in postmenopausal. British Journal of Nutrition 2004;91:245-252.

Soh JR, Cha YS. Gamma-Aminobutyric Acid and/or Carnitine Supplementation Alters Lipid and Some Immune Related Nutrient Levels in Mice. J. Food Sci Nutr 2004;9:58-64.

Soh JS, Hong S, Kim MK. Effect of Glutinous Barley Intake on Lipid Metabolism in Middle-Aged Rats Fed a High-Fat Diet. Food Sci. Biotechnol. 2007;16(6):1023-1028.

Son MJ, Rico CW, Nam SH, Kang MY. Influence of Oryzanol and Ferulic Acid on the Lipid Metabolism and Antioxidative Status in High Fat-Fed Mice. J Clin Biochem Nutr 2010 Mar;46:150-156.

Song JK, Stebbins CL, Kim TK, Kim HB, Kang HJ, Chai JH. Effects of 12 weeks of aerobic exercise on body composition and vascular compliance in obese boys. J Sports Med Phys Fitness 2012 Oct;52(5):522-9.

Song JY, Park SY, Kim JY, Won KC, Kim YD, Choi YJ, Zheng MS, Son JK, Kim YW. *Orthosiphon stamineus* Reduces Appetite and Visceral Fat in Rats. J. Korean Soc. Appl. Biol. Chem. 2011;54(2):200-205.

Song KH, Lee SH, Kim BY, Park AY, Kim JY. Extracts of Scutellaria baicalensis Reduced Body Weight and Blood Triglyceride in db/db Mice. Phytother Res. 2012 Apr 25.

Song MY, Lv N, Kim EK, Kwon KS, Yoo YB, Kim JH, Lee SW, Song JH, Lee JH, Lee SK, Shin BC, Ryu DG, Park BH, Kwon KB. Antiobesity activity of aqueous extracts of Rhizoma Dioscoreae Tokoronis on high-fat diet-induced obesity in mice. J Med Food 2009 Apr;12(2):304-9.

Song WY, Yang JA, Ku KH, Choi JH. Effect of Red Pepper Seeds Powder on Antioxidative System and Oxidative Damage in Rats Fed High-Fat High-Cholesterol Diet. J. Korean Soc Food Sci Nutr 2009;38(9):1161-1166.

Song WY, Chun SS, Ku KH, Choi JH. Effect of Red Pepper Seeds Powder on Lipid Composition in Rats Fed High-Fat High-Cholesterol Diets. J. Food Sci. Nutr 2010;15:184-188.

Song WY, Sung BH, Kang SK, Choi JH. Effect of Water Extracts from *Phellinus linteus* on Lipid Composition and Antioxidative System in Rats Fed High Fat High Cholesterol Diet. J Korean Soc Food Sci Nutr 2010;39(1):71-77.

Song WY, Kim YN, Chun SS, Ku KH, Choi JH. Effects of Ethanol Extracts from Red Pepper *(Capsicum annuum* L.) Seeds on Cholesterol Adsorption Capacity and UDP-Glucuronyl Transferase Activity. Journal of Life Science 2011;21(6):829-837.

Song YB, An YR, Kim SJ, Park HW, Jung JW, Kyung JS, Hwang SY, Kim YS. Lipid metabolic effect of Korean red ginseng extract in mice fed on a high-fat diet. J Sci Food Agric 2012 Jan 30;92(2):388-96.

Soriguer F, Almaraz MC, Ruiz-de-Adana MS, Esteva I, Linares F, García-Almeida JM, Morcillo S, García-Escobar E, Olveira-Fuster G, Rojo-Martínez G. Incidence of obesity is lower in persons who consume olive oil. European Journal of Clinical Nutrition 2009;63:1371-1374.

Sotaniemi EA, Haapakoski E, Rautio A. Ginseng Therapy in Non-Insulin-Dependent Diabetic Patients. Diabetes Care 1995;18(10):1373-1375.

Souza GA, Ebaid GX, Seiva FRF, Rocha KHR, Galhardi CM, Mani F, Novelli ELB. N-Acetylcysteine an *Allium* Plant Compound Improves High-Sucrose Diet-Induced Obesity and Related Effects. Evidence-Based Complementary and Alternative Medicine 2011:1-7.

Speechly DP, Rogers GG, Buffenstein R. Acute appetite reduction associated with an increased frequency of eating in obese males. Int J Obes Relat Metab Disord 1999 Nov;23(11):1151-9.

Speechly DP, Buffenstein R. Greater appetite control associated with an increased frequency of eating in lean males. Appetite 1999 Dec;33(3):285-97.

Spielmann J, Stangl GI, Eder K. Dietary pea protein stimulates bile acid excretion and lowers hepatic cholesterol concentration in rats. Journal of Animal Physiology and Animal Nutrition 2008;92:683-693.

Spillane M, Schwarz N, Leddy S, Correa T, Minter M, Longoria V, Willoughby DS. Effects of 28 days of resistance exercise while consuming commercially available pre- and post-workout supplements, NO-Shotgun® and NO-Synthesize® on body composition, muscle strength and mass, markers of protein synthesis, and clinical safety markers in males. Nutr Metab (Lond) 2011 Nov 3;8(78):1-11.

Spradley BD, Crowley KR, Tai CY, Kendall KL, Fukuda DH, Esposito EN, Moon SE, Moon JR. Ingesting a pre-workout supplement containing caffeine, B-vitamins, amino acids, creatine, and beta-alanine before exercise delays fatigue while improving reaction time and muscular endurance. Nutr Metab (Lond) 2011 Mar 30;9(28):1-9.

Srinivasan MR, Satyanarayana MN. Influence of capsaicin, curcumin and ferulic acid in rats fed high fat diets. J Biosci. 1987 Jun;12(2):143-152.

Sriplang K, Adisakwattana S, Rungsipipiat A. Effects of *Orthosiphon stamineus* aqueous extract on plasma glucose concentration and lipid profile in normal and stretozotocin-induced diabetic rats. J Ethnopharmacol 2007;109:510-514.

St-Onge MP, Ross R, ParsonsWD, Jones PJ. Medium-chain triglycerides increase energy expenditure and decrease adiposity in overweight men. Obes Res. 2003 Mar;11(3):395-402.

St-Onge MP, Bosarge A. Weight-loss diet that includes consumption of medium-chain triacylglycerol oil leads to a greater rate of weight and fat mass loss than does olive oil. Am J Clin Nutr 2008 March;87(3):621-626.

Stanhope KL, Schwarz JM, Keim NL, Griffen SC, Bremer AA, Graham JL, Hatcher B, Cox CL, Dyachenko A, Zhang W, McGahan JP, Seibert A, Krauss RM, Chiu S, Schaefer EJ, Aim M, Otokozawa S, Nakajima K, Nakano T, Beysen C, Hellerstein MK, Berglund L, Havel PJ. Consuming fructose-sweetened, not glucose-sweetened, beverages increases visceral adiposity and lipids and decreases insulin sensitivity in overweight/obese humans. J Clin Invest 2009 May;119(5):1322-34.

Stanko RT, Tietze DL, Arch JE. Body composition, energy utilization, and nitrogen metabolism with a 4.25-MJ/d low-energy diet supplemented with pyruvate. Am J. Clin. Nutr. 1992;56:630-5.

Stanko RT, Reynolds HR, Lonchar KD, Arch JE. Plasma lipid concentrations in hyperlipidemic patients consuming a high-fat diet supplemented with pyruvate for 6 wk. Am J. Clin. Nutr. 1992;56:950-4.

Stanko RT, Reynolds HR, Hoyson R, Janosky JE, Wolf R. Pyruvate supplementation of a low-cholesterol, low-fat diet: effects on plasma lipid concentrations and body composition in hyperlipidemic patients. Am J. Clin. Nutr. 1994;59:423-7.

Stark M, Lukaszuk J, Prawitz A, Salacinski A. Protein timing and its effects on muscular hypertrophy and strength in individuals engaged in weight-training. J Int Soc Sports Nutr 2012 Dec 14;9(1):54.

Stewart I, McNaughton L, Davies P, Tristram S. Phosphate loading and the effects on VO2max in trained cyclists. Res Q Exerc Sport 1990 Mar;61(1):80-4.

Stisen AB, Stougaard O, Langfort J, Helge JW, Sahlin K, Madsen K. Maximal fat oxidation rates in endurance trained and untrained women. Eur J Appl Physiol 2006 Nov;98(5):497-506.

Stomati M, Rubino S, Spinetti A, Parrini D, Luisi S, Casarosa E, Petraglia F, Genazzani AR. Endocrine, neuroendocrine and behavioral effects of oral dehydroepiandrosterone sulfate supplementatin in postmenopausal women. Gynecol Endocrinol 1999 Feb;13(1):15-25.

Stomati M, Monteleone P, Casarosa E, Quirici B, Puccetti S, Bernardi F, Genazzani AD, Rovati L, Luisi M, Genazzani AR. Six-month oral dehydroepiandrosterone supplementation in early and late postmenopause. Gynecol Endocrinol 2000 Oct;14(5):342-63.

Stookey JD, Constant F, Popkin BM, Gardner CD. Drinking water is associated with weight loss in overweight dieting women independent of diet and activity. Obesity (Silver Spring) 2008 Nov;16(11):2481-8.

Stoppani J, Scheett T, Pena J, Rudolph C, Charlebois D. Consuming a supplement containing branched-cain amino acids during a resistance-trainin program increases lean mass, muscle strength and fat loss. Journal of the International Society of Sports Nutrition 2009;6(1).

Strasser B, Schobersberger W. Evidence for Resistance Training as a Treatment Therapy in Obesity. Journal of Obesity 2011:1-9.

Sui Y, Zhao HL, Wong VC, Brown N, Li XL, Kwan AK, Hui HL, Ziea ET, Chan JC. A systematic review on use of Chinese medicine and acupuncture for treatment of obesity. Obes Rev. 2012 May;13(5):409-430.

Sugiyama K, Ohishi A, Ohnuma Y, Muramatsu K. Comparison between the Plasma Cholesterol-lowering Effects of Glycine and Taurine in Rats Fed on High Cholesterol Diets. Agric Biol. Chem. 1989;53(6):1647-1652.

Suliburska J, Bogdanski P, Szulinska M, Stepien M, Pupek-Musialik D, Jablecka A. Effects of Green Tea Supplementation on Elements, Total Antioxidans, Lipids, and Glucose Values in the Serum of Obese Patients. Biol Trace Elem Res. 2012 May 15.

Sultan MT, Butt MS, Anjum FM. Safety assessment of black cumin fixed and essential oil in normal Srague dawley rats: Serological and hematological indices. Food and Chemical Toxicology 2009;47:2768-2775.

Sumiyoshi M, Kimura Y. Hop (Humulus lupulus L.) extract inhibits obesity in mice fed a high-fat diet over the long term. Br J Nutr 2012 Apr 3:1-11.

Sumon MH, Mostofa M, Jahan MS, Kayesh MEH, Haque MA. Comparative Efficacy of powdered form of Stevia *(Stevia Rebaudiana Bertoni)* leaves and glimepiride in induced diabetic rats. Bangl. J. Vet. Med. 2008;6(2):211-215.

Sun BS, Chen YP, Wang YB, Tang SW, Pan FY, Li Z, Sung CK. Anti-obesity effects of mogrosides extracted from the fruits of *Siraitia grosvenorii* (Cucurbitaceae). African Journal of Pharmacy and Pharmacology 2012 May;6(20):1492-1501.

Sun C, Wang L, Yan J, Liu S. Calcium ameliorates obesity induced by high-fat diet and its potential correlation with p38 MAPK pathway. Mol Biol Rep. 2012 Feb;39(2):1755-63.

Sun X, Zemel MB. Calcium and Dairy Products Inhibit Weight and Fat Regain during Ad Libitum Consumpton Following Energy Restriction in A2-Agouti Transgenic Mice. J. Nutr. 2004 Nov;134(11):3054-60.

Sun YS, Chen SF, Zhu W. Effects and Mechanism of Resveratrol on Body weight and Adipose Tissue Distribution of KKAy Mice. J. Food Science 2011;32(13):289-292.

Sundaresan A, Harini R, Pugalendi KV. Ursolic acid and rosiglitazone combination alleviates metabolic syndrome in high fat diet fed C57BL/6J mice. Gen Physiol Biophys 2012 Sep;31(3):323-33.

Sung YY, Yoon T, Kim SJ, Yang WK, Kim HK. Anti-obesity of *Allium fistulosum* L. extract by down-regulation of the expression of lipogenic genes in high-fat diet-induced obese mice. Molecular medicine reports 2011;4:431-435.

Sung YY, Yoon T, Yang WK, Kim SJ, Kim HK. Anti-obesity effects of *Geranium thunbergii* extract via improvement of lipid metabolism in high-fat diet-induced obese mice. Molecular medicine reports 2011;4:1107-1113.

Sung YY, Yoon T, Yang WK, Kim SJ, Kim HK. Inhibitory Effects of *Elsholtzia ciliata* Extract on Fat Accumulation in High-fat Diet-induced Obese Mice. J. Korean Soc. Appl. Biol. Chem. 2011;54(3):388-394.

Supriya K, Sarita Kotagiri, Vrushabendra Swamy BM, Archana Swamy P, Vishwanath KN. Anti-Obesity Activity of *Shorea robusta* G. Leaves Extract on Monosodium Glutamate Induced Obesity in Albino Rats. Research Journal of Pharmaceutical, Biological and Chemical Sciences 2012;3(3):555-565.

Suter PM, Schutz Y, Jequier E. The effect of ethanol on fat storage in healthy subjects. N Engl J Med. 1992 Apr 9;326(15):983-7.

Suter PM, Jéquier E, Schutz Y. Effect of ethanol on energy expenditure. Am J Physiol. 1994 Apr;266(4 Pt 2):1204-12.

Suwannaphet W, Meeprom A, Yibchok-Anun S, Adisakwattana S. Preventive effect of grape seed extract against high-fructose diet-induced insulin resistance and oxidative stress in rats. Food and Chemical Toxicology 2010;48:1853-1857.

Suzuki Y, Unno T, Ushitani M. Antiobesity Activity of Extracts from *Lagerstroemia speciosa* L. Leaves on Female KK-A Mice. J Nutr Sci Vitaminol 1999;45:791-795.

Svendsen PF, Jensen FK, Holst JJ, Haugaard SB, Nilas L, Madsbad S. The effect of a very low calorie diet on insulin sensitivity, beta cell function, insulin clearance, incretin hormone secretion, androgen levels and body composition in obese young women. Scand J Clin Lab Invest 2012 Jun 18.

Sy M, Yang H, Seo SG, Shin SH, Chung MY, Kim J, Lee SJ, Lee HJ, Lee KW. Cocoa polyphenols suppress adipogenesis in vitro and obesity in vivo by targeting insulin receptor. Int J Obes (Lond) 2012.

Tajik N, Keshavarz SA, Masoudkabir F, Djalali M, Sadrzadeh-Yeganeh HH, Eshraghian MR, Chamary M, Ahmadivand Z, Yazdani T, Javanbakht MH. Effect of diet-induced weight loss on inflammatory cytokines in obese women. J Endocrinol Invest 2012 Jun 25.

Taing MW, Pierson JT, Hoang VL, Shaw PN, Dietzgen RG, Gidley MJ, Roberts-Thomson SJ, Monteith GR. Mango fruit peel and flesh extracts affect adipogenesis in 3T3-L1 cells. Food Funct. 2012 Aug 25;3(8):828-36.

Takada R, Saitoh M, Mori T. Dietary gamma-linolenic acid-enriched oil reduces body fat content and induces liver enzyme activities relating to fatty acid beta-oxidation in rats. J Nutr. 1994 Apr;124(4):469-74.

Takahashi S, Tamai M, Nakajima S, Kato H, Johno H, Nakamura T, Kitamura M. Blockade of adipocyte differentiation by cordycepin. Br J Pharmacol 2012 Apr 27.

Takahashi Y, Ide T, Fujita H. Dietary gamma-linolenic acid in the form of borage oil causes less body fat accumulation accompanying an increase in uncoupling protein 1 mRNA level in brown adipose tissue. Comparative Biochemstry and Physiology 2000;127:213-222.

Takayanagi K, Morimoto SI, Shirakura Y, Mukai K, Sugiyama T, Tokuji Y, Ohnishi M. Mechanism of Visceral Fat Reduction in Tsumura Suzuki Obese Diabetes (TSOD) Mice Orally Administered β-Cryptoxanthin from Satsuma Mandarin Oranges *(Citrus unshiu* Marc). J. Agric. Food Chem. 2011;59(23):12342-12351.

Takayanagi K. Prevention of adiposity by the oral administration of β-cryptoxanthin. Frontiers in Neurology 2011;2(67):1-6.

Takeuchi H, Tanaka T, Muramatsu K. Effects of Arginine and Methionine on the Growth Depression of Rats Fed Diets High in Glycine. Agr. Biol. Chem. 1969;33(8):1161-1168.

Takeuchi H, Sekine S,Kojima K, Aoyama T. The application of medium-chain fatty acids: edible oil with a suppressing effect on body fat accumulation. Asia Pac J Clin Nutr 2008;17:320-323.

Takikawa M, Inoue S, Horio F, Tsuda T. Dietary anthocyanin-rich bilberry extract ameliorates hyperglycemia and insulin sensitivity via activation of AMP-activated protein kinase in diabetic mice. J Nutr 2010 Mar;140(3):527-33.

Talanian JL, Galloway SDR, Heigenhauser GJF, BonenA, Spriet LL. Two weeks of high-intensity aerobic interval training increases the capacity for fat oxidation during exercise in women. J Appl Physiol 2007;102:1439-1447.

Tamer G, Mesci B, Tamer I, Kilic D, Arik S. Is vitamin D deficiency an independent risk factor for obesity and abdominal obesity in women?. Endokrynol Pol 2012;63(3):196-201.

Tan B, Yin Y, Liu Z, Li X, Xu H, Kong X, Huang R, Tang W, Shinzato I, Smith SB, Wu G. Dietary L-arginine supplementation increases muscle gain and reduces body fat mass in growing-finising pigs. Amino Acids 2009;37:169-175.

Tan B, Yin Y, Liu Z, Tang W, Xu H, Kong X, Li X, Yao K, Gu W, Smith SB, Wu G. Dietary L-arginine supplementation differentially regulates expression of lipid-metabolic genes in porcine adipose tissue and skeletal muscle. Journal of Nutritional Biochemistry 2011;22:441-445.

Tan Y, Kamal MA, Wang ZZ, Xiao W, Seale JP, Qu X. Chinese herbal extracts (SK0506) as a potential candidate for the therapy of the metabolic syndrome. Clinical Science 2011;120:297-305.

Tanaka K, Nishizono S, Tamaru S, Kondo M, Shimoda H, Tanaka J, Okada T. Anti-Obesity and Hypotriglyceridemic Properties of Coffee Bean Extract in SD Rats. Food Sci. Technol. Res. 2009;15(2):147-152.

Tanaka K, Tamaru S, Nishizono S, Miyata Y, Tamaya K, Matsui T, Tanaka T, Echizen Y, Ikeda I. Hypotriacylglycerolemic and Antiobesity Properties of a New Fermented Tea Product Obtained by Tea-Rolling Processing of Third-Crop Green Tea *(Camellia sinensis)* Leaves and Loquat *(Eriobotrya japonica)* Leaves. Biosci. Biotechnol. Biochem. 2010;74(8):1606-1612.

Tanaka Y, Sasaki R, Fukui F, Waki H, Kawabata T, Okazaki M, Hasegawa K, Ando S. Acetyl-L-carnitine supplementation restores decreased tissue carnitine levels and impaired lipid metabolism in aged rats. J Lipid Res. 2004 Apr;45(4):729-35.

Taniguchi H, Kobayashi-Hattori K, Tenmyo C, Kamei T, Uda Y, Sugita-Konishi Y, Oishi Y, Takita T. Effect of Japanese radish (Raphanus sativus) sprout (Kaiware-daikon) on carbohydrate and lipid metabolisms in normal and streptozotocin-induced diabetic rats. Phytother Res. 2006 Apr;20(4):274-8.

Taniguchi H, Muroi R, Kobayashi-Hattori K, Uda Y, Oishi Y, Takita T. Differing Effects of Water-Soluble and Fat-Soluble Extracts from Japanese Radish *(Raphanus sativus)* Sprouts on Carbohydrate and Lipid Metabolism in Normal and Streptozotocin-Induced Diabetic Rats. J Nutr Sci Vitaminol 2007;53:261-266.

Tanida M, Tsuruoka N, Shen J, Horii Y, Beppu Y, Kiso Y, Nagai K. Effects of Flavangenol on Autonomic Nerve Activities and Dietary Body Weight Gain in Rats. Biosci. Biotechnol. Biochem. 2009;73(90196):1-5.

Tang CL, Dai DC, Zhao GF, Zhu WF, Mei LF. Clinical observation on electroacupuncture combined with catgut implantation at acupoints for treatment of simple obesity of heart and spleen deficiency type. Zhongguo Zhen Jiu 2009 Sep;29(9):703-7.

Tang JJ, Li JG, Qi W, Qiu WW, Li PS, Li BL, Song BL. Inhibition of SREBP by a small molecule, betulin, improves hyperlipidemia and insulin resistance and reduces atherosclerotic plaques. Cell Metab. 2011 Jan 5;13(1):44-56.

Tanquilut NC, Tanquilut MRC, Estacio MAC, Torres EB, Rosario JC, Reyes BAS. Hypoglycemic effect of *Lagerstroemia speciosa* (L.) Pers. On alloxan-induced diabetic mice. Journal of Medicinal Plants Research 2009 Dec;3(12):1066-1071.

Taylor CG, Noto AD, Stringer DM, Froese S, Malcolmson L. Dietary Milled Flaxseed and Flaxseed Oil Improve N-3 Fatty Acid Status and Do Not Affect Glycemic Control in Individuals with Well-Controlled Type 2 Diabetes. Journal of the American College of Nutrition 2010;29(1):72-80.

Teff KL, Elliott SS, Tschöp M, Kieffer TJ, Rader D, Heiman M, Townsend RR, Keim NL, D'Alessio D, Havel PJ. Dietary fructose reduces circulating insulin and leptin, attenuates postprandial suppression of ghrelin, and increases triglycerides in women. J Clin Endocrinol Metab. 2004 Jun;89(6):2963-72.

Teff KL, Grudziak J, Townsend RR, Dunn TN, Grant RW, Adams SH, Keim NL, Cummings BP, Stanhope KL, Havel PJ. Endocrine and metabolic effects of consuming fructose- and glucose-sweetened beverages with meals in obese men and women: influence of insulin resistance on plasma triglycerides responses. J Clin Endocrinol Metab. 2009 May;94(5):1562-9.

Tembhurne SV, Sakarkar DM. Biochemical and physiological responses of fruit juice of *Murraya koenigii* (L) in 28 days repeated dose toxicity study. International Journal of PharmTech Research 2009;1(4):1568-1575.

Terra X, Pallarés V, Ardèvol A, Bladé C, Fernández-Larrea J, Pujadas G, Salvadó J, Arola L, Blay M. Modulatory effect of grape-seed procyanidins on local and systemic inflammation in diet-induced obesity rats. Journal of Nutritional Biochemistry 2011;22:380-387.

Tews JK. Dietary GABA decreases body weight of genetically obese mice. Life Sciences 1981 Dec 14;29(24):2535-2542.

Thabet SS. Assessment of the effect of lipoi acid administratio on hemostatic and lipid parameters in ovariectomized rats. JASMR 2009;4(2):149-156.

Thayalini K, Shanmugavelun S, Saminathan PM, Siti Masidayu MS, Nor Idayusni Y, Zainuddin H, Nurul Akmal CA, Wong HK. Effects of *Cymbopogon citratus* leaf and *Zingiber officinale* rhizome supplementation on growth performance, ileal morphology and lactic acid concentration in broilers. Mal. J. Anim. Sci. 2011;14:43-49.

Thayyil AH, Surulivel MK, Ahmed MF, Ahamed GSS, Sidheeq A, Rasheed A, Ibrahim M. Hypolipidemic activity of *Luffa aegiptiaca* fruits in choesterol fed hypercholesterolemic rabbits. International Journal of Pharmaceutical Applications 2011;2(1):81-88.

Thom E, Wadstein J, Gudmundsen O. Conjugated Linoleic Acid Reduces Body Fat in Healthy Exercising Humans. The Journal of International Medical Research 2001;29:392-396.

Thom E. The Effect of Chlorogenic Acid Enriched Coffee on Glucose Absorption in Healthy Volunteers and Its Effect on Body Mass When Used Long-term in Overweight and Obese People. The Journal of International Medical Research 2007;35:900-908.

Thomas DT, Wideman L, Lovelady CA. Effects of a dairy supplement and resistance training on lean mass and insulin-like growth factor in women. Int J Sport Nutr Exerc Metab 2011 Jun;21(3):181-8.

Thorsdottir I, Tomasson H, Gunnarsdottir I, Gisladottir E, Kiely M, Parra MD, Bandarra NM, Schaafsma G, Martinéz JA. Randomized trial of weight-loss-diets for young adults varying in fish and fish oil content. International Journal of Obesity 2007;31:1560-1566.

Thounaojam M, Jadeja R, Ansarullah, Devkar R, Ramachandran AV. Dysregulation of Lipid and Cholesterol Metabolism in High

Fat Diet Fed Hyperlipidemic Rats: Protective Effect of *Sida rhomboidea. Roxb* Leaf Extract. Journal of Health Science 2009;55(3):413-420.

Thounaojam MC, Jadeja RN, Ansarullah, Patel VB, Devkar RV, Ramachandran AV. Potential of *Sida rhomboidea Roxb* Leaf Extract in Controlling Hypertriglyceridemia in Experimental Models. Pharmacognosy Research 2009;1(4):208-212.

Thounaojam MC, Jadeja RN, Ansarullah, Devkar RV, Ramachandran AV. Prevention of High Fat Diet Induced Insulin Resistance in C57BL/6J Mice by *Sida rhomboidea* Roxb. Extract. Journal of Health Science 2010;56(1):92-98.

Thounaojam MC, Jadeja RN, Ramani UV, Devkar RV, Ramachandran AV. *Sida rhomboidea.* Roxb Leaf Extract Down-Regulates Expression of PPARγ2 and Leptin Genes in High Fat Diet Fed C57BL/6J Mice and Retards *in Vitro* 3T3L1 Pre-Adipocyte Differentiation. Int. J. Mol. Sci. 2011;12:4661-4677.

Thurmond DC, Tang AB, Nakamura MT, Stern JS, Phinney SD. Time-dependent effects of progressive gamma-linolenate feeding on hyperphagia, weight gain, and erythrocyte fatty acid composition durin growth of Zucker obese rats. Obes Res. 1993 Mar;1(2):118-25.

Thyagarajan-Sahu A, Lane B, Sliva D. ReishiMax, mushroom based dietary supplement, inhibits adipocyte differentiation, stimulates glucose uptake and activates AMPK. BMC Complementary and Alternative Medicine 2011;11:74.

Tian J, Dang HN, Yong J, Chui WS, Dizon MPG, Yaw CKY, Kaufman DL. Oral Treatment with γ-Aminobutyric Acid Improves Glucose Tolerance and Insulin Sensitivity by Inhibiting Inflammation in High Fat Diet-Fed Mice. PloS ONE 2011 Sep;6(9):1-7.

Tian WX, Li CH, Wu XD, Chen CC. Weight reduction by Chinese medicinal herbs may be related to inhibition of fatty acid synthase. Life Sciences 2004;74:2389-2399.

Titta L, Trinei M, Stendardo M, Berniakovich I, Petroni K, Tonelli C, Riso P, Porrini M, Minucci S, Pelicci PG, Rapisarda P, Recupero GR, Giorgio M. Blood orange juice inhibits fat accumulation in mice. International Journal of Obesity 2009;1-11.

Tjønna AE, Lee SJ, Rognmo Ø, Stølen TO, Bye A, Haram PM, Loennechen JP, Al-Share QY, Skogvoll E, Slørdahl SA, Kemi OJ, Najjar SM, Wisløff U. Aerobic interval training versus continuous moderate exercise as a treatment for the metabolic syndrome: a pilot study. Circulation 2008 Jul 22;118(4):346-54.

Tominaga S, Nishi K, Nishimoto S, Akiyama K, Yamauchi S, Sugahara T. Secoisolariciresinol attenuates high-fat diet-induced obesity in C57BL/6 mice. Food Funct. 2012 Jan;3(1):76-82.

Tominaga Y, Mae T, Kitano M, Sakamoto Y, Ikematsu H, Nakagawa K. Licorice Flavonoid Oil Effects Body Weight Loss by Reduction of Body Fat Mass in Overweight Subjects. Journal of Health Science 2006;52(6):672-683.

Tominaga Y, Nakagawa K, Mae T, Kitano M, Yokota S, Arai T, Ikematsu H, Inoue S. Licorice flavonoid oil reduces total body fat and visceral fat in overweight subjects: A randomized, double-blind, placebo-controlled study. Obesity Research & Clinical Practice 2009 Aug;3(3):169-178.

Tomita K, Okuhara Y, Shigematsu N, Suh H, Lim K. (-)-Hydroxycitrate Ingestion Increases Fat Oxidaton during Moderate Intensity Exercise in Untrained Men. Biosci. Biotechnol. Biochem. 2003;67(9):1999-2001.

Tomotake H, Yamamoto N, Yanaka N, Ohinata H, Yamazaki R, Kayashita J, Kato N. High protein buckwheat flour suppresses hypercholesterolemia in rats and gallstone formation in mice by hypercholesterolemic diet and body fat in rats because of its low protein digestibility. Nutrition 2006;22:166-173.

Tomonori N, Ryuji O, Takuya W, Kiyoshi K, Masanori K, Ichiro T. Visceral Fat-reducing Effect of Continuous Coffee Beverage Consumption in Obese Subjects. Yakuri to chiryo 2009;37(4):333-344.

Tong J, Chen JX, Zhang ZQ, Liu CS, Pan Y, Zheng J, Yao H. Clinical observation on simple obesity treated by acupuncture. Zhongguo Zhen Jiu 2011 Aug;31(8):697-701.

Tonstad S, Butler T, Yan R, Fraser GE. Type of vegetarian diet, body weight, and prevalence of type 2 diabetes. Diabetes Care 2009 May;32(5):791-6.

Torres MRSG, Ferreira TS, Carvalho DC, Sanjuliani AF. Dietary calcium intake and its relationship with adiposity and metabolic profile in hypertensive patients. Nutrition 2011;27:666-671.

Torres-Leal FL, Fonseca-Alaniz MH, Teodoro GFR, de Capitani MD, Vianna D, Pantaleão LC, Matos-Neto EM, Rogero MM, Jr Donato J, Tirapegui J. Leucine supplementation improves adiponectin and total cholesterol concentrations despite the lack of changes in adiposity or glucose homeostatis in rats previously exposed to a high-fat diet. *Nutrition & Metabolism* 2011;8:62.

Torres-Rovira L, Astiz S, Caro A, Lopez-Bote C, Ovilo C, Pallares P, Perez-Solana ML, Sanchez-Sanchez R, Gonzalez-Bulnes A. Diet-induced swine model with obesity/leptin resistance for the study of metabolic syndrome and type 2 diabetes. ScientificWorldJournal 2012.

Tourkostani R, Al Balouni I, Moselhy SS, Kumosani TA. A Diet Rich Fiber Improves Lipid Profile in Rats Fed on High Fat Diet. Türk Biyokimya Dergisi [Turkish Journal of Biochemistry – Turk J Biochem] 2009;34(2):105-111.

Trevisan MC, Souza JMP, Marucci MFN. Influence of soy protein intake and weight training on the resting energy expenditure of postmenopausal women. Rev Assoc Med Bras 2010;56(5):572-8.

Trilk JL, Singhal A, Bigelman KA, Cureton KJ. Effect of sprint interval training on circulatory function during exercise in sedentary, overweight/obese women. Eur J Appl Physiol 2011 Aug;111(8):1591-7.

Tsuchida T, Mukai K, Mizuno Y, Masuko K, Minagawa K. The comparative study of β-cryptoxanthin derived from Satsuma mandarin for fat of human body. Jpn. Pharmacol. Ther. 2008;36:247-253.

Tsuda T, Horio F, Uchida K, Aoki H, Osawa T. Dietary cyanidin 3-O-beta-D-glucoside-rich purle corn color prevents obesity and ameliorates hyperglycemia in mice. J Nutr 2003 Jul;133(7):2125-30.

Tsuji H, Kasai M, Takeuchi H, Nakamura M, Okazaki M, Kondo K. Dietary medium-chain triacylglycerols suppress accumulation of body fat in a double-blind, controlled trial in healthy men and women. J Nutr. 2001 Nov;131(11):2853-9.

Tsujita T, Takaku T. Lipolysis Induced by Segment Wall Extract from Satsuma Mandarin Orange *(Citrus unshu* Mark). J Nutr Sci Vitaminol 2007;53:547-551.

Tsukui T, Konno K, Hosokawa M, Maeda H, Sashima T, Miyashita K. Fucoxanthin and fucoxanthinol enhance the amount of docosahexaenoic acid in the liver of KKAy obese/diabetic mice. J Agric Food Chem 2007 Jun 27;55(13):5025-9.

Tsuruta Y, Nagao K, Kai S, Tsuge K, Yoshimura T, Koganemaru K, Yanagita T. Polyphenolic extract of lotus root (edible rhizome of *Nelumbo nucifera)* alleviates hepatic steatosis in obese diabetic *db/db* mice. Lipids in Health and Disease 2011;10:202.

Tsuruta Y, Nagao K, Shirouchi B, Nomura S, Tsuge K, Koganemaru K, Yanagita T. Effects of Lotus Root (the Edible Rhizome of *Nelumbo nucifera*) on the Development of Non-Alcoholic Fatty Liver Disease in Obese Diabetic *db/db* Mice. Biosci. Biotechnol. Biochem. 2012;76(3):462-466.

Tuomilehto J, Voutilainen E, Huttunen J, Vinni S, Homan K. Effect of Guar Gum on Body Weight and Serum Lipids in Hypercholesterolemic Females. Acta Medica Scandinavica 1980;208(1-6):45-48.

Tzeng TF, Lu HJ, Liou SS, Chang CJ, Liu IM. Vinegar-Baked Radix Bupleuri Regulates Lipid Disorders via a Pathway Dependent on Peroxisome-Proliferator-Activated Receptor-α in High-Fat-Diet-Induced Obese Rats. Evidence-Based Complementary and Alternative Medicine 2012.

Tzeng TF, Lu HJ, Liou SS, Chang CJ, Liu IM. *Cassia tora* (Leguminosae) seed extract alleviates high-fat diet-induced nonalcoholic fatty liver. Food and Chemistry Toxicology 2013;51:194-201.

Tzeng TF, Lu HJ, Liou SS, Chang CJ, Liu IM. Reduction of lipid accumulatio in white adipose tissues by *Cassia tora* (Leguminosae) seed extract is associated with AMPK activation. Food and Chemistry Toxicology 2013;136:1086-1094.

Udani J, Singh BB. Blocking carbohydrate absorption and weight loss: a clinical trial using a proprietary fractionated white bean extract. Altern Ther Health Med 2007 Jul-Aug;13(4):32-7.

Udani JK, Singh BB, Barrett ML, Singh VJ. Evaluation of Mangosteen juice blend on biomakers of inflammation in obese subjects: a pilot, dose finding study. Nutr J 2009 Oct 20;8:48.

Ugwu CE, Olajide JE, Alumana EO, Ezeanyika LUS. Comparative effects of the leaves of *Vernonia amygdalina* and *Telfairia occidentalis* incorporated diets on the lipid profile of rats. African Journal of Biochemistry Research 2011 Jan;5(1):28-32.

Uemura T, Hirai S, Mizoguchi N, Goto T, Lee JY, Taketani K, Nakano Y, Shono J, Hoshino S, Tsuge N, Narukami T, Takahashi N, Kawada T. Diosgenin present in fenugreek improves glucose metabolism by promoting adipocyte differentiation and inhibiting inflammation in adipose tissues. Mol Nutr Food Res. 2010 Nov;54(11):1596-608.

Ukwuani AN, Abukakar MG, Shehu RA, Hassan LG. Antiobesity Effects of Pulp Extract *Tamarindus indica* in Albino Rat. Asian Journal of Biochemistry 2008;3(4):221-227.

Vafa M, Mohammadi F, Shidfar F, Sormaghi MS, Heidari I, Golestan B, Amiri F. Effects of Cinnamon Consumption on Glycemic Status, Lipid Profile and Body Composition in Type 2 Diabetic Patients. International Journal of Preventive Medicine 2012;3(8):531-536.

Valdecantos MP, Pérez-Matute P, González-Muniesa P, Prieto-Hontoria PL, Moreno-Aliaga MJ, Martine JA. Lipoic acid administration prevents nonalcoholic steatosis linked to long-term high-fat feeding by modulating mitochondrial function. Journal of Nutritional Biochemistry 2012.

Van Walleghen EL, Orr JS, Gentile CL, Davy BM. Pre-meal water consumption reduces meal energy intake in older but not younger subjects. Obesity (Silver Spring). 2007 Jan;15(1):93-9.

Vaneeta J, Dhingra D, Sharma S, Parle M, Harna RK. Hypolipidemic and weight reducing activity of the ethanol extract of *Tamarindus indica* fruit pulp in cafeteria diet- and sulpiride-induced obese rats. J Pharmacol Pharmacother 2011 Apr-Jun;2(2): 80-84.

Vaquero MR, Yáñez-Gascón MJ, Villalba RG, Larrosa M, Fromentin E, Ibarra A, Roller M, Tomás-Barberán F, de Gea JCE, Garcia-Conesa MT. Inhibition of Gastric Lipase as a Mechanism for Body Weight and Plasma Lipids Reduction in Zucker Rats Fed a Rosemary Extract Rich in Carnosic Acid. PloS one 2012 Jun;7(6):39773.

Vartika J, Verma SK, Katewa SS. Therapeutic validation of *Ipomoea digitata* tuber *(Ksheervidari)* for its effect on cardio-vascular risk parameters. Indian Journal of Traditional Knowledge 2011;10(4):617-623.

Vasudeva N, Sharma SK, Rani N. Quality assessment and anti-obesity activity of Stellaria media (Linn.) Vill. BMC Complementary and Alternative Medicine 2012;12:145.

Vembu S, Sivanasan D, Prasanna G. Effect of *Phoenix deactylifera* on high fat diet induced obesity. Journal of Chemical and Pharmaceutical Research 2012;4(1):348-352.

Verma PR, Deshpande SA, Kamtham YN, Vaidya LB. Hypolipidemic and antihyperlipidemic effects from an aqueous extract of *Pachyptera hymenaea* (DC.) leaves in rats. Food Chemistry 2012;132:1251-1257.

Vermunt SH, Pasman WJ, Schaafsma G, Kardinaal AF. Effects of sugar intake on body weight: a review. Obes Rev. 2003 May;4(2):91-9.

Venkatalakshmi P, Vedha VN, Sangeetha S. Hypolipidemic effect of *Achyranthes aspera* on High fat diet induced atherogenic rats. Research Journal of Pharmaceutical, Biological and Chemical Sciences 2012 Jul - Sep;3(3):75-84.

Vianna D, Resende GFT, Torres-Leal FL, Pantaleão LC, Jr Donato J, Tirapegui J. Long-term leucine supplementation reduces fat mass gain without changing body protein status of aging rats. Nutrition 2012;28:182-189.

Vijaimohan K, Jainu M, Sabitha KE, Subramaniyam S, Anandhan C, Devi CSS. Beneficial effects of alpha linolenic acid rich flaxseed oil on growth performance and hepatic cholesterol metabolism in high fat diet fed rats. Life Sciences 2006;79:448-454.

Vijayakumar MV, Pandey V, Mishra GC, Bhat MK. Hypolipidemic effect of fenugreek seeds is mediated through inhibition of fat accumulation and upregulation of LDL receptor. Obesity (Silver Spring) 2010 Apr;18(4):667-74.

Vikøren LA, Nygård OK, Lied E, Rostrup E, Gudbrandsen OA. A randomised study on the effects of fish protein supplement on glucose tolerance, lipids and body composition in overweight adults. Br J Nutr. 2012 May 31:1-10.

Villareal DT, Holloszy JO, Kohrt WM. Effects of DHEA replacement on bone mineral density and body composition in elderly women and men. Clin Endocrinol (Oxf) 2000 Nov;53(5):561-8.

Vincent M, Philippe E, Everard A, Kassis N, Rouch C, Denom J, Takeda Y, Uchiyama S, Delzenne NM, Cani PD, Migrenne S, Magnan C. Dietary Supplementation With Agaricus Blazei Murill Extract Prevents Diet-Induced Obesity and Insulin Resistance in Rats. Obesity (Silver Spring) 2012 Jun 7.

Vinson JA, Burnham BR, Nagendran MV. Randomized, double-blind, placebo-controlled, linear dose, crossover study to evaluate the efficacy and safety of a green coffee bean extract in overweight subjects. Diabetes, Metabolic Syndrome and Obesity: Targets and Therapy 2012;5:21-27.

Vogels N, Nijs IMT, Westerterp-Plantenga MS. The effect of grape-seed extract on 24h energy intake in humans. European Journal of Clinical Nutrition 2004;58:667-673.

Volpato GT, Calderon IMP, Sinzato S, Campos KE, Rudge MVC, Damasceno DC. Effect of *Morus nigra* aqueous extract treatment on the maternal-fetal outcome, oxidative stress status and lipid profle of streptozotocin-induced diabetic rats. Journal of Ethnopharmacology 2011;138:691-696.

Volpe SL, Kobusingye H, Bailur S, Stanek E. Effect of Diet and Exercise on Body Composition, Energy Intake and Leptin Levels in Overweight Women and Men. Journal of the American College of Nutrition 2008;27(2):195-208.

Vosough-Ghanbari S, Rahimi R, Kharabaf S, Zeinali S, Mohammadirad A, Amini S, Yasa N, Salehnia A, Toliat T, Nikfar S, Larijani B, Abdollah M. Effects of *Satureja khuzestanica* on Serum Glucose, Lipids and Markers of Oxidative Stress in Patients with Type 2 Diabetes Mellitus: A Double-Blind Randomized Controlled Trial. ECAM 2010;7(4):465-470.

Vukovich MD, Stubbs NB, Bohlken RM. Body composition in 70-year-old adults responds to dietary beta-hydroxy-beta-methylbutyrate similarly to that of young adults. J Nutr. 2001 Jul;131(7):2049-52.

Vuong T, Benhaddou-Andaloussi A, Brault A, Harbilas D, Martineau LC, Vallerand D, Ramassamy C, Matar C, Haddad PS. Antiobesity and antidiabetic effects of biotransformed blueberry juice in KKAʸ mice. International Journal of Obesity 2009:1-8.

Vuyyuru AB, Kotagiri S, Vrushabendra SBM, Swamy A. Antihyperlipidemic Activity of *Ananas Comosus* L. Leaves Extract in Albino Rats. RJPBCS 2012 Jul - Sep;3(3):1229-1242.

Wahl P, Zinner C, AchtzehnS,BlochW,Mester J. Effect of high- and low-intensity exercise and metabolic acidosis on levels of GH, IGF-I, IGFBP-3 and cortisol. Growth Horm IGF Res. 2010 Oct;20(5):380-5.

Walczewska B, Trzewikowska M. Influence of glutamic acid, histidine and arginine on dietary intake. Chemical structure and body mass composition of rats. Rocz Panstw Zakl Hig 1993;44(2-3):181-9.

Wall BT, Stephens FB, Constantin-Teodosiu D, Marimuthu K, Macdonald IA, Greenhaff PL. Chronic oral ingestion of L-carnitine and carbohydrate increases muscle carnitine content and alters muscle fuel metabolism during exercise in humans. J Physiol 2011;589(4):963-973.

Wang J, Zhang W, Zhu D, Zhu X, Pang X, Qu W. Hypolipidaemic and hypoglycaemic effects of total flavonoids from seed residues of Hippophae rhamnoides L. in mice fed a high-fat diet. J Sci Food Agric 2011 Jun;91(8):1446-51.

Wang J, Rong X, Li W, Yamahara J, Li Y. *Salacia oblonga* ameliorates hypertriglyceridemia and excessive ectopic fat accumulation in laying hens. Journal of Ethnopharmacology 2012.

Wang L, Yamasaki M, Katsube T, Sun X, Yamasaki Y, Shiwaku K. Antiobesity effect of polyphenolic compounds from molokheiya (*Corchorus olitorius* L.) leaves in LDL receptor-deficient mice. Eur J Nutr 2011;50:127-133.

Wang L, Sun J, Yi Q, Wang X, Ju X. Protective Effect of Polyphenols Extact of Adlay *(Coix lachryma-jobi* L. var *ma-yuen Stapf)* on Hypercholesterolemia-Induced Oxidative Stress in Rats. Molecules 2012;17:8886-8897.

Wang SH, Wang WJ, Wang XF. Effects of salidroside on carbohydrate metabolism and differentiation of 3T3-L1 adipocytes. Journal of Chinese Integrative Medicine 2004;2(3):193-195.

Wang T, Wang Y, Kontani Y, Kobayashi Y, Sato Y, Mori N, Yamahita H. Evodiamine Improve Diet-Induced Obesity in a Uncoupling Protein-1-Independent Manner: Involvement of Antiadipogenic Mechanism and Extracellularly Regulated Kinase/Mitogen-Activated Protein Kinase Signaling. Endocrinology 2008;149(1):358-366.

Wang T, Takikawa Y, Satoh T, Yoshioka Y, Kosaka K, Tatemichi Y, Suzuki K. Carnosic acid prevents obesity and hepatic steatosis in ob/ob mice. Hepatol Res. 2011 Jan;41(1):87-92.

Wang W, Wang WX, Sun BH, Zhao DZ, Gao P. Effect of haidonghua powder(HDHP) on hypothalamic obesity in rats. Zhongguo Zhong Yao Za Zhi 2000 Aug;25(8):490-2.

Wang Y, Li X, Guo Y, Chan L, Guan X. Alpha-Lipoic acid increases energy expenditure by enhancing adenosine monophosphate-activated protein kinase-peroxisome proliferator-activated receptor-gamma coactivator-1alpha signaling in the skeletal muscle of aged mice. Metabolism 2010 Jul;59(7):967-76.

Wang Z, Xue L, Guo C, Han B, Pan C, Zhao S, Song H, Ma Q. Stevioside ameliorates high-fat diet-induced insulin resistance and adipose tissue inflammation by downregulating the NF-κB pathway. Biochemical and Biophysical Research Communication 2012;417:1280-1285.

Wang ZH, Hsu CC, Yin MC. Aqueous Extract from Pepino *(Solanum muricatum* Ait.) Attenuated Hyperlipidemia and Cardiac Oxidative Stress in Diabetic Mice. International Scholarly Research Network ISRN Obesity 2012.

Wang ZQ, Zuberi AR, Zhang XH, Macgowan J, Qin J, Ye X, Son L, Wu Q, Lian K, Cefalu WT. Effects of dietary fibers on weight gain, carbohydrate metabolism, and gastric ghrelin gene expression in ice fed a high-fat diet. Metabolism Clinical and Experimental 2007;56:1635-1642.

Wang ZQ, Zhang XH, Yu Y, Poulev A, Ribnicky D, Floyd ZE, Cefalu WT. Bioactives from bitter melon enhance insulin signaling and modulate acyl carnitine content in skeletal muscle in high-fat diet-fed mice. Journal of Nutritional Biochemistry 2011;22: 1064-1073.

Wang ZQ, Yu Y, Zhang XH, Ribnicky D, Cefalu WT. Ecdysterone enhances muscle insulin signaling by modulating acylcarnitine profile and mitochondrial oxidative phosphorylation complexes in mice fed a high-fat diet. Diabetes 2011 May;60(5):1645.

Wannamethee SG, Shaper AG. Alcohol, body weight and weight gain in middle-aged men. Am J Clin Nutr. 2003 May;77(5):1312-7.

Watanabe K, Arozal W, Tanaka H, Ma M, Satoh S, Veeraveedu PT, Kobayashi T, Oyama H, Sakaguchi Y. Beneficial Effect of Food Substitute Containing L-Arginine, ω-3 Poly Unsaturated Fatty Acid, and Ribonucleic Acid in Preventing or Improving Metabolic Syndrome: A Study in 15 Overweight Patients and a Study of Fatty Acid Metabolism in Animals. J. Clin. Biochem. Nutr. 2009;44:266-274.

Wei X, Wang D, Yang Y, Xia M, Li D, Li G, Zhu Y, Xiao Y, Ling W. Cyanidin-3-O-β-glucoside improves obesity and triglyceride metabolism in KK-Ay mice by regulating lipoprotein lipase activity. J Sci Food Agric 2011 Apr;91(6):1006-13.

Weigle DS, Sande KJ, Iverius PH, Monsen ER, Brunzell JD. Weight loss leads to a marked decrease in nonresting energy expenditure in ambulatory human subjects. Metabolism 1988 Oct;37(10):930-6.

Weisberg SP, Leibel R, Tortoriello DV. Dietary Curcumin Significantly Improves Obesity-Associated Inflammation and Diabetes in Mouse Models of Diabesity. Endocrinology 2008;149(7):3549-3558.

Weiss EP, Villareal DT, Fontana L, Han DH, Holloszy JO. Dehydroepiandrosterone (DHEA) replacement decreases insulin resistance and lowers inflammatory cytokines in aging humans. AGING 2011 May;3(5):533-542.

274

Whelan K, Efthymiou L, Judd PA, Preedy VR, Taylor MA. Appetitw during consumption of enteral formula as a sole source of nutrition: the effect of supplementing pea-fibre and fructo-oligosaccharides. British Journal of Nutrition 2006;96:350-356.

Whyte LJ, Gill JMR, Cathcart AJ. Effect of 2 weeks of sprint interval training on health-related outcomes in sedentary overweight/obese men. Metabolism Clinical and Experimental 2010;59:1421-1428.

Willi SM, Oexmann MJ, Wright NM. The Effects of a High-protein, Low-fat, Ketogenic Diet on Adolescents With Morbid Obesity: Body Composition, Blood Chemistries, and Sleep Abnormalities. Pediatrics 1998 Jan 1;101(1):61-67.

Willis LH, Slentz CA, Bateman LA, Shields AT, Piner LW, Bales CW, Houmard JA, Kraus WE. Effects of aerobic and/or resistance training on body mass and fat mass in overweight or obese adults. J Appl Physiol 2012;113:1831-1837.

Wisløff U, Støylen A, Loennechen JP, Bruvold M, Rognmo Ø, Haram PM, Tjønna AE, Helgerud J, Slørdahl SA, Lee SJ, Videm V, Bye A, Smith GL, Najjar SM, Ellingsen Ø, Skjaerpe T. Superior cardiovascular effect of aerobic interval training versus moderate continuous training in heart failure patients: a randomized study. Circulation 2007 Jun 19;115(24):3086-94.

Wolden-Hanson T, Mitton DR, McCants RL, Yellow SM, Wilkinson CW, Matsumoto AM, Rasmussen DD. Daily Melatonin Administration to Middle-Aged Male Rats Suppresses Body Weight, Intraabdominal Adiposity, and Plasma Leptin and Insulin Independent of Food Intake and Total Body Fat. Endocrinology 2000;141(2):487-497.

Woo MN, Jeon SM, Shin YC, Lee MK, Kang MA, Choi MS. Anti-obese property of fucoxanthin is partly mediated by altering lipid-regulating enzymes and uncoupling proteins of visceral adipose tissue in mice. Mol Nutr Food Res 2009 Dec;53(12):1603-11.

Woo MN, Jeon SM, Kim HJ, Lee MK, Shin SK, Shin YC, Park YB, Choi MS. Fucoxanthin supplementation improves plasma and hepatic lipid metabolism and blood glucose concentration in high-fat fed C57BL/6N mice. Chemico-Biological Interactions 2010;186:316-322.

Wood RJ, Fernandez ML, Sharman MJ, Silvestre R, Greene CM, Zern TL, Shrestha S, Judelson DA, Gomez AL,Kraemer WJ, Volek JS. Effects of a carbohydrate-restricted diet with and without supplemental soluble fiber on plasma low-density lipoprotein cholesterol and other clinical markers of cardiovascular risk. Metabolism Clinical and Experimental 2007;56:58-67.

Woodgate DE, Conquer JA. Effects of a Stimulant-Free Dietary Supplement on Body Weight and Fat Loss in Obese Adults: A Six-Week Exploratory Study. Current Therapeutic Research 2003 Apr;64(4):248-262.

Wu CH, Lin MC, Wang HC, Yang MY, Jou MJ, Wang CJ. Rutin inhibits oleic acid induced lipid accumulation via reducing lipogenesis and oxidative stress in hepatocarcinoma cells. J Food Sci. 2011 Mar;76(2):65-72.

Wu CH, Yang MY, Chan KC, Chung PJ, Ou TT, Wang CJ. Improvement in high-fat diet-induced obesity and body fat accumulation by a Nelumbo nucifera leaf flavonoid-rich extract in mice. J Agric Food Chem 2010 Jun 9;58(11):7075-81.

Wu G, Collins JK, Perkins-Veazie P, Siddiq M, Dolan KD, Kelly KA, Heaps CL, Meininger CJ. Dietary supplementation with watermelon pomace juice enhances arginine availability and ameliorates the metabolic syndrome in Zucker diabetic fatty rats. J Nutr. 2007 Dec;137(12):2680-5.

Wu H, Pan A, Yu Z, Qi Q, Lu L, Zhang G, Yu D, Zong G, Zhou Y, Chen X, Tang L, Feng Y, Zhou H, Chen X, Li H, Demark-Wahnefried W, Hu FB, Lin X. Lifestyle Counseling and Supplementation with Flaxseed or Walnuts Influence the Management of Metabolic Syndrome. The Journal of Nutrition 2010;140:1937-1942.

Wu Y, Ou-Yang JP, Wu K, Wang Y, Zhou YF, Wen CY. Hypoglycemic effect of *Astragalus* polysaccharide and its effect on PTP1B. Acta Pharmacologica Sinica 2005 Mar;26(3):345-352.

Wu ZH. Effects of the multiple needling with shallow insertion for simple obesity: a clinical observation on lipid metabolism and on the chest, waist and hip circumferences. J Tradit Chin Med. 2009 Sep;29(3):179-81.

Wutzke KD, Lorenz H. The Effect of L-Carnitine on Fat Oxidation, Protein Turnover, and Body Composition in Slightly Overweight Subjects. Metabolism 2004 Aug;53(8):1002-1006.

Wycherley TP, Noakes M, Clifton PM, Cleanthous X, Keogh JB, Brinkworth GD. A high-protein diet with resistance exercise training improves weight loss and body composition in overweight and obese patients with type 2 diabetes. Diabetes Care 2010 May;33(5):969-76.

Wyss V, Ganzit GP, Rienzi A. Effects of L-carnitine administration on VO2max and the aerobic-anaerobic threshold in normoxia and acute hypoxia. Eur J Appl. Physiol Occup Physiol. 1990;60(1):1-6.

Xi L, Qian Z, Xu G, Zheng S, Sun S, Wen N, Sheng L, Shi Y, Zhang Y. Beneficial impact of crocetin, a carotenoid from saffron, on insulin sensitivity in fructose-fed rats. Journal of Nutritional Biochemistry 2007;18:64-72.

Xia DZ, Yu XF,Wang HM, Ren QY, Chen BM. Anti-obesity and hypolipidemic effects of ethanolic extract from Alpinia officinarum Hance (Zingiberaceae) in rats fed high-fat diet. J Med Food 2010 Aug;13(4):785-91.

Xia M, Wang JY, Ma XY, Lu YS, Tian QS, Liu X. Effects and mechanism of Sibiraea angustata on lipid metabolism in high-fatted rats. Zhong Yao Cai 2011 Jun;34(6):922-6.

Xio L, Zhang J, Li H, Liu J, He L, Zhang J, Zhai Y. Inhibition of adipocyte differentiation and adipogenesis by the traditional Chinese herb *Sibiraea angustata*. Experimental Biology and Medicine 2010;235:1442-1449.

Xie JT, Chang WT, Wang CZ, Mehendale SR, Li J, Ambihaipahar R, Ambihaipahar U, Fong HH, Yuan CS. Curry Leaf *(Murraya koenigii* Spreng.) Reduces Blood Cholesterol and Glucose Levels in *ob/ob* Mice. Am. J. Chin. Med. 2006;34:279.

Xie N, CuiY, Yin YN, Zhao X, Yang JW, Wang ZG, Fu N, Tang Y, Wang XH, Liu XW, Wang CL, Lu FG. Effects of two *Lactobacillus* strains on lipid metabolism and intestinal microflora in rats fed a high-cholesterol diet. BMC Complementaryand Alternative Medicine 2011;11(53):1-11.

Xie W, Xing D, Sun H, Wang W, Ding Y, Du L. The effects of Ananas comosus L. leaves on diabetic-dyslipidemic rats induced by alloxan and a high-fat/high-cholesterol diet. Am J Chin Med 2005;33(1):95-105.

Xie W, Wang W, Su H, Xing D. Hypolipidemic Mechanisms of *Ananas comosus* L. Leaves in Mice: Different From Fibrates but Similar to Statins. J Pharmacol 2007;103:267-274.

Xie W, Gu D, Li J, Cui K, Zhang Y. Effects and action mechanisms of berberine and Rhizoma coptidis on gut microbes and obesity in high-fat diet-fed C57BL/6J mice. PloS One 2011;6(9):1-10.

Xiong Y, Shen L, Liu KJ, Tso P, Xiong Y, Wang G, Woods SC, Liu M. Antiobesity and Antihyperglycemic Effects of Ginsenoside Rb1 in Rats. Diabetes 2010 Oct;59:2505-2512.

Xiong ZD, Li PG, Mu TH. The Differentiation- and Proliferation-Inhibitory Effects of Sporamin from Sweet Potato in 3T3-L1

Preadipocytes. Agricultural Sciences in China 2009;8(6):671-677.

Xiping L, Xianqiong F. Clinical Effects of Tartary Buckwheat on Senile Hyperlipemia. Current Advances in Buckwheat Research 1995:947-950.

Xu A, Wang H, Hoo RLC, Sweeney G, Vanhoutte PM, Wang Y, Wu D, Chu W, Qin G, Lam KSL. Selective Elevation of Adiponectin Production by the Natural Compounds Derived from a Medicinal Herb Alleviates Insulin Resistance and Glucose Intolerance in Obese Mice. Endocrinology 2009 Feb;150(2):625-633.

Xue C, Liu Y, Wang J, Zheng Z, Zhang Y, Zhang Y, Zhang R, Yu X, Jin H, Nosaka N, Arai C, Kasai M, Aoyama T,Wu J. Chinese Hypertrigylcideamic Subjects of Different Ages Respond Differently to Consuming Oil with Medium- and Long-Chain Fatty Acids. Biosci. Biotechnol. Biochem.2009;73(8):1711-1717.

Xue C, Liu Y, Wang J, Zhang R, Zhang Y, Zhang J, Zhang Y, Zheng Z, Yu X, Jing H, Nosaka N, Arai C, Kasai M, Aoyama T, Wu J. Consumption of medium- and long-chain triacylgycerols decreases body fat and blood triglyceride in Chinese hypertriglyceridemic subjects. Eur J Clin Nutr 2009 Jul;63(7):879-86.

Yaghoobi N, Al-Waili N, Ghayour-Mobarhan M, Parizadeh SMR, Abasalti Z, Yaghoobi Z, Yaghoobi F, Esmaeili H, Kazemi-Bajestani SMR, Aghasizadeh R,Saloom KY, Ferns GAA. Natural Honey and Cardiovascular Risk Factors; Effects on Blood Glucose, Cholesterol, Triacylglycerole, CRP, and Body Weight Compared with Sucrose. The Scientific World Journal 2008;8: 463-469.

Yagnik B, Nilesh K, Rameshvar P, Natavarlal P, Jitendra V, Nurudin J. Antihyperlipidemic and antioxidant activity of *Benincasa cerifera* on high fat diet induced hyperlipidemic rat. Journal of Pharmacy Research 2009 March;2(3):363-366.

Yajima H, Noguchi T, Ikeshima E, Shiraki M, Kanaya T, Tsuboyama-Kasaoka N, Ezaki O, Oikawa S, Kondo K. Prevention of diet-induced obesity by dietary isomerized hop extract containing isohumulones, in rodents. International Journal of Obesity 2005;29:991-997.

Yamada K, Hosokawa M, Yamada C, Watanabe R, Fujimoto S, Fujiwara H, Kunitomo M, Miura T, Kaneko T, Tsuda K, Seino Y, Inagaki N. Dietary Corosolic Acid Ameliorates Obesity and Hepatic Steatosis in KK-Ay Mice. Biol. Pharm. Bull. 2008;31(4): 651-655.

Yamagishi K, Oita S, Kimura T, Iwashita K, Shinmoto H. Suppressive Effect of Extract from Raw Mushroom *Auricularia auricularia (Kikurage)* on Differentiation of Mouse Preadipocytes. Nippon Shokuhin Kagaku Kogaku Kaishi 2007;54(10):456-458.

Yamamoto M, Shimura S, Itoh Y, Ohsaka T, Egawa M, Inoue S. Anti-obesity effects of lipase inhibitor CT-II, an extract from edible herbs, Nomame Herba, on ratsfed a high-fat diet. International Journal of Obesity 2000;24:758-764.

Yamamoto N, Kanemoto Y, Ueda M, Kawasaki K, Fukuda I, Ashida H. Anti-obesity and anti-diabetic effects of ethanol extract of Artemisia princeps in C57BL/6 mice fed a high-fat diet. Food Funct 2011 Jan;2(1):45-52.

Yamamoto Y, Aoyama S, Hamaguchi N, Rhi GS. Antioxidative and Antihypertensive Effects of Welsh Onion on Rats Fed ith a High-Fat High-Sucrose Diet. Biosci. Biotechnol. Biochem. 2005;69(7):1311-1317.

Yamamoto Y, Oue E. Antihypertensive Effect of Quercetin in Rats Fed with a High-Fat High-Sucrose Diet. Biosci. Biotechnol. Biochem. 2006;70(4):933-939.

Yamashita H, Fujisawa K, Ito E, Idel S, Kawaguchi N, Kimoto M, Hiemori M, Tsuji H. Improvement of Obesity and Glucose Tolerace by Acetate in Type 2 Diabetic Otsuka Long-Evans Tokushima Fatty (OLETF) Rats. Biosci. Biotechnol. Biochem. 2007;71(5):1236-1243.

Yamashita H, Maruta H, Jozuka M, Kimura R, Iwabuchi H, Yamato M, Saito T, Fujisawa K, Takahashi Y, Kimoto M, Hiemori M, Tsuji H. Effects of Acetate on Lipid Metabolism in Muscles and Adipose Tissues of Type 2 Diabetic Otsuka Long-Evans Tokushima Fatty (OLETF) Rats. Biosci. Biotechnol. Biochem. 2009;73(3):570-576.

Yamashita Y, Okabe M, Natsume M, Ashida H. Prevention mechanisms of glucose intolerance and obesity by cacao liquor procyanidin extract in high-fat diet-fed C57BL/6 mice. Archives of Biochemistry and Biophysics 2012.

Yang CY, Xie ZG, Cheng WB, Jiang X, Chen ZH. Effects of Panax notoginseng saponins on anti-hyperglycemic, anti-obese and prevention from kidney pathological changes in KK-Ay mice. Zhong Yao Cai 2009 Oct;32(10):1571-6.

Yang CY, Wang J, Zhao Y, Shen L, Jiang X, Xie ZG, Liang N, Zhang L, Chen ZH. Anti-diabetic effects of *Panax notoginseng* saponins and its major anti-hyperglycemic components. Journal of Ethnopharmacology 2010;130:231-236.

Yang G, Lee J, Jung ED, Ham I, Choi HY. Lipid lowering activity of Citri unshii pericarpium in hyperlipemic rats. Immunopharmacol Immunotoxicol 2008;30(4):783-91.

Yang J, Yin J, Gao H, Xu L, Wang Y, Xu L, Li M. Berberine Improves Insulin Sensitivity by Inhibiting Fat Store and Adjusting Adipokines Profile in Human Preadipocytes and Metabolic Syndrome Patients. Evidence-Based Complementary and Alternative Medicine Volume 2012.

Yang JH, Han JS. Effect of Mulberry Leaf Extract Supplement on Blood Glucose, Glycated Hemoglobin and Serum Lipids in Type II Diabetic Patients. J Korean Soc. Food Sci. Nutr. 2006;35(5):549-556.

Yang JH, Lim HS, Heo YR. *Sasa borealis* leaves extract improves insulin resistance by modulating inflammatory cytokine secretion in high fat diet-induced obese C57/BL6J mice. Nutrition Research and Practice (*Nutr Res Pract*) 2010;4(2):99-105.

Yang JJ, Xing HJ, Wang SJ, Xiao HL, Li M, Li Q. Effects of acupuncture combined with dietary adjustments and aerobic exercise on body weight, body mass index and serum leptin level in simple obesity patients. Zhen Ci Yan Jiu 2010 Dec;35(6):453-7.

Yang JY, Lee SJ, Park HW, Cha YS. Effect of genistein with carnitine administration on lipid parameters and obesity in C57BI/6J mice fed a high-fat diet. J Med Food 2006 Winter;9(4):459-67.

Yang L, Chen JH, Lv J, Wu Q, Xu T, Zhang H, Liu QH, Yang HK. Rice protein improves adiposity, body weight and reduces lipids level in rats through modification of triglyceride metabolism. Lipids in Health and Disease 2012;11:24.

Yang MY, Peng CH, Chan KC, Yang YS, Huang CN, Wang CJ. The hypolipidemic effect of Hibiscus sabdariffa polyphenols via inhibiting lipogenesis and promoting hepatic lipid clearance. J Agric Food Chem 2010 Jan 27;58(2):850-9.

Yang X, Yang L, Zheng H. Hypolipidemic and antioxidant effects of mulberry *(Morus alba* L.) fruit in hyperlipidaemia rats. Food and Chemical Toxicology 2010;48:2374-2379.

Yang XY, Qu WJ, Xu ZL, Shao GM, Zhang W, Yang YX. Effect of flavonoids from seed residues and oil of hippophae rhamnoides L. on serum lipid of female aged rats with obesity. Acta Nutrimenta Sinica 2007.

276

Yang Y, Zhou L, Gu Y, Zhang Y, Tang J, Li F, Shang W, Jiang B, Yue X, Chen M. Dietary chickpeas reverse visceral adiposity, dyslipidaemia and insulin resistance in rats induced by a chronic high-fat diet. British Journal of Nutrition 2007;98:720-726.

Yazdanparast R, Bahramikia S. Evaluation of the effect of *Anethum graveolens* L. crude extracts on serum lipids and lipoproteins profiles in hypercholesterolaemic rats. DARU 2008;16(2).

Yin J, Zhang Q, Liu A, Du W, Wang X, Hu X, Ma G. Calcium supplementation for 2 years improves bone mineral accretion and lean body mass in Chinese adolescents. Asia Pac J Clin Nutr 2010;19(2):152-160.

Yoneshiro T, Aita S, Kawai Y, Iwanaga T, Saito M. Nonpungent capsaicin analogs (capsinoids) increase energy expenditure through the activation of brown adipose tissue in humans. Am J Clin Nutr 2012 Apr;95(4):845-50.

Yoon JY, Jung KO, Kil JH, Park KY. Antiobesity Effect of Major Korean Spices (Red Pepper Powder, Garlic and Ginger) in Rats Fed High Fat Diet. J Food Sci Nutr 2005;10:58-63.

Yoon KN, Alam N, Lee JS, Cho HJ, Kim HY, Shim MJ, Lee MW, Lee TS. Antihyperlipidemic Effect of Dietary *Lentinus edodes* on Plasma, Feces and Hepatic Tissues in Hypercholesterolemic Rats. Mycobiology 2011;39(2):96-102.

Yoon KN, Alam N, Shim MJ, Lee TS. Hypolipidemic and antiatherogenesis effect of culinary-medicinal pink oyster mushroom, Pleurotus salmoneostramineus L. Vass. (higher Basidiomycetes), in hypercholesterolemic rats. Int J Med Mushrooms 2012;14(1):27-36.

Yoon SS, Rhee YH, Lee HJ, Lee EO, Lee MH, Ahn KS, Lim HT, Kim SH. Uncoupled protein 3 and p38 signal pathways are involved in anti-obesity activity of *Solanum tuberosum* L. cv. Bora Valley. Journal of Ethnopharmacology 2008;118:396-404.

Yoon TS, Sung YY, Jang JY, Yang WK, Ji Y, Kim HK. Anti-obesity Activity of Extract from *Saussurea lappa*. Korean J. Medicinal Crop Sci 2010;18(3):151-156.

Yoshiaki I, Satoshi K, Samir KS, Takashi O, Masami I, Yoshihiro K. Structure of New Monoterpene Glycoside from *Sibiraea angustata* Rchd. And Its Anti-obestic Effect. Chem. Pharm. Bull. 2009;57(3):294-297.

Yoshida T, Rikimaru K, Sakai M, Nishibe S, Fujikawa T, Tamura Y. *Plantago lanceolata* L. leaves prevent obesity in C57BL/6J mice fed a high-fat diet. Natural Product Research 2012:1-6.

Yoshikawa M, Shimoda H, Nishida N, Takada M, Matsuda H. Salacia reticulata and its polyphenolic constituents with lipase inhibitory and lipolytic activities have mild antiobesity effects in rats. J Nutr. 2002 Jul;132(7):1819-24.

Yoshimatsu H, Tsuda K, Niijima A, Tatsukawa M, Chiba S, Sakata T. Histidine induces lipolysis through sympathetic nerve in white adipose tissue. Eur J Clin Invest 2002 Apr;32(4):236-41.

Yoshinari O, Shiojima Y, Igarashi K. Anti-Obesity Effects of Onion Extract in Zucker Diabetic Fatty Rats. Nutrients 2012;4: 1518-1526.

Yoshioka M, Sylvie SP, Masashige S, Angelo T. Effects of red pepper added to high-fat and high-carbohydrate meals on energy metabolism and substrate utilization in Japanese women. British Journal of Nutrition 1998;80:503-510.

Yoshioka M, Doucet E, St-Pierre S, Alméras N, Richard D, Labrie A, Després JP, Bouchard C, Tremblay A. Impact of high-intensity exercise on energy expenditure,lipid oxidation and body fatness. Int J Obes Relat Metab Disord 2001 Mar;25(3):332-9.

Yoshioka Y, Tamesada M, Tomi H. A repeated dose 28-day oral toxicity study of extract from cultured *Lentinula edodes* mycelia in Wistar rats. The Journal of Toxicological Sciences 2010;35(5):785-791.

Yu L, Shirai N, Suzuki H. Effects of Some Chinese Spices on Body Weights, Plasma Lipids, Lipid Peroxides, and Glucose, and Liver Lipids in Mice. Food Sci. Technol. Res. 2007;13(2):155-161.

Yu L, Shirai N, Suzuki H, Hosono T, Nakajima Y, Kajiwara M, Takatori K. Effect of Lipid Extracted from Tsao-ko (*Amomum tsao-ko* Crevost et Lemaire) on Digestive Enzyme Activity, Antioxidant Activity, Plasma and Liver Lipids, and Blood Glucose Levels of Mice. J Nutr Sci Vitaminol 2008;54:378-383.

Yu L, Shirai N, Suzuki H, Sugane N, Hosono T, Nakajima Y, Kajiwara M, Takatori K. The Effect of Methanol Extracts of Tsao-ko (*Amomum tsao-ko* Crevost et Lemaire) on Digestive Enzyme and Antioxidant Activity in Vitro, and Plasma Lipids and Glucose and Liver Lipids in Mice. J Nutr Sci Vitaminol 2010;56:171-176.

Yu MH, Lee HJ, Im HG, Bo MHH, Kim HJ, Lee IS. The Effects of *Kimchi* with *Monascus purpureus* on the Body Weight Gain and Lipid Metabolism in Rats Fed High Fat Diet. Journal of Life Science 2005;15(4):536-541.

Yu Q, Wang Y, Yu Y, Li Y, Zhao S, Chen Y, Waqar AB, Fan J, Liu E. Expression of TRPV1 in rabbits and consuming hot pepper affects its body weight. Mol Biol Rep 2012 Jul;39(7):7583-9.

Yu YM, Chang WC, Liu CS, Tsai CM. Effect of Young Barley Leaf Extract and Adlay on Plasma Lipids and LDL Oxidation in Hyperlipidemic Smokers. Biol. Pharm. Bull. 2004;27(6):802-805.

Yu YT, Lu TJ, Chiang MT, Chiang W. Physicochemical Properties of Water-soluble Polysaccharide Enriched Fractions of Adlay and Their Hypolipidemic Effect in Hamsters. Journal of Food and Drug Analysis 2005;13(4):361-367.

Yuan HD, Kim SJ, Quan HY, Huang B, Chung SH. Ginseng Leaf Extract Prevents High Fat Diet-Induced Hyperglycemia and Hyperlipidemia through AMPK Activation. J. Ginseng Res. 2010;34(4):369-375.

Yuan Z, He P, Takeuchi H. Ameliorating Effects of Water-Soluble Polysaccharides from Woody Ear (*Auricularia auricula-judae* Quel.) in Genetically Diabetic KK-A Mice. J Nutr. Sci. Vitaminol. 1998;44:829-840.

Yun SN, Moon SJ, Ko SK, Im BO, Chung SH. Wild ginseng prevents the onset of high-fat diet induced hyperglycemia and obesity in ICR mice. Arch Pharm Res. 2004 Jul;27(7):790-6.

Yunoki K, Sasaki G, Tokuji Y, Kinoshita M, Naito A, Aida K, Ohnishi M. Effect of dietary wine pomace extract and oleanolic acid on plasma lipids in rats fed high-fat diet and its DNA microarray analysis. J Agric Food Chem 2008 Dec 24;56(24):12052-8.

Zaid SSM, Sulaiman SA, Sirajudeen KNM, Othman NH. The effects of tualang honey on female reproductive organs, tibia bone and hormonal profile in ovariectomised rats – animal model for menopause. BMC Complementary and Alternative Medicine 2010;10:82.

Zamami Y, Takatori S, Koyama T, Goda M, Iwatani Y, Doi S, Kawasaki H. Effect of Propolis on Insulin Resistance in Fructose-drinking Rats. Yakugaku Zasshi 2007;127(12):2065-2073.

Zarrouki B, Pillon NJ, Kalbacher E, Soula HA, Nia N'Jomen G, Grand L, Chambert S, Geloen A, Soulage CO. Cirsimarin, a potent antilipogenic flavonoid, decreases fat deposition in mice intra-abdominal adipose tissue. Int J Obes (Lond) 2010 Nov;34(11): 1566-75.

277

Zemel MB, Bruckbauer A. Effects of a Leucine and Pyridoxine-Containing Nutraceutical on Fat Oxidation, and Oxidative and Inflammatory Stress in Overweight and Obese Subjects. Nutrients 2012;4:529-541.

Zhang G, Shirai N, Suzuki H. Relationship between the effect of dietary fat on swimming endurance and energy metabolism in aged mice. Ann Nutr Metab 2011 Oct;58(4):282-9.

Zhang H, Cao P, Agellon LB, Zhai CK. Wild rice *(Zizania latifolia* (Griseb) Turcz) improves the seru lipid profile and antioxidant status of rats fed with a high fat/cholesterol diet. British Journal of Nutrition 2009;102:1723-1727.

Zhang H, Peng Y, Liu Z, Li S, Lv Z, Tian L, Zhu J, Zhao X, Chen M. Effects of acupuncture therapy on abdominal fat and hepatic fat content in obese children: a magnetic resonance imaging and proton magnetic resonance spectroscopy study. J Altern Complement Med. 2011 May;17(5):413-20.

Zhang J, Zhang YN, Han LK. Studies on chemical constituents of leaves of Salix matsudana Koidz and their influence on lipolysis. Zhongguo Zhong Yao Za Zhi 2000 Sep;25(9):538-41.

Zhang M, Wang J, Zhang S. Study on the composition of Lycium barbarum polysaccharides and its effects on the growth of weanling mice. Wei Sheng Yan Jiu 2002 Apr;31(2):118-9.

Zhang M, Bi LF, Fang JH, Su XL, Da GL, Kuwamori T, Kagamimori S. Beneficial effects of taurine on serum lipids in overweight or obese non-diabetic subjects. Amino Acids 2004 Jun;26(3):267-71.

Zhang N, Wang XH, Mao SL, Zhao F. Astragaloside IV improves metabolic syndrome and endothelium dysfunction in fructose-fed rats. Molecules 2011 May10;16(5):3896-907.

Zhang W, Liu CQ, Wang PW, Sun SY, Su WJ, Zhang HJ, Li XJ, Yang SY. Puerarin improves insulin resistance and modulates adipokine expression in rats fed a high-fat diet. European Journal of Pharmacology 2010;649:398-402.

Zhang W, Fujikawa T, Mizuno K, Ishida T, Ooi K, Hirata T, Wada A. Eucommia Leaf Extract (ELE) Prevents OVX-Induced Osteoporosis and Obesity in Rats. Am J Chin Med. 2012;40(4):735-52.

Zhang Y, Guo K, LeBlanc RE, Loh D, Schwartz GJ, Yu YH. Increasing Dietary Leucine Intake Reduces Diet-Induced Obesity and Improves Glucose and Cholesterol Metabolism in Mice via Multimechanisms. Diabetes 2007 Jun;56:1647-1654.

Zhang Y, Liu Y, Wang J, Zhang R, Jing H, Yu X, Zhang Y, Xu Q, Zhang J, Zheng Z, Nosaka N, Arai C, Kasai M, Aoyama T, Wu J, Xue C. Medium- and long-chain triacylglycerols reduce body fat and blood triacylglycerols in hypertriacylglycerolemic, overweight but not obese, Chinese individuals. Lipids 2010 Jun;45(6):501-10.

Zhang Y, Zhang Z, Yang Y, Zu X, Guan D, Wang Y. Diuretic Activity of *Rubus idaeus L* (Rosaceae) in Rats. Tropical Journal of Pharmaceutical Research Jun 2011;10(3):243-248.

Zhang YH, Liu YH, Zheng ZX, Wang J, Zhang Y, Zhang RX, Yu XM, Jing HJ, Xue CY, Wu J. Medium- and long-chain fatty acid triacylglycerol reduce body fat and serum triglyceride in overweight and hypertriglyceridemic subjects. Zhonghua Yu Fang Yi Xue Za Zhi 2009 Sep;43(9):765-71.

Zhang Z, Li Q, Liu F, Sun Y, Zhang J. Prevention of diet-induced obesity by safflower oil: insights at the levels of PPARalpha, orexin, and ghrelin gene expression of adipocytes in mice. Acta Biochim Biophys (Shanghai) 2010 Mar 15;42(3):202-8.

Zhao HL, Sim JS, Shim SH, Ha YW, Kang SS, Kim YS. Antiobese and hypolipidemic effects of platycodin saponins in diet-induced obese rats: evidences for lipase inhibition and calorie intake restriction. International Journal of Obesity 2005;29:983-990.

Zhao R, Li Q, Xiao B. Effect of *Lycium barbarum* Polysaccharide on the Improvement of Insulin Resistance in NIDDM Rats. Yakugaku Zasshi 2005;125(12):981-988.

Zhao Y, Li F, Yang J, An X, Zhou M. Effect of phillyrin on the anti-obesity in nutritive obesity mice. Zhong Yao Cai 2005 Feb;28(2):123-4.

Zhu X, Zhang W, Zhao J, Wang J, Qu W. Hypolipidaemic and hepatoprotective effects of ethanolic and aqueous extracts from Asparagus officinalis L. by-products in mice fed a high-fat diet. J Sci Food Agric 2010 May;90(7):1129-35.

Zhu X, Zhang W, Pang X, Wang J, Zhao J, Qu W. Hypolipidemic effect of n-butanol Extract from Asparagus officinalis L. in mice fed a high-fat diet. Phytother Res. 2011 Aug;25(8):1119-24.

Zhu Y, Zhang FX, Li B, Zhang P, Song P. Clinical observation on therapeutic effect of electric-heat needle combined with acupoint sticking therapy for treatment of simple obesity. Zhongguo Zhen Jiu 2010 Feb;30(2):103-6.

Zhou J, Zhao LJ, Watson P, Zhang Q, Lappe JM. The effect of calcium and vitamin D supplementation on obesity in postmenopausal women: secondary analysis for a large-scale, placebo controlled, double-blind, 4-year longitudinal clinical trial. Nutrition & Metabolism 2010;7:62.

Zhou J, Keenan MJ, Losso JN, Raggio AM, Shen L, McCutcheon KL, Tulley RT, Blackman MR, Martin RJ. Dietary whey protein decreases food intake and body fat in rats. Obesity (Silver Spring) 2011 Aug;19(8):1568-73.

Ziegenfuss TN, Hofheins JE, Mendel RW, Landis J, Anderson RA. Effects of a Water-Soluble Cinnamon Extract on Body Composition and Features of the Metabolic Syndrome in Pre-Diabetic Men and Women. Journal of the International Society of Sports Nutrition 2006;3(2):45-53.

Zong W, Zhao G. Corosoli acid isolation from the leaves of *Eriobotrta japonica* showing the effects on carbohydrate metabolism and differentiation of 3T3-L1 adipocytes. Asia Pac J Clin Nutr 2007;16(1):346-352.

Zwiauer KFM, Widhalm KM. Effect of a Very Low Calorie Diet on Lipoproteins and Various Serum Proteins in Grossly Obese Adolescent Patients. Clinical Nutrition 1987;6:137-142.

Zyla K, Mika M, Fortuna T, Szymczyk B, Czubak M. Effect of sesame seeds germination on phytate degradation, *in vitro* nutrient digestibility and plasma lipid profile in rats. Electronic journal of polish agricultural universities 2005;8(4)..